SBAs for the Final FRCA

Dr James Nickells FRCA
Dr Tobias Everett FRCA
Dr Benjamin Walton FRCA
North Bristol NHS Trust
Bristol

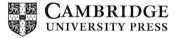
CAMBRIDGE
UNIVERSITY PRESS

CAMBRIDGE UNIVERSITY PRESS
Cambridge, New York, Melbourne, Madrid, Cape Town, Singapore,
São Paulo, Delhi, Dubai, Tokyo

Cambridge University Press
The Edinburgh Building, Cambridge CB2 8RU, UK

Published in the United States of America by Cambridge University Press, New York

www.cambridge.org
Information on this title: www.cambridge.org/9780521139489

First published 2010

Printed in the United Kingdom at the University Press, Cambridge

A catalogue record for this publication is available from the British Library

Library of Congress Cataloguing in Publication data
Nickells, James.
SBAs for the final FRCA / James Nickells, Toby Everett, Benjamin Walton.
    p.   cm.
ISBN 978-0-521-13948-9 (pbk.)
1. Anesthesia – Examinations, questions, etc.   I. Everett, Toby.   II. Walton,
Benjamin.   III. Title.   IV. Title: Single best answers for the final FRCA.
RD82.3.N53   2010
617.9′6076–dc22

                                                                2010000378

ISBN 978-0-521-13948-9 Paperback

From James
To my lovely girls, Jasna, Kasia and Roxy

From Toby
To my magnificent wife, Claire, for her consistent love and support and our wonderful daughters, Iris and Coralie

From Ben
To my children, Joseph and Isabella, and my grandfathers, Samuel Basil Turner and George Walton

Contents

Preface

We have written *SBAs for the Final FRCA* with a number of aims in mind. Our first aim was to provide a set of questions as examples of the single best answer (SBA) style of multiple choice question (MCQ), allowing the candidate approaching the Final FRCA to practise exam style questions under exam conditions. We wanted to cover a fairly broad range of the Final FRCA syllabus, so, unlike the examples posted by The Royal College of Anaesthetists (the College), we have covered some of the non-clinical knowledge areas within the syllabus. We have also written explanations that contain useful information that we hope the owner of this book will wish to refer back to for years to come. We have usually set most questions with a specific educational goal in mind and have included vignettes in the explanations that are often difficult to find elsewhere.

For a number of years we have been teaching and lecturing on MCQs for the Final FRCA. Up to 2008, this included an hour-long lecture on our Crammer Course on good tactics for answering negatively marked MCQs that concluded with the advice

'Answer all the questions'.

Following removal of negative marking, the advice session on answering MCQs reduced in time from one hour to two sentences. They are:

'Answer all the questions. Errmmm, that's it!'

This may seem fairly simplistic, and obviously expanding the sentence to 'Answer all the questions correctly' would be more accurate, if less helpful, advice. From discussions with trainees and in compiling this book, we have tried to come up with useful tips in response to frequently asked questions (FAQs) about the SBA questions in the Final FRCA MCQ exam.

SBA FAQs

The Final FRCA: what is the point?
What are SBAs?
What does the MCQ paper consist of?
How many marks will I get for a correct SBA question?
When is the paper set?
Why has the College adopted this question style?
What do SBAs test?
What structure do SBAs have?
Aren't SBAs just longer true/false questions?
How do I answer SBAs?
How are the sub-specialties represented in the paper?
Will the College increase the proportion of SBA questions in the examination?
How much time should I allocate to these questions?
Should I answer the questions in order?
Are there clues in the way the question is worded?
If guessing, should I always answer 'd'?
Are questions repeated?
How should I revise for this exam?
How should I prepare for this exam?
How should I use this book?

The Final FRCA: what is the point?

The College has a number of duties when it is examining anaesthetists for the Final FRCA. It has to:

- assess whether you have the knowledge, mental processing power and, to a lesser degree, the ability to handle a stressful situation. They are testing everyone to see whether you have reached a threshold level that is sufficient to allow you to cope with the clinical world beyond completion of the Certificate of Completion of Training. In education speak, this means that the exam is criterion referenced. It is designed to assess what you can do rather than where you sit within the exam-sitting cohort. This should mean that, in theory, everyone could pass any given sitting of the Final FRCA. Now there's a happy thought (although, equally, everyone could fail!).
- determine whether you can think about anaesthesia beyond pure recall of the facts. The College wants you to demonstrate an understanding of the concepts and

principles, to be able to think 'on your feet' and appreciate different sides of an argument. In addition to the knowledge base you amassed for the Primary examination, you should have a good grasp of the current literature and an opinion on areas of controversy. Traditionally, the other phases of the Final FRCA exam have been used for testing higher level learning such as concepts and principles, with the MCQ paper testing a large number of individual knowledge points. With SBAs, the College is now looking to test processing power as well as pure recall in this phase of the exam.

- show that the College is relevant. Hence the focus on safety and up-to-date, topical, scientific, widely accepted subjects.
- be in line with current trends in medical education.

What are SBAs?

The 2009 MCQ papers consisted entirely of multiple true/false (MTF) questions. These questions had a stem followed by five options, all of which may be true or false. From September 2010, the College will replace 30 of the MTF questions with SBAs. In these questions, there is also a stem followed by five options. These options include a best answer and four distractors. The candidate has to weigh up which is the best answer.
    To illustrate:

Example MTF question – stem and five true/false branches
The following are types of chocolate bar:

a) Wispa   T/F
b) Triple Trecker   T/F
c) Yorkie   T/F
d) Opal Fruits   T/F
e) Winalot   T/F

Answers a) True b) False c) True d) False e) False

Example SBA question
Which one of the following has the lowest proportion of chocolate?

a) Galaxy
b) Kit Kat
c) Dairy Crunch
d) Cadbury Dairy Milk
e) Ripple

Answer: b

What does the MCQ paper consist of?

We can say with some certainty what the MCQ paper will consist of in September 2010 and for a few cycles thereafter. In its 2009 form, the paper consisted of 90 MTF questions to be answered in three hours. This gave 450 knowledge point tests. From September 2010, the College will replace 30 of the MTF questions with SBAs. This will provide 300 knowledge point tests from MTF and 30 from SBAs. The two styles will run in a combined paper for some time while the College gathers data comparing performance across the two paper styles. This will allow a standard to be created for the SBA question bank. (See 'Are questions repeated?')

How many marks will I get for a correct SBA question?

With the mixed MTF/SBA paper, the College has stated that it will give one mark for each correct true/false answer in the MTF section. However, it has not yet announced how many marks you will receive for a correct SBA question. The implication is that it would be more than one but less than five marks.

When is the paper set?

By the time the first exam containing SBAs starts, in September 2010, the Working Party for the Examiners Board will have spent at least 18 months on developing a bank of SBA questions. The final paper will be agreed upon two months prior to the examination date.

Why has the College adopted this question style?

There are a number of suggested reasons why SBAs have been adopted.

SBAs are thought to be a better test of the learning required to work as an effective anaesthetist. Multiple true/false questions are an adequate tool to test pure factual recall. SBAs are thought to be better at testing the application or processing of knowledge. They therefore would seem more 'fit for purpose' when testing a clinician. Workplace conundrums usually involve 'What would I do if...?' questions rather than purely remembering an isolated fact.

Single best answers help to spread the range of marks in the exam, making it easier to separate good and bad candidates and in the absence of negative marking reduces the power of guessing.

Using MTFs, with random guessing the candidate would score a mark of approximately 50%.

In a 90-question MTF paper (450 knowledge point tests), random guessing would give 225 right and 225 wrong answers, and a mark of 50%.
A poor candidate would score about 65%
The pass mark would be at around 75%
An outstanding candidate would score 85%

In a 200-question SBA paper, random guessing would give 40 right and 160 wrong answers, and a mark of 20%.
If we assume the candidates' contributions to the marks scored above the random guessing baseline remain the same.
The poor candidate would score 44%
The pass mark would be 60%
The outstanding candidate would score 76%

While we are in this area we should discuss a third question type, the extended matching question (EMQ).

Example extended matching question

a) Spangles
b) Space Dust
c) Aero (mint)
d) Cadbury Cream Egg
e) Mars Bar
f) Flake
g) Kinder Egg
h) Fry's Turkish Delight
i) Lion Bar
j) Snickers

Which of the above:

1) Is made from only milk chocolate?
2) Is a sweet, a toy and a surprise?
3) 'Helps you work, rest and play'?

Answer: 1) f   2) g   3) e

In reality, colleges adopting EMQs have mainly mixed them in with SBAs in papers of around 200 questions in three hours. However if we consider an EMQ only exam, random guessing would give 20 right and 180 wrong answers, and a mark of 10% if all the EMQs had ten options.

If we assume the candidates' contributions to the marks scored above the random guessing baseline remain the same:

The poor candidate would score 37%
The pass mark would be 55%
The outstanding candidate would score 73%

The MTFs were popular because they produced five questions per topic area; but had the problem that they gave a 50/50 chance of correct guessing.

The SBA is less economical to write, with only one question per stem, but only produces a 20% chance of getting the correct answer by guessing. The EMQs are becoming increasingly popular with other colleges. An answer can usually be used once, or not at all, so the number of questions per topic is substantial. The chance of a correct guess in this example is only 10%. Many colleges are now adopting this format. The College has not yet announced adopting EMQs, but in our opinion it is only a matter of time before this happens.

What do SBAs test?

Single best answers can test a wide range of levels of understanding:

- They can test knowledge. This is usually in the form of the pure facts that the candidate may have read. A typical question would start with 'What' or 'Select'. There is usually only one correct answer.
- They can test comprehension. This is a test of understanding and goes beyond simple recall. Typical lead-ins start with 'Why' or 'How'. There is usually only one correct answer.
- They can test application. In this case the candidate may be asked to apply knowledge to a new situation. Typical lead-ins start with 'Choose', 'Select' or 'Identify'. There is usually only one correct answer.
- They can test analysis. This requires the candidate to demonstrate judgement based on the information presented. Typical lead-ins start with 'Determine', 'Evaluate', or 'Prioritise'. There may appear to be a number of answers that would work with the stem. It is the candidate's job to find the single best answer.

What structure do SBAs have?

If the SBA is just testing knowledge, it usually has a simple form with a question, followed by five options. One of the options will be correct and the other four are called distractors. In well written questions the distractors should all seem plausible, and look roughly similar to the correct option. For example, they should not all be double the length of the correct option.

For tests of comprehension, application or analysis, the question will be preceded by a stem. For a clinical question, this will usually involve a clinical scenario. The stem should be fairly short (around 60 words), should not contain a question and should not have content that is repeated in the options. The stem is then followed by the lead-in, which is the sentence asking the question. This might be, for example, 'What is the likely diagnosis?' This is again followed by the five options.

Aren't SBAs just longer true/false questions?

In some cases this assertion is correct, except that the guessing candidate has worse odds of success. However, the clue to these questions is in the name. 'Single best answers' means that often you are being asked to work out which answer is the best. Several of the options may work, but only one is the best.

How do I answer SBAs?

This will sound like an echo from your earliest days of education, but it doesn't hurt for us to say 'make sure you read the question carefully'.

A good tactic is to read the stem and lead-in, cover up the options and ask yourself what the correct answer would be. If you are 100% confident of the answer and this answer appears in the options, it is most likely to be correct.

If you are not in the lucky position of definitely knowing the answer and are trying to work it out, it is very important to not just settle on the first option you see that looks correct. Read all the options against the lead-in and ask yourself: 'Which one fits best?'

In trials of SBAs with trainees we have noticed that they often find that two of the options can be discounted immediately, leaving two or three options to whittle down to one. If this happens to you, go back and read the stem, looking to see if there is anything within the detail that will allow you to reduce the options further. It may end up with a wild guess between two final options, but at least your odds of guessing correctly have increased from 20% to 50%.

Even if you only have the vaguest notion about the subject area, apply any knowledge you have and make an educated guess. Do not leave a blank.

It is also important to state that only one mark per question should be made on the answer sheet. More than one mark and the candidate will score zero for that question.

How are the sub-specialties represented in the paper?

The initial samples produced by the College, and the corresponding information, stated that the SBA questions would be used to test 20 questions in clinical anaesthesia, 5 in intensive care medicine and 5 in pain management. This ties in with the College stating that it is using SBAs to test clinical decision-making. The other areas of the MCQ paper, such as the basic sciences and clinical measurement, are not represented in the College's initial examples. We have included some questions in these areas in this book. The SBA question is enormously flexible and works well with certain lines of enquiry about most subjects. We predict that the College will progressively increase the proportion of SBAs in the Final FRCA MCQ paper. Even if just testing an area of knowledge that a good candidate would find easy to spot the correct answer, one of the great advantages of an SBA question is that, with four distractors, the chances of a successful wild guess by a candidate without the required knowledge drops from 50% to 20%.

Will the College increase the proportion of SBA questions in the examination?

For the foreseeable future the College has stated that it will persist with the MTF questions to test pure knowledge recall. With time, once the College has enough data and experience with SBAs we predict that the MTF-type questions will be phased out.

The plan for 2010 is 30 SBA questions to fill an equivalent of one hour of the paper. We would also predict that the number of SBAs per unit time will increase. Typically other colleges experienced with this question style have asked 200 SBAs in a three-hour paper. This may well be where the paper is heading in a few years' time. However, the College has generally given 18 months to two years warning of any major changes to the exam system, so if you are planning on sitting the exam within the next nine months and you have not heard that anything is changing for your exam, do not worry about last-minute changes to the exam structure.

How much time should I allocate to these questions?

At the time of writing this book, answering this question involves a little guess-work. The experience with other colleges, such as the Royal College of General Practitioners, adopting SBAs was that a single question took just under a minute to answer and that answering 200 questions in 180 minutes was tough but achievable. For the initial introduction, our College has been rather more generous, replacing one hour of the exam with just 30 SBAs. Our advice would have to be, divide the time evenly, stick to time and whatever you do ensure that you answer all the questions. Running out of time and leaving out questions is exam suicide. If the College turns the heat up by reducing the time or increasing the number of SBAs, it will become imperative to practise your skills at nailing down the best answer in the shortest time possible.

Should I answer the questions in order?

Some people like to wander around an MCQ paper, answering the ones they know first while trying to recall information on the ones they are unsure about. If this is the only tactic that works for you, then you should stick with it. However, we would strongly recommend that you avoid this plan if you have a choice. Wandering around is a bit of a hangover from negative marking where some people would use the (flawed) tactic of answering only the questions they were absolutely sure about. In this exam you have to answer all the questions, so start at the beginning and carry on through to the end. This is the most time-efficient tactic and helps to minimise transcription errors on your answer sheet. Some colleges use computer input centres where the computer does not let you flit around the paper, and this may be a path the College follows in the future.

Are there clues in the way the question is worded?

If the question is well written, the answer to this question is 'No'. Occasionally, poorly written questions may slip through and may be identified by some of the following signs:

- Distractors of different length to the correct answer: this usually takes the form of a long correct answer with short distractors.
- Distractors of different style to the correct answer: for example, this could be numerical data presented in a different style.
- Options that overlap should not occur and would usually be distractors.
- Options containing double negatives should not occur and would usually be distractors.
- Options that contain some of the stem should not occur and would usually be distractors.
- Emphatic statements or absolute terms such as 'always' or 'never' are often incorrect in medicine and would usually indicate a false statement.
- Grammatical errors: the option should grammatically follow the stem. Failure to do this would imply that it was written as an afterthought and is more likely to be a distractor.

- Only one option contains all the common variables. For example:
  a) Give low flow oxygen, 1000 mL fluid challenge, hydrocortisone 200 mg iv, chlorpheniramine 10 mg iv
  b) Give high flow oxygen, 2000 mL fluid challenge, hydrocortisone 200 mg iv, chlorpheniramine 10 mg iv
  c) Give high flow oxygen, 1000 mL fluid challenge, hydrocortisone 200 mg iv, chlorpheniramine 10 mg iv
  d) Give high flow oxygen, 1000 mL fluid challenge, hydrocortisone 100 mg iv, chlorpheniramine 10 mg iv
  e) Give high flow oxygen, 1000 mL fluid challenge, hydrocortisone 200 mg iv, chlorpheniramine 1 mg iv

  By eliminating factors that occur only once, you come up with the correct answer 'c'.

If you are having a complete wild guess, some of these clues may guide you, but do not let them put you off if you have knowledge that indicates a specific answer.

If guessing, should I always answer 'd'?

When we first started writing SBAs we noticed a preponderance for putting the correct option in the 'Option d' slot. We thought this was because we wanted the candidates to work through all the options before spotting the correct one, but didn't want to make it so obvious by putting all 'e's. We noticed then that when reading each others' questions you would start by reading Options 'd' and 'e' first. Once identified, we made sure that the correct answer was randomly sprinkled through the options. Each letter is fairly evenly represented throughout the book as the correct option and this should be the case in any well written paper.

Are questions repeated?

From paper to paper, the College will definitely repeat MCQ questions. In particular, we think it is likely that they will repeat SBA questions as their question bank will be smaller for SBAs compared to the MTF questions, and they need to repeat a minimum proportion of good discriminator questions (the questions that the good candidates get right and the worse candidates get wrong) across a number of exams to maintain temporal validity. This is the process of standard setting whereby the pass mark is shifted to take into account how today's cohort of candidates performed compared to previous years answering the same questions. The need to test the same questions on subsequent cohorts is also required to allow the performance between the MTF and SBA sections to be reviewed over a number of exam cycles to test the robustness of the new SBA assessment tool.

How should I revise for this exam?

Revision tactics are highly individual so you are the only person who knows what's best for you. We can only give general advice, but there are some universal truths. The biggest of these is that the best way to bullet-proof yourself against failure is to know loads. You cannot pass this exam without chewing a certain volume of cardboard. Some people work best by sitting down and reading 2500-page anaesthetic reference books from cover to cover three times. Other people prefer darting in and out of smaller books. Some people like to keep connected to e-learning resources via their mobile phone. If a particular system has previously proven successful for you, then stick with it. We feel that having a plan that ensures you cover as much of the syllabus as possible is very important. This will give you much greater confidence that you are not going to get rolled over in the exam by a difficult SAQ or viva question. As long as you cover all the important topics, a variety of revision tactics is our preference as it will maintain a fresh feeling when learning. Do not waste opportunities to revise. This may involve a question and answer session in theatre with a consultant, listening to a podcast while cycling to work or reading a study guide chapter in the bath. Do not underestimate the value of reading the journals. Examiners love visiting the journals as sources for exam question topics. This is because the journal articles are usually, relevant, up to date, scientific and peer reviewed. Remember, this was one of the College's missions under 'The Final FRCA: what is the point?' Revising from journals is a skill, but a fairly easy one to acquire. People often get put off by approaching the journals as the exam looms because the content is not so readily laid out as it would be in a textbook. The keys are to be able quickly to work out what not to read and to avoid getting distracted by trivia. Editorials, review articles and the introductions or abstracts of clinical research papers are where the best material is usually found.

How should I prepare for this exam?

In addition to revising, it is very important to practise answering MCQ questions. Forming a study group will help pool resources of MCQ questions. If you get an answer wrong, work out why. Good MCQ practice resources should explain their answers and give you guidance as to why you may have got an answer wrong. Sometimes this may have been because the question was poorly written. Sometimes it may have been that you misread the question. More often than not, it is because you are short on knowledge in that area. If you think the question was relevant, use a failed question to guide you as to where you should revise next.

How should I use this book?

This book has been laid out as four papers with 75 questions in each paper. If the College adopts the 200 SBAs in three hours format, a 75-question paper would take 67.5 minutes. If the College persists with its projected 30 questions per hour, then you have a slightly more luxurious 2 hours 30 minutes to complete a 75-question paper from this book. We would recommend that you choose a practice experience that mirrors current practice by the College and see how you perform under exam conditions. Although this book would also be suitable for learning by dipping in and out of a few questions and looking up the answers, the most useful experience would be gained by repeatedly testing yourself to hunt out the best answer under exam conditions and time constraints. In addition to providing exam practice, the question papers are followed by a section with focused explanations that contain invaluable information about the topic areas covered and give some insight into how questions are constructed. We have tried to cover a broad sweep of the syllabus and address questions that cover important educational points.

Know plenty, practise loads and always be lucky.
James Nickells
Toby Everett
Ben Walton

Question Papers

Paper A

Question 1

Regarding albumin, the following statements are true except which one?

a) Albumin is a negative acute phase protein
b) A common cause of hypoalbuminaemia is starvation or malnutrition
c) In health the liver produces approximately 10 g per day of albumin
d) The circulation half-life of albumin is approximately 18 days
e) The majority of total body albumin is found in the extravascular compartment

Question 2

Which of the following statements regarding sugammadex is true?

a) It is a modified α-cyclodextrin
b) The drug forms complexes with steroidal neuromuscular blocking drugs with a ratio of 1:2
c) Following sugammadex administration to reverse rocuronium-induced neuromuscular blockade the measured total plasma rocuronium concentration will rise
d) The majority of the drug is metabolised and excreted by the kidneys
e) Sugammadex exerts its effect by binding with rocuronium at the neuromuscular junction

Question 3

Pulmonary vasoconstriction may be caused by

a) Hypothermia
b) Smoking 'Crack' cocaine
c) Volatile anaesthetic agents
d) Calcium channel blockers
e) Positive end expiratory pressure

Question 4

Regarding central neuraxial blocks, which one of the following is most likely to cause permanent neurological injury?

a) An epidural sited for obstetric indications
b) An epidural sited for adult general surgical indications

c) An epidural sited for paediatric general surgical indications
d) A spinal sited rather than an epidural
e) An epidural sited for chronic pain indications

Question 5

A nasogastric tube is sited in a patient ventilated on the critical care unit. Which one of the following is considered the most accurate way of confirming correct positioning?

a) Measurement of the aspirate using pH indicator strips
b) Auscultation of air insufflated through the nasogastric tube (the 'whoosh' test)
c) Testing the acidity/alkalinity of aspirate from the nasogastric tube using litmus paper
d) Observing the appearance of the aspirate from the nasogastric tube
e) Chest radiograph

Question 6

Which of the following patient groups is not thought to be at increased risk of infective endocarditis and therefore does not require prophylaxis against infective endocarditis when undergoing an interventional procedure?

a) Moderate mitral regurgitation
b) A patient with a history of previous endocarditis but a structurally normal heart
c) Isolated atrial septal defect
d) Hypertrophic cardiomyopathy
e) Pulmonary stenosis

Question 7

A 40-year-old woman known to have myasthenia gravis presents to the emergency department with severe global weakness. She is pale, sweaty and cyanosed. Her partner explains that she was diagnosed some time ago and she is, to the best of his knowledge, compliant with her oral pyridostigmine therapy. She is a smoker and has been coughing more than usual recently. He has been worried about her low mood in past months. In order to distinguish between an excess or inadequacy of her myasthenia treatment, which one of the following features is likely to be the most helpful?

a) Rapid onset of ventilatory failure
b) Response to dose of cholinesterase inhibitor
c) Flaccid muscle paralysis
d) Presence of bronchospasm
e) Loss of deep tendon reflexes

Question 8

Which of the following is not a recognised cause of the toxic effects of tricyclic antidepressant drugs taken in overdose?

a) Inhibition of noradrenaline reuptake at nerve terminals
b) A myocardial membrane stabilising effect
c) An anticholinergic action
d) Indirect activation of $GABA_A$ receptors
e) Direct alpha adrenergic action

Question 9

Regarding the use of tourniquets in the theatre environment, the following statements are true except which one?

a) Exsanguination and tourniquet inflation is associated with immediate rise in central venous pressure, arterial blood pressure and heart rate
b) After two hours' inflation time, a significant decrease in core temperature can be expected on deflation of the tourniquet
c) Pre-inflation, ketamine 0.25 mg/kg intravenously can prevent the hypertensive response to tourniquets
d) When using a double-cuff tourniquet for intravenous regional anaesthesia the proximal cuff is the first to be used
e) If the continuous tourniquet inflation time exceeds two hours, the ischaemic cell damage and lesions associated with acidosis are irreversible

Question 10

You are called to the resuscitation room where an unwell, 34-year-old man is undergoing assessment. You agree to take the venous blood sample for investigations. The bottles and syringes required are all listed below. Select the sample that you would draw and fill third.

a) Standard gold-topped sample bottle containing gel activator (SST) for urea and electrolyte
b) Standard grey-topped sample bottle containing fluoride oxalate for glucose
c) Standard blue-topped sample bottle containing citrate coagulation screen
d) Standard purple-topped sample bottle containing EDTA for full blood count
e) Blood culture bottles

Question 11

A 55-year-old male smoker presents with lethargy, cough and intermittent chest pains. He requires assessment because of progressive respiratory failure. On examination he has a central trachea and reduced chest expansion. On the right he has a dull percussion note, easily audible breath sounds and whispering pectoriloquy. On the left his breath sounds seem less audible but there are no added sounds and vocal resonance is normal. Which of the following is the most likely diagnosis?

a) Right pleural effusion
b) Left pneumothorax
c) Right pneumonic consolidation
d) Left lobar collapse with patent major bronchi
e) Right bronchial proximal obstructing lesion

Question 12

Regarding meta-analysis, which one of the following statements is true?

a) Is analagous to a systematic review
b) The size of a 'blob' in a 'blobbogram' reflects the degree of significance found in the individual study
c) If the centre line is crossed by the confidence interval of the combined result, there is no association between the variables
d) The 'x' axis of the results graph is usually expressed as relative risk
e) The funnel plot helps to identify selection bias

Question 13

Negative pressure may be applied to the chest drainage tube of the affected hemithorax in the following circumstances except which one?

a) Post-pneumonectomy
b) Known bronchopleural fistula
c) Known haemothorax
d) Known empyema
e) Post-oesophagectomy

Question 14

The following are direct or indirect measurements of acute phase proteins except which one?

a) C-reactive protein
b) Plasma viscosity
c) Haptoglobin
d) Rheumatoid factor
e) Erythrocyte sedimentation rate

Question 15

A patient has a CT-confirmed retroperitoneal haemorrhage. He is on warfarin for atrial fibrillation. His international normalised ratio (INR) is usually stable between two and three. It is now eight, and this may be explained by the recent commencement of a new drug. Of the following drugs, which is the least likely to be responsible for the derangement?

a) Clopidogrel
b) Paracetamol
c) Amiodarone
d) Fluconazole
e) Metronidazole

Question 16

A horse rider falls at a jump and sustains a closed head injury without impairment of consciousness at any stage and a femoral shaft fracture, which is internally fixated with an intramedullary nail soon after admission. At 48 hours post-injury she becomes confused, tachypnoeic, hypoxaemic and pyrexial (38.2 °C). An atypical rash is also noted. Which one of the following statements is most appropriate?

a) Immediately alert the orthopaedic surgeons
b) Based on these features, anticoagulation is indicated
c) Transfusion of packed red cells is indicated
d) A chest X-ray will contribute to resolving the situation
e) An urgent CT head scan is highest priority

Question 17

A 54-year-old male requires emergency laparotomy. He has long-standing depression and is taking a monoamine oxidase inhibitor. Which one of the following monoamine oxidase inhibitors is least likely to cause incident during conduct of general anaesthesia?

a) Moclobemide
b) Phenelzine
c) Isocarboxazid
d) Tranylcypromine
e) Iproniazid

Question 18

You are asked to see a 65-year-old patient on the ICU who had been admitted 24 hours previously following emergency laparotomy for a bleeding duodenal ulcer. He had been extubated 24 hours previously. His haematology, coagulation and biochemistry profiles are normal and he was on 30% oxygen but has suddenly become very short of breath with some pleuritic central chest pain. He is cardiovascularly stable. You suspect a possible pulmonary embolism (PE) and start him on high-flow oxygen. Which of the following statements represents your best immediate management plan?

a) 12-lead electrocardiogram (ECG), blood for cardiac troponin, computerised tomography pulmonary angiogram (CTPA) and therapeutic dose unfractionated heparin if the CTPA shows a significant PE
b) 12-lead ECG, CTPA and thrombolytic therapy if the CTPA shows a significant PE
c) 12-lead ECG, CTPA and therapeutic dose unfractionated heparin if the CTPA shows a significant PE
d) CTPA and therapeutic dose enoxaparin sodium if the CTPA shows a significant PE
e) 12-lead ECG, D-dimer and if both are normal no further immediate interventions

Question 19

Regarding electrical equipment designed to optimise patient safety, which one of the following statements is true?

a) Under single fault conditions, type I, CF equipment should have a leakage current in the order of 5 mA
b) Type BF equipment is safe because the patient circuit is earthed
c) To promote patient safety a theatre suite should have a UPS
d) Class III equipment is defined as that which operates at 'safety extra-low voltage' of less than 12 V
e) A current-operated earth-leakage circuit breaker relies on an unacceptable current causing disintegration of a fuse that then breaks the circuit

Question 20

A 57-year-old woman is listed for elective abdominal surgery. She has a history of rheumatoid arthritis. On auscultation of her praecordium, a murmur is detected. Regarding this patient, the following statements are true except for which one?

a) If this murmur is related to a left-sided valve abnormality it will be heard louder in expiration than inspiration
b) The most likely murmurs would be an apical pansystolic murmur radiating to the axilla or a diastolic murmur heard best at the left sternal edge
c) If this murmur was secondary to aortic stenosis then a grade one sounding murmur is of less significance than a grade five sounding murmur
d) If this murmur was secondary to mitral regurgitation, a quiet first heart sound would be not altogether unsurprising
e) Atrial fibrillation would prompt suspicion of a mitral source of the murmur

Question 21

Regarding colloid preparations for intravenous infusion, which one of the following statements is correct?

a) Gelofusine® consists of urea-linked gelatin component molecules
b) Regarding pentastarches, the 'pent' refers to 50% esterification with succinyl groups
c) Dextran 70 and 110 interfere with platelet aggregation and have an anticoagulant action, whereas Dextran 40 does not
d) Gelatin used for medical colloids is derived from exposing collagen from sheep bones to a strong alkali then boiling water
e) Hetastarch contains molecules with a mean molecular weight of 450 kDa

Question 22

During an emergency in the hospital you are evacuated with an anaesthetised patient into the hospital car park. You want to measure the patient's blood pressure and are handed a stethoscope and a sphygmomanometer. What sounds on auscultation would you use to identify the systolic and diastolic blood pressure?

a) The peak of the first Korotkoff sound and the muffling of the fourth Korotkoff sound
b) The start of the first Korotkoff sound and the start of the fifth Korotkoff sound
c) The start of the first Korotkoff sound and the muffling of the fourth Korotkoff sound
d) The peak of the first Korotkoff sound and the peak of the fifth Korotkoff sound
e) The start of the first Korotkoff sound and the peak of the fifth Korotkoff sound

Question 23

You are told to draw up a new inotrope for infusion to be administered to an 80 kg patient. The drug comes as an ampoule containing 200 mg in 20 mL. You are instructed to draw the whole ampoule up with water for injection to make a final volume of 50 mL. You only have a basic syringe driver that runs in mL/h. The product information recommends starting the infusion at 20 mcg/kg/min. How many mL/h would you set the syringe driver to?

a) 9.6 mL/h
b) 12.0 mL/h
c) 16.7 mL/h
d) 18.0 mL/h
e) 24.0 mL/h

Question 24

Of the following techniques, which one may be used to measure residual volume?

a) Carbon monoxide dilution
b) Total body plethysmography
c) Bohr's method
d) Pendelluft analysis
e) Wet spirometry

Question 25

Listed below are five descriptions of a cardiotocograph trace. With regards to signs of foetal distress, which one of the following is the second most concerning trace?

a) Heart rate 90 beats/min, late decelerations, variability 5 beats/min
b) Heart rate 145 beats/min, early decelerations, variability 25 beats/min

c) Heart rate 40 beats/min, no decelerations, variability 2 beats/min
d) Heart rate 160 beats/min, variable decelerations, variability 30 beats/min
e) Heart rate 100 beats/min, early decelerations, variability 20 beats/min

Question 26

A 25-year-old female presents with significant haemorrhage secondary to a ruptured ectopic pregnancy. Which blood component transfusion practice is most likely to cause harm?

a) Transfusion of A +ve packed red cells to an AB −ve recipient
b) Transfusion of A −ve packed red cells to an AB +ve recipient
c) Transfusion of AB +ve fresh frozen plasma to an AB −ve recipient
d) Transfusion of B +ve cryoprecipitate to an O −ve recipient
e) Transfusion of AB −ve platelets to an O +ve recipient

Question 27

Regarding malignant carcinoid syndrome, the following statements are true except which one?

a) Malignant carcinoid syndrome occurs in around 50% of those patients with a carcinoid tumour
b) Fibrosis of heart valves is more commonly seen on the right side of the heart than the left
c) Carcinoid tumours can produce insulin
d) For a patient to have malignant carcinoid syndrome they are likely to have liver metastases
e) Carcinoid tumours originating in the appendix are likely to be benign

Question 28

Regarding asthma in pregnancy, which one of the following statements is true?

a) Asthma attacks in brittle asthmatics are more common during labour than at any other stage of the pregnancy
b) Theophyllines are contraindicated for treating asthmatics in pregnancy
c) Oral steroid therapy should be avoided in gravid patients with acute severe asthma
d) Intravenous magnesium sulphate should not be administered to an asthmatic in labour
e) Uncontrolled asthma is associated with pre-eclampsia

Question 29

A lactic acidosis will be accompanied by a normal anion gap in the presence of which one of the following circumstances?

a) Concurrent diabetic ketoacidosis
b) Hypoalbuminaemia
c) Lithium poisoning
d) Intractable vomiting
e) Hypoaldosteronism

Question 30

Regarding the calculation of number needed to treat (NNT), which one of the following formulae is used?

a) 1/absolute risk reduction
b) 1/the odds ratio
c) The odds ratio/absolute risk reduction
d) Relative risk reduction/absolute risk reduction
e) 1/relative risk reduction

Question 31

Based on their associated biochemical derangements, which one of the following surgical pathologies is the odd one out?

a) Pyloric stenosis
b) Enteric fistula
c) Ureterosigmoidostomy
d) Toxic megacolon
e) Villous adenoma of the rectum

Question 32

The FLACC scale is a commonly used tool for assessing pain in a population who may not be able to verbalise postoperative pain or discomfort. Which one of the following statements is correct?

a) The tool is applicable to the age range: two months to seven years
b) The 'A' in FLACC stands for 'Arms'
c) The maximum score, indicating the worst possible pain, is 15
d) A child who is kicking with their legs drawn up would score 1 for legs
e) The nature of the child's crying has no impact on the score

Question 33

Regarding normal physiological changes in a healthy pregnancy, which one of the following changes would not be consistent with expected changes?

a) 10% increase in heart rate by 12 weeks gestation
b) 20% increase in stroke volume by 12 weeks gestation
c) 20% increase in red cell volume by 28 weeks gestation
d) 20% increase in anatomical dead space by 28 weeks gestation
e) 50% increase in glomerular filtration rate by 12 weeks gestation

Question 34

You are providing general anaesthesia to a 47-year-old patient having an open hemi-colectomy. You have been infusing all fluids through a fluid warmer but notice that the patient's temperature has dropped to 35 °C. The patient will be losing most heat by which one of the following processes?

a) Conduction into the patient's general surroundings
b) Convection with the room air
c) Radiation to the patient's general surroundings
d) Evaporation from wound and skin
e) Respiratory losses from conduction, convection and evaporation

Question 35

Which one of the following statements regarding antimicrobials is true?

a) Carbapenems are not β-lactam antibacterial drugs

b) Action against Gram-negative bacteria was superior with the earlier generations of cephalosporins but Gram-positive cover has been sequentially improved
c) Fluoroquinolones include norfloxacin, ofloxacin and lomefloxacin
d) Tazocin® is the trade name for the generic antimicrobial tazobactam
e) Aminoglycoside antibacterial drugs include gentamicin, netilmicin, vancomycin and tobramycin

Question 36

Regarding misplacement of limb leads prior to recording a 12-lead electrocardiogram, the following misplacements would mimic the stated condition except which one?

a) Left-arm electrode and right-arm electrode switch – dextrocardia
b) Right-leg electrode and right-arm electrode switch – pericardial effusion
c) Left-arm electrode and left-leg electrode switch – inferior myocardial infarction
d) Right-leg electrode and left-leg electrode switch – true posterior myocardial infarction
e) Clockwise rotated limb leads (with right leg correctly sited) – extra-nodal atrial rhythm

Question 37

Regarding intraocular pressure and drugs used in anaesthesia, the following statements are true except which one?

a) Intravenous midazolam reduces intraocular pressure
b) Metoclopramide causes an increase in intraocular pressure
c) Atracurium has no effect on intraocular pressure
d) Rocuronium reduces intraocular pressure
e) All intravenous induction agents reduce intraocular pressure, except ketamine

Question 38

A 58-year-old male patient is recovering on the cardiac intensive care unit following first-time coronary bypass grafting. The surgeon is concerned that the drain output is greater than acceptable. You take a blood sample for thromboelastography. Which of the following findings would be consistent with a diagnosis of thrombocytopaenia?

a) A prolonged r time, an increased k time, a decreased alpha angle, a decreased MA
b) A normal r time, an increased k time, a normal alpha angle, an extremely decreased MA
c) A decreased r time, a decreased k time, an increased alpha angle, an increased MA
d) A normal r time, a normal k time, an increased alpha angle, a continuously decreasing MA
e) A prolonged r time, a normal k time, an increased alpha angle, a normal MA

Question 39

In an anaesthetised, intubated patient various neurophysiological monitors may be used. Of the following monitors, which one is least likely to be affected by a concurrent remifentanil infusion?

a) Auditory evoked potentials
b) Electroencephalography
c) Bispectral index
d) Spectral entropy
e) Somatosensory evoked potentials

Question 40

Which one of the following options is a function performed by the lung?

a) Conversion of angiotensinogen to angiotensin I
b) Secretion of immunoglobulin E into bronchial mucus
c) Uptake and metabolism of histamine
d) Deactivation of prostaglandin E_2
e) Manufacture of phosphatidylinositol biphosphate, the phospholipid component of surfactant

Question 41

The following antihypertensive agents are linked with well recognised side effects except which one?

a) Lisinopril may cause angioedema
b) Metoprolol may cause impotence
c) Diltiazem may cause insulin resistance
d) Bendroflumethiazide may cause hyperuricaemia
e) Losartan may cause a dry cough

Question 42

Regarding antiemetics, which one of the following statements is true?

a) Dexamethasone has been shown to downregulate $5\text{-}HT_3$ receptors in the chemoreceptor trigger zone
b) As an anticholinergic, glycopyrrolate has useful antiemetic properties
c) Cyclizine acts as an antiemetic by antagonism of muscarinic acetylcholine receptors
d) Ondansetron exerts antagonism at $5\text{-}HT_3$ receptors only in the chemoreceptor trigger zone and the nucleus tractus solitarius
e) Nabilone is an antagonist at endogenous cannabinoid receptors

Question 43

A heat moisture exchanger incorporating a standard high efficiency particulate air (HEPA) filter has a pore size as small as or smaller than all of the following pathogens, except which one?

a) *Mycobacterium tuberculosis*
b) *Staphylococcus aureus*
c) *Legionella pneumophilia*
d) *Mycoplasma pneumoniae*
e) *Pseudomonas aeruginosa*

Question 44

A previously fit and well 52-year-old patient develops a regular narrow-complex tachycardia in recovery, but is otherwise stable with a blood pressure of 125/85 mmHg. You apply oxygen on high flow via a facemask, perform a 12-lead ECG and start carotid sinus massage, which fails to correct the tachycardia. You give adenosine 6 mg intravenously, which fails to alter the rhythm, followed by a further adenosine 12 mg intravenously, again with no improvement. What would you do next?

a) Give digoxin 500 mc/g intravenously
b) Give amiodarone 300 mg loading dose intravenously

c) Give verapamil 2.5 mg intravenously over two minutes
d) Give adenosine 12 mg intravenously
e) Perform synchronised DC cardioversion

Question 45

During arterial blood gas analysis, representation of quantity of hydrogen ions present in the sample may be displayed as pH, hydrogen ion concentration or both. The following statements are correct equivalences except which one?

a) pH 7.6 = 25 nanomol/L
b) pH 7.4 = 40 nanomol/L
c) pH 7.3 = 50 nanomol/L
d) pH 7.2 = 63 nanomol/L
e) pH 7.0 = 114 nanomol/L

Question 46

There are a number of absolute contraindications to tissue donations. These include the following circumstances except for which one?

a) A patient with a family history of Creutzfeldt–Jacob disease (CJD)
b) A patient with Alzheimer's disease
c) A patient with multiple sclerosis
d) A patient who has had a previous transplant requiring immunosuppressive treatment even if that treatment was not being received at the time of death
e) Donation of corneas and sclera from a patient who has died with a proven diagnosis of metastatic carcinoma of the colon

Question 47

The following are eponymous cardiovascular reflexes except which one?

a) Anrep effect: acute increase in afterload causes reduction in stroke volume then reflex restitution
b) Cushing's reflex: raised intracranial pressure causes hypertension and reflex bradycardia
c) Bainbridge reflex: an increase in venous pressure causes tachycardia
d) Bowman effect: as heart rate increases, contractility increases
e) Bezold–Jarish reflex: seen in myocardial ischaemia – stimulation of ventricular receptors cause bradycardia and hypotension

Question 48

Regarding mixed venous oxygen saturations, which one of the following statements is correct?

a) In septic shock, SvO_2 is unlikely to be normal or supranormal
b) With a ventricular septal defect, a reduction in SvO_2 will be observed
c) If oxygen flux is fixed, elevated oxygen consumption results in increased SvO_2
d) If arterial oxygen saturation, haemoglobin and oxygen consumption are constant, SvO_2 varies directly with cardiac output
e) Cyanide toxicity causes a reduction in SvO_2

Question 49

Which one of the following options is a true statement regarding the intrinsic muscles of the larynx?

a) The cricothyroids are the only muscles to tense the cords
b) The posterior cricoarytenoids, supplied by the recurrent laryngeal nerve, adduct the cords
c) Vocalis is supplied by the recurrent laryngeal nerve but is not considered an intrinsic muscle of the larynx
d) Thyrohyoid elevates the larynx
e) The internal laryngeal nerve supplies only one of these muscles

Question 50

A 30-year-old woman presents for elective surgery. She is 170 cm tall, weighs 35 kg and has a long history of an eating disorder. The following statements about this patient are true except for which one?

a) She is more likely to have mitral valve prolapse than a similar patient with a normal body mass index (BMI)
b) She is more likely to be bradypnoeic and bradycardic than a similar patient with a normal BMI
c) She is likely to be anaemic and leucopaenic
d) Her gastric emptying time is likely to be slower compared to a similar patient with a normal BMI
e) Common electrocardiogram (ECG) findings in this patient would include atrioventricular block, QT prolongation, ST segment depression and T-wave inversion

Question 51

Regarding the Acute Physiology and Chronic Health Evaluation II (APACHE II) scoring system, which one of the following statements is true?

a) There are 15 physiological variables incorporated within the APACHE II scoring system
b) The maximum number of age points that can be assigned is ten
c) A similar patient will score fewer chronic health points if they are a non-operative critical care admission than if they are admitted following elective surgery
d) Points for the Glasgow Coma Score (GCS) are calculated by subtracting the actual GCS from 15
e) The scores for the physiological variables are obtained by recording the most abnormal variable in each category within the first 12 hours of admission to the critical care unit

Question 52

A 25-year-old man requires urgent assessment in the emergency department. Recently admitted following a fall of 20 m while climbing, he has suddenly become hypotensive (BP 55/30 mmHg), hypoxaemic (SpO$_2$ 88% on 15 L/min O$_2$ via a non-rebreathe mask) and tachycardic (HR 160 bpm) having been cardiovascularly stable with good saturations on admission 60 minutes earlier. He has sustained multiple bilateral rib fractures, a sternal fracture, bilateral fractured scapulae and a mid-shaft femoral fracture but no pelvic fracture. Auscultation of his lung fields reveals bilateral air entry, his trachea is midline, his abdomen is soft and non-distended and there has been no response to administration of 3000 mL of crystalloid. Which of the following is the most likely diagnosis to explain the sudden deterioration?

a) Blood loss secondary to multiple fractures
b) Cardiac tamponade

c) Severe, bilateral pulmonary contusions
d) Tension pneumothorax
e) Liver laceration

Question 53

Regarding aspects of acute stridor in children, which one of the following statements is correct?

a) Respiratory syncytial virus (RSV) most commonly causes laryngotracheobronchitis
b) Because of the potential for complete airway obstruction, an intravenous cannula should be sited as a priority
c) Steroids no longer have a place in the treatment of croup
d) Once intubated, patients with a diagnosis of croup tend to have longer time to extubation than those with epiglottitis
e) A two day history of high fever and barking cough in a 4-year-old is typical for a diagnosis of croup

Question 54

Regarding the magnetic resonance imaging (MRI) contrast medium gadolinium, which one of the following statements is true?

a) Gadolinium is usually administered as the soluble salt, gadolinium chloride
b) Unlike X-ray contrast media, gadolinium is safe to administer to patients with stage 3 chronic kidney disease
c) Gadolinium is paramagnetic in its Gd^{3+} state
d) The main role in MRI for gadolinium is to enhance the brightness of neural tissue
e) Gadolinium produces a similar incidence of severe allergic reactions compared to X-ray contrast media

Question 55

A 55-year-old, 75 kg male sustains 40% body surface area (BSA) burns in a house fire. Using the Parkland formula, in addition to maintenance fluids, the extra intravenous fluid he should receive in the first eight hours following injury is:

a) 3000 mL of crystalloid
b) 3000 mL of colloid
c) 750 mL colloid and 2250 mL of crystalloid
d) 4000 mL of crystalloid
e) 6000 mL of crystalloid

Question 56

Regarding opioids, which one of the following statements is correct?
Compared to fentanyl, morphine has:

a) A higher lipid solubility, a lower potency and a higher proportion bound to plasma protein
b) A lower lipid solubility, a higher potency and a higher proportion bound to plasma protein
c) A higher lipid solubility, a higher potency and a lower proportion bound to plasma protein
d) A lower lipid solubility, a lower potency and a higher proportion bound to plasma protein
e) A lower lipid solubility, a lower potency and a lower proportion bound to plasma protein

Question 57

Regarding making the diagnosis of autonomic neuropathy, which one of the following statements is correct?

a) Anhydrosis is the most common presenting symptom
b) A normal sinus arrhythmia involves mild elevation of heart rate during expiration and mild depression during inspiration
c) A Valsalva manoeuvre is of no use as a bedside test
d) During a sustained handgrip, a normal response would be an increase in diastolic blood pressure of >16 mmHg in the opposite arm
e) The patient's ability to perform mental arithmetic may aid diagnosis at the bedside

Question 58

A 45-year-old male presents for microlaryngoscopy following the development of a persistent hoarse voice. He mentions that when he had an appendicectomy, at age 12, the anaesthetist told him he had struggled to place his breathing tube. Which one of the following would most predict a potential difficulty with tracheal intubation?

a) Thick beard and moustache
b) Maximal mouth opening of 4 cm
c) Sternomental distance of 12 cm
d) Patel's distance of 6.5 cm
e) Wilson score 1

Question 59

In peri-operative care, which one of the following interventions reduces the risk of wound infections by 80%, the risk of requiring secondary surgery by 70% and the risk of pulmonary complications by 80%?

a) Screening for and treating MRSA colonisation
b) Avoiding inadvertent peri-operative hypothermia
c) Stopping smoking eight weeks pre-operatively
d) Intraoperative goal directed therapy
e) Preoperative safety briefing

Question 60

A 78-year-old male with advanced dementia presents with a large incarcerated inguinal hernia. He is extremely confused, agitated and combative. He is being physically violent and despite his age and weighing only 60 kg he is requiring four theatre staff to prevent him from falling off the theatre table. He has already kicked one theatre support worker and attempts to secure venous access have failed, prompting further violent outbursts from the patient. It is your judgement that he requires a rapid sequence induction but that he currently poses a risk of harm to himself and others. It is your intention to provide sedation sufficient to tolerate intravenous cannulation whereupon you will pre-oxygenate and perform an intravenous rapid sequence induction. You request ketamine, 100 mg/mL, which you plan to deliver intramuscularly. Which one of the following is the most suitable volume to administer?

a) 0.6 mL
b) 1.2 mL
c) 2.4 mL
d) 4.2 mL
e) 6.0 mL

Question 61

A 55-year-old man requires cerebral angiography and possible coiling of a large basilar aneurysm. He is diabetic with impaired renal function. Which of the following has been shown to reduce most the chances of the patient developing a contrast-induced nephropathy (CIN)?

a) An infusion of isotonic sodium bicarbonate commenced prior to contrast infusion
b) An N-acetylcysteine infusion commenced prior to contrast infusion
c) The use of the lowest dose of an iso-osmolar contrast medium possible
d) Commencement of an aminophylline infusion prior to contrast infusion
e) An infusion of 0.9% sodium chloride commenced prior to contrast infusion

Question 62

In severe anaphylaxis under anaesthesia, which of the following is most commonly the first to be detected?

a) Flushing of the skin
b) Facial oedema
c) Desaturation
d) Difficulty in ventilating
e) Decrease in arterial pressure

Question 63

An Ohmeda Isotec 5 vaporiser filled correctly with isoflurane has a 1 L/min fresh gas flow delivered to it at sea level and 20 °C. The control dial is set such that the splitting ratio is 5%. What is the resulting concentration of isoflurane at the outlet of the vaporiser?

a) 0.8%
b) 1.6%
c) 2.4%
d) 3.2%
e) 5.0%

Question 64

An 82-year-old female is awaiting a hip hemiarthroplasty having sustained a fractured neck of femur. She has mild dementia and is unable to relate her medical history. Her old notes are currently unavailable and as she has recently moved from out of the region her computer records are unhelpful. On examination she has a small volume, regular pulse. Her blood pressure is 136/72 mmHg and her JVP is not raised. She has an undisplaced, tapping apex beat. On auscultation, she has a short rumbling diastolic murmur audible all over the praecordium. Which one of the following is the most likely valve lesion?

a) Mitral stenosis
b) Aortic regurgitation
c) Mixed aortic valve disease
d) Tricuspid stenosis
e) Pulmonary regurgitation

Question 65

Regarding acute liver failure, which one of the following statements is true?

a) Subacute liver failure carries a better prognosis than hyperacute liver failure

b) Acute liver failure refers to 'jaundice to encephalopathy time' of one to four weeks
c) The commonest cause in the UK is infective hepatitis
d) Hyperglycaemia and hypokalaemia is the common metabolic derangement at presentation
e) Deliberate self-harm patients cannot be considered for liver transplantation

Question 66

Regarding normal coronary artery blood flow, the following statements are true except which one?

a) Total left coronary artery flow is initially decreased by tachycardia
b) At rest, right coronary artery blood flow is greater than left coronary artery blood flow at the beginning of systole
c) Flow in the left coronary artery at rest may be as high as 100 mL/min
d) Right coronary flow is at its lowest at the beginning of diastole
e) At rest, peak left coronary artery flow may be six times higher than peak right coronary artery flow

Question 67

Which one of the following statements regarding the anatomy of the brachial plexus is true?

a) The median nerve derives contributions from spinal nerve roots C5 to C8
b) The upper, middle and lower trunks each have divisions that unite to form the posterior cord
c) The axillary and radial nerves are both derived from the lateral cord
d) The medial cutaneous nerves of the arm and forearm are branches of the ulnar nerve
e) The lateral cutaneous nerve of the forearm is a terminal branch of the radial nerve

Question 68

Regarding oxygenation indices the following statements are correct except for which one?

a) Calculating venous admixture requires a pulmonary artery flotation catheter
b) A PaO_2:FIO_2 ratio <26.6kPa is a criterion for diagnosis of ARDS
c) $P(A-a)O_2$ is the respiratory index
d) Ideally an oxygenation index should not vary with changes in FIO_2
e) The alveolar gas equation is required for a number of oxygenation indices

Question 69

Regarding the diagnosis and management of peptic ulcer disease, which one of the following statements is correct?

a) In the UK, gastric ulcers are, overall, more common than duodenal ulcers
b) Alcohol consumption is an independent risk factor for peptic ulcer disease
c) Peptic ulcers, almost universally, present with pain as one of the clinical features
d) The presence of night-pain tends to suggest a duodenal rather than gastric ulcer
e) A perforated peptic ulcer necessitates urgent laparotomy

Question 70

Regarding urinary chemical reagent dipstick testing, the following are true except which one?

a) The presence of leucocytes with no nitrites is more common than the presence of nitrites with no leucocytes
b) Urine specific gravity measurements may need to be adjusted upwards if the urine is strongly acidic
c) If the stick is left with a coating of excess urine after dipping, errors are most likely to be found in the pH reading
d) Concurrent nephrotic syndrome may lead to overdiagnosing the syndrome of inappropriate antidiuretic hormone (SIADH) when analysing dipstick specific gravity
e) If the urine is allowed to stand for one hour, glucose testing may produce a false negative

Question 71

According to the product information leaflets, which one of the following statements is true?

a) Albumin solution should not be used in patients with known egg allergy
b) The use of 20% Intralipid is safe in patients with a known peanut allergy
c) Gelofusine® may be unacceptable for the management of a Hindu patient
d) Propofol should not be used in patients with a known egg allergy
e) The use of hydroxyl ethyl starch solutions in patients with gluten-sensitive enteropathy should be avoided

Question 72

A patient on the intensive care unit develops offensive diarrhoea following treatment for ventilator-associated pneumonia. *Clostridium difficile* toxin has been detected in the stool. Which one of the following statements regarding *C. difficile* infection is true?

a) Following initial treatment of *C. difficile* colitis recurrence is uncommon
b) Over 50% of adults carry *C. difficile* asymptomatically
c) The pathogenesis of *C. difficile* is secondary to the production of two types of exotoxin
d) Treatment with broad spectrum cephalosporins carries the highest risk of developing *C. difficile* colitis compared with treatment with other antibiotic types or groups
e) Non-toxin producing strains of *C. difficile* may cause pseudomembranous colitis

Question 73

According to the CEMACH report (2003–5) published in 2007, which one of the following is true?

a) The leading cause of indirect maternal death is psychiatric
b) There has been a significant rise in direct deaths due to amniotic fluid embolism
c) A third of the women who died from direct or indirect causes were overweight or obese
d) Thromboembolism is the second highest cause of direct maternal death
e) The time frame applied to late maternal death is >30 days and <1 year from the end of the pregnancy

Question 74

Regarding cranial nerve examination during testing for brain-stem death, the following cranial nerves are examined except which one?

a) Cranial nerve VIII
b) Cranial nerve V
c) Cranial nerve XI
d) Cranial nerve IX
e) Cranial nerve X

Question 75

Regarding implantable cardiac defibrillators, which one of the following statements is true?

a) An implantable defibrillator must be turned off before surgery involving diathermy
b) If the indifferent grounding pad is greater than 15 cm from the defibrillator, the risk from unipolar diathermy electrocautery is eliminated
c) An internal cardioversion shock of two joules will cause painful skeletal and diaphragmatic contraction in the awake patient
d) External cardiac pacing is contraindicated in the presence of implantable defibrillator leads
e) In approaching 90% of cases, a functioning implantable defibrillator will successfully terminate a malignant arrhythmia within 15 seconds

Paper B

Question 76

Regarding the use of phenylephrine following central neuraxial block in obstetric anaesthesia, the following statements are true except which one?

a) Continuous infusion produces fewer periods of hypotension than intermittent boluses
b) It results in less umbilical artery acidaemia than ephedrine
c) It produces less bradycardia compared to ephedrine
d) It produces less supraventricular tachycardia compared to ephedrine
e) It has not been shown to exhibit tachyphylaxis

Question 77

Refeeding syndrome can manifest with the following derangements except which one?

a) Hypophosphataemia
b) Hyperkalaemia
c) Hypomagnesaemia
d) An increase in the minute volume and respiratory quotient
e) Increased extracellular fluid volume

Question 78

A 29-year-old multiparous woman suffers an antepartum haemorrhage secondary to placental abruption and in the course of the resuscitation and subsequent emergency caesarean section receives twelve units of packed red blood cells and four units of fresh frozen plasma. The following laboratory results would be expected in acute disseminated intravascular coagulation except which one?

a) Reduced soluble fibrin
b) Moderate thrombocytopenia
c) Decreased factor VII levels
d) Gradual decrease in fibrinogen
e) Prolonged activated partial thromboplastin time

Question 79

Regarding peri-operative fluid management, which one of the following statements is most correct?

a) In patients with acute kidney injury, potassium-containing balanced electrolyte solutions should be avoided
b) Higher molecular weight hydroxyethyl starch solutions should be avoided in severe sepsis
c) For patients with acute kidney injury, if free water is required 5% dextrose solution should be avoided
d) In patients without gastric emptying disorders, oral water is acceptable pre-operatively except in the last hour prior to induction of anaesthesia
e) Elderly patients are more likely to benefit from 4% dextrose/0.18% saline fluid as maintenance

Question 80

After cessation of smoking 20 cigarettes a day for 20 years, which one of the following takes the longest to show signs of significant improvement?

a) Small airway function
b) The negative inotropic effect of smoking
c) Excess sputum production
d) Polycythaemia
e) Risk of chest infection

Question 81

In a patient having cortical somatosensory evoked potentials monitoring of spinal cord integrity during spinal surgery, the following may produce important inaccuracies except which one?

a) Blood pressure variations
b) Temperature variations
c) Neuromuscular blocking drugs
d) Haemorrhage down to a haemoglobin of 5.5 g/dL
e) Maintenance of anaesthesia with sevoflurane

Question 82

A 30-year-old Chinese woman who has been in the United Kingdom for the last year is scheduled to have a laparoscopic cholecystectomy. She has no significant past medical history other than rheumatoid arthritis for which she takes occasional analgesia only. She has been feeling tired over the last few months. Clinical examination is consistent with rheumatoid arthritis but otherwise unremarkable. She has a microcytic, hypo-chromic anaemia with a haemoglobin of 9.6 g/dL. Which of the following is least likely to be the cause?

a) HbH disease
b) Alpha-thalassaemia trait
c) Anaemia secondary to rheumatoid arthritis
d) Beta-thalassaemia minor
e) Anaemia secondary to menorrhagia

Question 83

Regarding a person with acromegaly presenting for transsphenoidal hypophysec-tomy, which of the following statements is most likely to be true?

a) The patient is more likely to be male than female
b) Males with acromegaly are as likely to suffer from obstructive sleep apnoea as females

c) Patients with acromegaly are more likely to have a distal rather than a proximal myopathy
d) They are likely to have raised adrenocorticotrophic hormone (ACTH) levels
e) They are likely to have raised levels of insulin-like growth factor-1 (IGF-1)

Question 84

A patient is brought into the resuscitation room with a reduced conscious level. He was recognised as having been admitted a week earlier with deliberate self-poisoning. His blood gases were as follows: pH 7.01; PaO_2 9.8 kPa; $PaCO_2$ 6.1 kPa; HCO_3^- 12 mEq/L; base excess −18; anion gap 9 mEq/L.
Which one of the following is the patient most likely to have been poisoned with?

a) Amitriptyline
b) Methadone
c) Paroxetine
d) Ethanol
e) Organophosphates

Question 85

Regarding systemic lupus erythematosus (SLE), the following statements are correct except which one?

a) There is a 10:1 female preponderance, particularly affecting women of child-bearing age
b) Patients with SLE and isolated lupus anticoagulant antibody are clinically coagulopathic contraindicating central neuraxial blockade
c) Peri-partum high dose steroid therapy may be necessary
d) Pregnant patients are at increased risk of pregnancy-induced hypertension, regardless of their pre-pregnancy renal status
e) More than 50% of patients with SLE have demonstrable psychiatric or neurological abnormalities including seizures and cerebrovascular events

Question 86

A patient with severe acute respiratory distress syndrome (ARDS) develops a pneumothorax requiring insertion of a chest drain. You decide to institute high-frequency oscillatory ventilation (HFOV). Regarding this case which of the following options is correct?

a) Positive end expiratory pressure (PEEP) levels during HFOV would be similar to those in an optimal conventional ventilator strategy
b) Tidal volumes employed in HFOV are generally only 1 to 2 mL/kg more than the physiological dead-space volume
c) Maximum ventilation frequency may be up to 300 per minute
d) On commencement of HFOV a drop in cardiac output and central venous pressure and a rise in pulmonary artery pressure would be expected
e) The tidal volume generated during HFOV is directly related to both the driving pressure and ventilator frequency, both of which are controlled by the operator

Question 87

The following are used by a laboratory to calculate an estimated glomerular filtration rate except for which one?

a) Age
b) Weight

c) Ethnic group
d) Local variations in serum creatinine measurement
e) Gender

Question 88

A 35-year-old male presents to the intensive care unit with respiratory failure requiring mechanical ventilation. His chest X-ray shows bilateral pulmonary infiltrates. Which of the following statements makes a diagnosis of non-cardiogenic pulmonary oedema most likely?

a) The presence of peribronchial cuffing
b) Even or central radiographic distribution of the pulmonary oedema
c) The presence of septal lines
d) The presence of an air bronchogram
e) The presence of pleural effusions

Question 89

Regarding xenon, the following statements are true except which one?

a) Xenon has analgesic as well as anaesthetic properties
b) Xenon may protect against hypoxic neuronal injury
c) A worldwide conversion to xenon use for anaesthesia would be beneficial with respect to climate change
d) Xenon's first reported use as an anaesthetic was in 1951
e) Xenon has a blood:gas partition coefficient of 0.115

Question 90

A previously fit and well 31-year-old male patient requiring ventilation for severe respiratory failure characterised by haemoptysis and hypoxia was found to have diffuse pulmonary haemorrhage. He also tested positive for haematuria and proteinuria. His tests for c-ANCAs (classical antineutrophil cytoplasmic antibodies) were positive, confirming the diagnosis of Wegener's granulomatosis. Once the diagnosis has been made, which one of the following would be the preferred drug therapy?

a) Cyclophosphamide i.v. 1 g/day
b) Methylprednisolone i.v. 30 mg/day
c) Ciclosporin i.v. 200 mg/day
d) Azathioprine i.v. 250 mg/day
e) Methotrexate i.v. 7.5 mg/week

Question 91

You are working in the developing world and a patient with known acute intermittent porphyria presents for emergency surgery. Which one of the following pharmaceuticals would it be best to avoid in this patient?

a) Suxamethonium
b) Halothane
c) Aspirin
d) Pancuronium
e) Ropivacaine

Question 92

Which one of the following statements is true regarding anaesthesia for routine elective neurosurgery?

a) Desflurane is the agent of choice for many neuroanaesthetists
b) Dense neuromuscular blockade is required for a craniotomy
c) Permissive hypothermia is usually employed for cerebral protection
d) Resection of cortex is profoundly stimulating
e) A central venous catheter is mandatory for a craniotomy in a head-up position

Question 93

The following drugs are correctly paired with their mechanism of action except which one?

a) Dopexamine – dopamine and beta-adrenergic agonist
b) Prenalterol – beta-adrenergic agonist
c) Digoxin – inhibition of sodium–potassium ATPase pump
d) Bucladesine – phosphodiesterase inhibitor
e) Istaroxime – calcium channel stimulator

Question 94

Amniotic fluid embolism (AFE) is an obstetric emergency. Which one of the following statements is true?

a) Polyhydramnios is a proven risk factor
b) AFE most commonly occurs during caesarean section
c) Regarding symptoms of AFE, headache is more common than chest pain
d) Presence of foetal squamous cells in the pulmonary vasculature is diagnostic
e) Delivery of the baby is not a priority in terms of improving maternal outcome

Question 95

A 38-year-old woman who is hypotensive and has severe abdominal pain requires review. She has a raised serum amylase. Which of the following is the least likely to explain her symptoms and biochemical findings?

a) Perforated duodenal ulcer
b) Ruptured ectopic pregnancy
c) Diabetic ketoacidosis
d) Myocardial infarction
e) Acute pyelonephritis

Question 96

Regarding hormone production in the adrenal cortex, the following statements are true except which one? (CRH: corticotropin releasing hormone; ACTH: adrenocorticotrophin hormone)

a) Secretion of cortisol is under the exclusive control of the hypothalamopituitary CRH–ACTH axis
b) ACTH stimulates aldosterone secretion
c) Hyperkalaemia is a major stimulus to aldosterone secretion
d) Etomidate inhibits 17α-hydroxylase in the zona glomerulosa
e) Urinary cortisol metabolites give a reliable representation of cortisol secretion

Question 97

At rest and during light, moderate or heavy exercise the distribution of cardiac output through specific vascular beds varies. For a typical 70 kg male, the following statements are true except which one?

a) During heavy exercise, the cerebral blood flow is 750 mL/min
b) At rest, renal blood flow is 450 mL/min per 100 g of tissue
c) At rest, skeletal muscle receives 20% of total cardiac output
d) During heavy exercise, coronary blood flow increases eight-fold
e) During heavy exercise, splanchnic blood flow falls to around 1% of total cardiac output

Question 98

You have collected data on the blood pressure of 40 patients both pre- and post-admission to the critical care unit. You now wish to analyse this data. Which of the following statistical tests would be the most appropriate?

a) Mann–Whitney U test
b) Spearman's rank correlation coefficient
c) Kruskal–Wallace one-way analysis of variance
d) Paired Student's t-test
e) Wilcoxon signed-rank test

Question 99

The following statements regarding intensive care unit (ICU)-acquired weakness are true except which one?

a) The incidence of critical illness polyneuropathy among septic shock patients on the ICU is 80%
b) Muscles of facial expression are spared by critical illness polymyopathy
c) Presence of normal deep tendon reflexes does not eliminate the diagnosis of critical illness polyneuropathy
d) Persistent hyperglycaemia is an independent risk factor for ICU-acquired weakness
e) Electrophysiological studies typically show a reduced nerve conduction velocity

Question 100

Multiple sclerosis relapse is more commonly found to occur in all of the following situations except which one?

a) Post-partum
b) Following influenza immunisation
c) In the spring and summer
d) Following periods of stress
e) Following hyperpyrexia

Question 101

A 23-year-old female presents on a Sunday evening with acute appendicitis and is booked for urgent appendicectomy. She is Caucasian and has been a UK resident all her life. She is 19 weeks pregnant. She was previously fit and well although has noticed some peripheral oedema and dyspnoea on exertion recently. On examination, she is found to be unwell, pyrexial (39.5 °C) and tachycardic. On praecordial auscultation, a mid- to late-systolic murmur at the left sternal edge is audible. Her electrocardiogram shows left axis deviation, some premature beats and some inconsistent T-wave changes. An echocardiogram cannot be performed until Monday morning. Her electrolytes are normal and she has been adequately volume resuscitated by the surgical team. Which one of the following statements regarding conduct of anaesthesia is true?

a) Surgery should not be delayed until a cardiology opinion can be given
b) Coagulopathy of pregnancy necessitates the availability of blood component therapy
c) Nitrous oxide should be avoided as there is evidence that, as a potent inhibitor of methionine synthetase, foetal detriment may be incurred
d) Awareness should be avoided by the use of slightly elevated concentrations of volatile anaesthetic agent, given the increased minimum alveolar concentration (MAC) associated with pregnancy
e) The prophylactic use of terbutaline, as a tocolytic, is recommended to avoid precipitating miscarriage

Question 102

Regarding the physics of ultrasound, which one of the following statements is correct?

a) Application of a direct current causes piezoelectric materials to vibrate
b) The speed of sound conduction through the human body is $940\,m/s$
c) Differences in acoustic impedence of different tissues causing refraction of the incident beam is the basis of ultrasound imaging in the body
d) For most applications in anaesthesia, e.g. vessel cannulation and regional anaesthesia, A-mode display format is employed
e) Anisotropy is an example of an ultrasound artefact where the echoic amplitude of a structure varies with the angle of insonation

Question 103

Regarding the clinical management of older patients with fractures of the femoral neck, the following are recognised targets except which one?

a) Surgical fixation should be within 24 hours of admission unless there are clear reversible medical conditions
b) Patients should be admitted to an appropriate ward area within four hours of presentation
c) A preoperative electrocardiogram is mandatory
d) Addressing analgesic need is a clinical priority
e) Patients with a normal plain radiograph but a strong clinical suspicion of a fracture should undergo urgent supplementary imaging (MRI, CT or bone isotope scan)

Question 104

Regarding spectrophotometric oximetry, which one of the following statements is correct?

a) $660\,nm$ is the wavelength of light emitted by one of the LEDs in the apparatus because this is one of the isobestic points of the pertinent absorption spectra
b) While placed on the ear, approximately 30% of absorbed energy is due to the pulsatile component of the tissue
c) Venous blood in the tissues does not contribute to the absorption of the red and infrared light
d) Of all the potential colours of nail varnish, red-coloured nail varnish will disrupt the pulse oximeter to the greatest extent
e) Oximetry may determine relative proportions of carboxyhaemoglobin and methaemoglobin

Question 105

Regarding drowning, the following statements are true except which one?

a) Absence of water in the lungs at post mortem confirms a diagnosis of 'dry drowning', usually caused by laryngospasm
b) In the UK, 25% of cases of drowning occur in salt water
c) Atypical drowning may involve a sudden stopping of the heart on immersion in cold water
d) The incidence of cervical spine injury in drowning events is 1 in 200
e) Aspiration of as little as 200 mL of water by an 80 kg man may increase intrapulmonary shunt from 10% to 75%

Question 106

A patient is admitted for incision and drainage of buttock abscesses. He is a 39-year-old professional bodybuilder who was competing in a national bodybuilding tournament four days ago. He is 185 cm tall and weighs 100 kg. He admits that his abscesses are due to long-term abuse of injected anabolic steroids administered into the buttock. Compared to a healthy male matched for age, height and weight who takes moderate exercise for 30 minutes three times a week, which of the following is least likely to be found in this patient?

a) A higher risk of developing atrial fibrillation
b) A higher anaerobic threshold
c) A higher risk of pressure sores
d) A faster emergence from volatile anaesthesia
e) A higher risk of venous thromboembolism

Question 107

From the *Serious Hazards of Transfusion Reports (SHOT) 1996–2008*, which one of the following conditions has resulted in the highest number of deaths in which a transfusion reaction was felt to be either causal or contributory?

a) Transfusion-related acute lung injury
b) Incorrect blood component transfused
c) Acute transfusion reaction
d) Transfusion-transmitted infections
e) Transfusion-associated graft versus host disease

Question 108

A patient is admitted to the intensive care unit following an out-of-hospital ventricular fibrillation cardiac arrest. He was sedated and cooled for 24 hours and is now 72 hours post event. Which of the following is not invariably associated with a poor outcome (i.e. a Glasgow Outcome Scale score of three or less)?

a) Absent bilateral N2O response from the primary somatosensory cortex at 72 hours post event
b) Extensor posturing to noxious stimulus at 72 hours post event
c) Absence of a corneal response at 72 hours post event
d) Myoclonic status epilepticus at 24 hours post event
e) Significantly elevated levels of S100 (glial protein) post cardiac arrest

Question 109

Regarding the anaesthetic considerations of patients with diabetes mellitus, the following are correct except which one?

a) The National Institute of Health and Clinical Excellence recommends preoperative urinalysis for ASA 2 patients with cardiovascular comorbidity
b) The Alberti regime initially involves 500 mL of 10% dextrose with 10 mmol of potassium chloride and 10 units of rapid acting soluble insulin infused at 100 mL/h
c) Patients with diabetes are prone to gastroparesis and thus pulmonary aspiration of gastric contents
d) Glycosylation of collagen in cervical and temporomandibular joints may render laryngoscopy difficult
e) Autonomic dysfunction is detectable in 40% of patients with diabetes mellitus Type 1

Question 110

All of the following drugs were withdrawn or had their licence removed because of cardiovascular adverse effects at therapeutic doses except which one?

a) Cisapride
b) Aprotinin
c) Droperidol
d) Co-proxamol
e) Rofecoxib

Question 111

Regarding rivaroxaban, which one of the following statements is true?

a) It is a new oral direct thrombin inhibitor
b) It is a pro-drug
c) At therapeutic doses it has a superior effect on venous thromboembolism rate compared to enoxaparin
d) At therapeutic doses it produces lower rates of bleeding complications compared to enoxaparin
e) It has a half-life of two to four hours

Question 112

In primary hyperaldosteronism (Conn's syndrome) which one of the following is most likely to be found on routine blood investigations?

a) High potassium, low sodium and high hydrogen ions
b) High potassium, low sodium and low hydrogen ions
c) Low potassium, low sodium and high hydrogen ions
d) Low potassium, high sodium and high hydrogen ions
e) Low potassium, high sodium and low hydrogen ions

Question 113

A 21-year-old woman has acute appendicitis and requires general anaesthesia for an appendicectomy. Thorough pre-oxygenation is undertaken and a rapid sequence induction of anaesthesia is performed using 5 mg/kg of thiopentone and 1.5 mg/kg of suxamethonium while a trained assistant applies 30 N of cricoid pressure. After three attempts at tracheal intubation it has not been possible to intubate the trachea.

According to the Difficult Airway Society guidelines, which one of the following options is the most appropriate action to be taken next?

a) Have one last (fourth) attempt at intubation
b) Check and optimise the patient's head and neck position
c) Request that the assistant performs backwards–upwards–rightwards pressure
d) Recognise that this is a failed intubation and move to 'Plan B'
e) Ventilate via a facemask

Question 114

The following methods can be used, clinically or experimentally, to detect carbon dioxide, except for which one?

a) Infrared light spectroscopy
b) Infrared photoacoustic spectroscopy
c) Raman spectroscopy
d) Polarography
e) Chromatography

Question 115

Regarding heparin-induced thrombocytopenia (HIT) the following statements are true except which one?

a) The patient receiving low molecular weight heparin is less likely to develop HIT than the patient receiving unfractionated heparin
b) A diagnosis of HIT is more likely if the platelet count falls to $50 \times 10^9/L$ than falls to $10 \times 10^9/L$
c) The assays used to make a diagnosis of HIT have a higher specificity than they do sensitivity
d) A patient with HIT is more likely to develop thrombosis than a similar patient without HIT
e) Prophylactic platelet transfusions should be avoided in a patient with HIT

Question 116

The preoperative administration of carbohydrate-rich beverages has been shown to reduce all the following except which one?

a) Risk of significant aspiration
b) Postoperative nausea and vomiting
c) Insulin resistance
d) Length of hospital stay
e) Anxiety

Question 117

The following are recognised causes of a U wave on an electrocardiogram except which one?

a) Congenital long QT syndrome
b) Hypercalcaemia
c) Flecainide
d) Thyrotoxicosis
e) Hypokalaemia

Question 118

The National Patient Safety Agency (NPSA) recommends a number of methods to reduce the risk of a throat pack (TP) being inadvertently left *in situ*. As part of these recommendations they suggest that one of two methods be used in all cases. Which of the following options contains both of these suggested methods?

a) Placing a visible label on the patient stating a TP is *in situ* and removing it when the TP is removed, or placing a label on the airway device (LMA or endotracheal tube) stating a TP is *in situ*
b) Tying one end of the TP to the airway device, or recording insertion and removal of the TP as part of the formal swab count
c) Recording insertion and removal of the TP as part of the formal swab count, or performing a formalised two-person check of the insertion and removal of the TP
d) Leaving part of the TP protruding externally, or putting a visible label or mark on the patient stating a TP is *in situ*
e) Recording insertion and removal of the TP as part of the formal swab count, or attaching the TP securely to the artificial airway device

Question 119

According to the British Thoracic Society guidelines on non-invasive ventilation (2002), essential features of a non-invasive ventilator include the following except which one?

a) A disconnection alarm
b) Internal battery with power for at least one hour
c) Sensitive flow triggers
d) Rate capability of at least 40 breaths/min
e) Pressure control

Question 120

Which one of the following clinical features is most likely to distinguish myasthenia gravis from Lambert–Eaton myasthenic syndrome?

a) Aged 55 at onset of symptoms
b) An improvement of strength with the administration of intravenous edrophonium
c) Involvement of facial muscles
d) Finding of immunoglobulin G antibodies to the nicotinic acetylcholine receptor
e) Presence of deep tendon reflexes

Question 121

Regarding the soda lime in a circle system, the following statements are true except which one?

a) The granule diameter is 3 to 4 mm
b) If it contains Titan Yellow, the colour change will be from deep pink when fresh to off-white when exhausted
c) It will contain water even in an unopened packet prior to use
d) It will always contain calcium hydroxide
e) As it is used there will be a steady decline in the amount of sodium hydroxide present

Question 122

A 15 kg 2-year-old boy is being anaesthetised, spontaneously breathing on a laryngeal mask airway, for exploration and repair of a small umbilical hernia. The child is otherwise fit and well. Thirty minutes into the procedure, for no apparent reason, the child develops a bradycardia of 30 bpm and end-tidal CO_2 falls to zero. With regard to the choice of uncuffed endotracheal tube (internal diameter in mm) for initial intubation attempt, the bolus dose of intravenous adrenaline, and setting for the manual monophasic defibrillator, which of the following options describes the best practice?

a) 4.0 endotracheal tube, 300 mcg adrenaline, defibrillator set to 30 joules
b) 4.5 endotracheal tube, 150 mcg adrenaline, defibrillator set to 60 joules
c) 4.0 endotracheal tube, 150 mcg adrenaline, defibrillator set to 60 joules
d) 4.5 endotracheal tube, 150 mcg adrenaline, defibrillator set to 30 joules
e) 4.0 endotracheal tube, 300 mcg adrenaline, defibrillator set to 60 joules

Question 123

Regarding methylene blue, the following statements are true except which one?

a) It has been used in cases of anaphylaxis previously unresponsive to standard treatment
b) It has been used in combination with light to treat psoriasis
c) It has been used to treat arsenic poisoning
d) It has been used to treat methaemoglobinaemia
e) It has been used to treat malaria

Question 124

Regarding the arterial supply of the spinal cord, the following statements are true except which one?

a) There are two posterior spinal arteries and one anterior spinal artery, all derived from the vertebral arteries
b) The great anterior radicular artery (spinal artery of Adamkiewicz) most often arises at T10 on the left
c) Some radicular arteries derive their supply from intercostal arteries
d) The pia mater does not cover the spinal vasculature
e) The anterior inferior spinal cord is more vulnerable to ischaemia than the posterior cord

Question 125

A 23-year-old severely asthmatic primigravida suffers a major post-partum haemorrhage due to uterine atony following a vaginal delivery. As well as appropriate therapy of major haemorrhage she receives syntometrine intramuscularly, syntocinon intravenously as a bolus and then by infusion. Which one of the following would be the most suitable agent for further pharmacological management of her condition?

a) Carboprost
b) Mifepristone
c) Misoprostol
d) Alprostadil
e) Dinoprostone

Question 126

Which of the following decreases the anticoagulant effect of warfarin?

a) Garlic
b) Glucosamine

c) Echinacea
d) Evening primrose oil
e) St John's wort

Question 127

Which one of the following statements regarding β-blockers is true?

a) When using esmolol, a loading dose of 0.1 mg/kg intravenously over one minute is reasonable
b) Propranolol has high oral bioavailability
c) Atenolol has high β_1 receptor selectivity
d) Metoprolol has low lipid solubility thus its absorption and bioavailability are limited
e) Labetalol antagonises α_1:β adrenoreceptors with a ratio of 1:7 when administered orally

Question 128

Which one of the following statements regarding approaches to the blocking of the brachial plexus is true?

a) The axillary approach alone is sufficient for all aspects of awake hand surgery
b) The interscalene approach blocks the plexus at the level of the trunks
c) The vertical infraclavicular approach has the highest rate of pneumothorax
d) An advantage of the supraclavicular approach is, being more distal, phrenic nerve block is not a complication
e) The subclavian perivascular approach relies on the plexus being immediately posterior to the subclavian artery as it crosses the first rib in between the scalenus anterior and medius

Question 129

Which one of the following gases is paramagnetic?

a) Nitrogen
b) Nitrous oxide
c) Nitric oxide
d) Nitrogen dioxide
e) Dinitrogen tetroxide

Question 130

While working abroad, at an altitude of 5000 m, it becomes necessary to administer a general anaesthetic with an F_IO_2 of 0.9, to a healthy patient who lives locally. The operating theatre is heated and equipped with an anaesthetic machine that uses variable orifice flowmeters and a Tec5 isoflurane vaporiser, out of circuit. Regarding your anaesthetic management, the following statements are true except for which one?

a) The delivered concentration of isoflurane will be more than that shown on the dial of the vaporiser
b) The oxygen rotameter will accurately read the delivered flow of oxygen
c) The alveolar concentration of isoflurane will need to be higher than at sea level to achieve the same degree of anaesthesia
d) The partial pressure of isoflurane in the vaporiser is the same as it would be if you returned with the same vaporiser to sea level
e) The patient's oxygen saturation is more likely to be 90% than 96%

Question 131

You are ventilating a patient in the theatre using a simple bag-in-bottle ventilator connected to the common gas outlet. You are using a fresh gas flow of 1 L/min, a circle breathing system and volume control ventilation mode. Using spirometry connected to your anaesthetic machine you note a tidal volume of 500 mL, a respiratory rate of 12 breaths per minute and an I:E ratio of 1:2. You need to rapidly affect a change in circuit concentration of volatile anaesthetic agent. You increase your fresh gas flow to 4 L/min. You leave all the ventilator settings unchanged. One minute later, what delivered minute volume would you expect the spirometry to be registering?

a) 5 L/min
b) 6 L/min
c) 7 L/min
d) 8 L/min
e) 9 L/min

Question 132

A 55-year-old man is awaiting a transjugular intrahepatic portosystemic shunt procedure. Considering the Child–Pugh classification of liver disease, of the following clinical features, which one does not score two points?

a) Ascites controlled with diuretics
b) Encephalopathy grade II
c) Bilirubin 42 micromol/L
d) Albumin 27 g/L
e) INR 2.4

Question 133

Regarding the anatomy and regional anaesthesia of the lumbar plexus, the following statements are true except which one?

a) The lumbar plexus is described as being derived from spinal nerve roots T12–L4
b) The genitofemoral nerve is of L1–2 spinal root origin
c) The lumbar plexus is embedded in the psoas major muscle
d) A lumbar plexus block combined with a proximal sciatic nerve block can provide complete anaesthesia for all leg and foot surgery
e) As the skin on the back is less sensitive, a lumbar plexus block is one which is better tolerated by patients without the need for sedation/analgesia

Question 134

The most common cause for an anaphylactic reaction under anaesthesia is which one of the following?

a) Antibiotics
b) Latex
c) Neuromuscular blocking drugs
d) Colloid solutions
e) Radiocontrast media

Question 135

A 30-year-old Jehovah's Witness presents for emergency surgery. Which of the following options is likely to be least acceptable to this patient during the peri-operative period?

a) Transfusion of pre-operatively donated autologous blood
b) Transfusion of human albumin solution
c) Epidural blood patch
d) Intraoperative cell salvage
e) Cardiac bypass

Question 136

A patient with known variegate porphyria presents with suspected acute appendicitis and requires a laparoscopy. The patient is fasted, in pain and extremely anxious. Which one of the following options describes the best peri-operative management?

a) Fluid: Hartmanns + 10% glucose; Premedication: Midazolam; Induction agent: Propofol; Maintenance anaesthetic agent: Isoflurane
b) Fluid: Hartmanns; Premedication: none; Induction agent: Thiopentone; Maintenance anaesthetic agent: Propofol
c) Fluid: Hartmanns + 10% glucose; Premedication: none; Induction agent: Propofol; Maintenance anaesthetic agent: Sevoflurane
d) Fluid: 5% dextrose; Premedication: none; Induction agent: Propofol; Maintenance anaesthetic agent: Isoflurane
e) Fluid: Hartmanns + 10% glucose; Premedication: none; Induction agent: Thiopentone; Maintenance anaesthetic agent: Isoflurane

Question 137

Regarding temperature measurement, the following statements are true except which one?

a) Rectal temperature tends to be higher than oesophageal temperature
b) Oesophageal probes most commonly incorporate a thermistor to transduce temperature to electrical changes
c) A thermopile is a collection of thermocouples connected in parallel
d) Tympanic membrane thermometers often employ the Seebeck effect
e) Miniaturised temperature measurement probes typically have response times of around one second

Question 138

The following nerves must be anaesthetised when performing regional anaesthesia of the foot. Which nerve is readily amenable to location using the peripheral nerve stimulator?

a) Superficial peroneal (fibular) nerve
b) Deep peroneal (fibular) nerve
c) Tibial nerve
d) Sural nerve
e) Saphenous nerve

Question 139

Regarding the measurement of biopotentials, which one of the following statements is true?

a) Signal-to-noise ratio must be minimised to optimise fidelity of displayed biopotential
b) Electrocardiogram electrodes generate potential as well as conduct current

c) Input impedance at the amplifier must be minimised in order to maximise the potential measured

d) The bandwidth of frequencies over which an electromyogram must consistently amplify is 0.5 to 100 Hz

e) Gain and common-mode rejection ratio are measured in Sone units

Question 140

A British anaesthetist working in the United Kingdom suffering a needle stick injury with a bloody, hollow sharp from a patient known to have hepatitis B, has serum tests at ten weeks post-inoculation. Which of the following is least likely to be found?

a) Positive for antibody to hepatitis B surface antigen
b) Positive for IgM for anti-hepatitis D virus
c) Positive for anti-hepatitis B surface antigen
d) Positive for hepatitis B virus DNA
e) Positive for hepatitis B e antigen

Question 141

Regarding the drug sodium nitroprusside (SNP), the following statements are correct except which one?

a) SNP ultimately causes vasodilation via increased concentration of intracellular cyclic guanylate monophosphate (cGMP)
b) Dicobalt edetate has a place in the management of toxicity induced by SNP
c) Vitamin B12 deficiency may predispose to SNP toxicity
d) SNP causes increased right-to-left intrapulmonary shunt
e) Thiocyanate, produced during one pathway of SNP metabolism, is non-toxic

Question 142

Regarding invasive arterial blood pressure monitoring, which one of the following statements is true?

a) An overdamped waveform underestimates diastolic pressure
b) An anacrotic notch is a sign of severe aortic stenosis
c) A rapid systolic upstroke is associated with a high systemic vascular resistance
d) The dicrotic notch appears later in the waveform complex if measured at the radial artery compared to the dorsalis pedis
e) Critical damping refers to the perfect level of damping and is the desired set-up for the system

Question 143

Which of the following scenarios would give you most concern that the patient lacked capacity to consent for the given procedure?

a) A 51-year-old understands the risks of delaying the surgery for her aggressive bowel cancer but still maintains that she does not want an operation that may cure her
b) For the fourth successive time a 63-year-old agrees to have surgery for a large incarcerated inguinal hernia, but on arriving in the anaesthetic room panics at the thought of the anaesthetic and refuses to have the operation
c) A 38-year-old woman who is 16 weeks pregnant with worsening signs and symptoms of acute appendicitis has the risks and benefits of surgery including the risks to the foetus explained. She refuses to have surgery as she believes any medicines, including anaesthetics, may damage her baby

d) An 87-year-old with mild dementia who is conversational and orientated but prone to being forgetful asks you twice to repeat the risks you have explained to him about the anaesthetic for his dynamic hip screw surgery

e) A 24-year-old with depression thought to be at high risk of suicide who has benefited from electroconvulsive therapy (ECT) in the past, refuses ECT against the recommendations of two senior psychiatrists. Six months earlier, the patient, during a period when considered by her mental health team to be of sound mind, had legally signed an advanced directive stating that she did not wish to ever have ECT again

Question 144

At preoperative assessment it is noticed that a patient's top teeth appear to be abnormally anterior to their bottom teeth. When asked to close their mouth, the tip of their top central incisors is 12 mm anterior to the tip of their bottom central incisors. Which one of the following terms best describes the patient's condition?

a) Overbite
b) Malocclusion
c) Micrognathia
d) Overjet
e) Overclosure

Question 145

A 69-year-old, 80 kg male is admitted to the intensive care unit with respiratory failure secondary to a lower respiratory tract infection. He has his trachea intubated and mechanical ventilation of the lungs is commenced. He has a PiCCO cardiac output monitor sited; an internal jugular central venous catheter and urinary catheter are also inserted. He receives antibiotics, intravenous fluid resuscitation and an infusion of noradrenaline. Three hours following admission to hospital, some of his clinical measurands are as follows: heart rate 110 bpm; mean arterial blood pressure 66 mmHg; central venous pressure 10 mmHg; arterial oxygen saturation 93%; central venous oxygen saturation 68%; cardiac index 2.5 L/min per m^2; urine output 30 mL/h; pH 7.23; PaCO$_2$ 6.0 kPa; PaO$_2$ 9.1 kPa; HCO$_3^-$ 19 mmol/L; base excess −6.2 mmol/L; lactate 3.2 mmol/L; haematocrit 0.31; FiO$_2$ 0.7; MV 7.2 L/min; plateau pressure 29 cmH$_2$O. Which one of the following should be prioritised for the patient to receive next?

a) Increased rate of noradrenaline infusion
b) Dobutamine infusion
c) Further intravenous fluid
d) Infusion of packed red cells
e) Increased minute ventilation

Question 146

The following statements regarding the features of local anaesthetic toxicity are true except which one?

a) Prilocaine toxicity may cause the pulse oximeter to read 85%
b) At a plasma lidocaine concentration of 5 mg/mL, tinnitus may be present
c) As toxicity develops, inhibitory pathway inhibition at first causes excitation
d) Unconsciousness may precede convulsions
e) Cardiac resting membrane potential is made more negative

Question 147

Which of the following is not a basic SI unit?

a) Candela
b) Kelvin
c) Mole
d) Newton
e) Ampere

Question 148

Following a day case procedure under general anaesthesia, which one of the following is not a criterion for approval of discharge from the day surgery unit?

a) Able to ambulate unassisted
b) No pain or mild pain controllable with oral analgesia
c) Agreed carer for 24 hours
d) No bleeding or minimal bleeding or wound drainage
e) Stable vital signs for one hour

Question 149

Which one of the following statements regarding calcium channel blocking drugs is true?

a) Most of these drugs act on the T-type calcium channel
b) Nifedipine acts mainly by negative inotropy
c) Nimodipine is a class III calcium channel blocking drug
d) Verapamil is a suitable treatment for supraventricular tachycardia
e) Heart block caused by calcium channel blocking drug overdose is treated with atropine

Question 150

A 31-year-old male with known haemophilia A presents with a fracture of his left tibia sustained while playing football. The orthopaedic surgeons propose operative application of an external fixation frame. The patient is unable to grade the severity of his haemophilia but has had two knee haemarthroses in the previous seven years. As part of the preoperative preparation of this patient, which one of the following should be administered intravenously?

a) Fresh frozen plasma
b) Cryoprecipitate
c) Recombinant factor VIII concentrate
d) Recombinant factor IX concentrate
e) Desmopressin

Paper C

Question 151

The following statements regarding the laws of physics applied to anaesthesia are true except which one?

a) Darcy's law is analogous to Ohm's law
b) Henry's law relates quantity of dissolved gases to their partial pressure
c) Laplace's law relates pressure, tension and radius of curvature of a tube, sphere or bubble
d) Hooke's law can be applied to the resonance witnessed in underdamped arterial blood pressure recording
e) Charles' law is often quoted in association with Boyle's law

Question 152

Regarding polycystic kidney disease the following statements are true except which one?

a) Autosomal dominant polycystic kidney disease is one of the most common inherited disorders in humans
b) Clinical manifestations usually present in the third or fourth decade of life
c) Hepatic cysts, diverticular disease and cardiac valvular abnormalities are associated with polycystic kidney disease
d) Flank pain is a recognised, although uncommon, complaint
e) Pregnancy in autosomal dominant polycystic kidney disease is not associated with higher rates of complications from extrarenal manifestations

Question 153

A 51-year-old man currently smokes 20 cigarettes a day, has a 40-pack-year history, asthma and is scheduled for elective inguinal hernia repair. Which of the following statements regarding the effects of his cigarette smoking is incorrect?

a) On average, compared to an identical non-smoker his morphine dose requirement will be increased
b) On average, compared to an identical non-smoker his vecuronium dose requirement will be increased
c) On average, compared to an identical non-smoker he is less likely to suffer postoperative nausea and vomiting

d) On average, compared to an identical non-smoker his paracetamol dose requirement will be increased
e) If he were to stop smoking, his therapeutic theophylline dose is likely to be reduced

Question 154

Regarding lactate metabolism, the following statements are true except which one?

a) A proportion of plasma lactate is produced by both erythrocytes and the heart
b) Ethanol excess produces a Type B lactic acidosis
c) Sepsis produces a Type B_1 lactic acidosis
d) Hyperlactaemia is variably associated with acidaemia
e) Lactate is metabolised by the liver, kidneys and skeletal muscle

Question 155

Regarding obstructive sleep apnoea (OSA), the following statements are true except which one?

a) Diagnosis is not dependent on polysomnography analysis
b) Hypopnoea is defined as >50% reduction in air flow for more than ten seconds
c) OSA syndrome is diagnosed by the presence of more than five episodes of apnoea or hypopnoea in every hour of sleep
d) Polysomnography may reveal arterial blood pressure of 240/120 mmHg during the arousal phase after an apnoeic episode
e) A neck circumference of greater than 17 inches (42 cm) is the most significant predictor for the presence of OSA

Question 156

Regarding awake tracheal intubation, the following statements are true except which one?

a) Xylometazoline is a useful agent for nasal vasoconstriction
b) During a translaryngeal block, remifentanil sedation, to minimise coughing, is desirable
c) For a 70 kg patient the maximum safe dose of cocaine is 1 mL of a 10% solution
d) Lidocaine applied topically has its potential plasma concentration reduced by first-pass metabolism
e) Superior laryngeal nerve block may be performed via a needle insertion point 1 cm inferior and 2 cm anterior to the prominent cornu of the hyoid

Question 157

A 61-year-old diabetic patient in the emergency department has developed signs of a systemic inflammatory response in the 90 minutes since she arrived with a painful, red, swollen ankle. She scratched her ankle yesterday. In the hour since triage, she has become rapidly unwell and the rash has spread up her leg to the knee, with the skin looking indurated, purple and blistering.

Along with resuscitating the patient, initial management should involve which of the following options?

a) Administer intravenous imipenem and arrange a computerised tomography (CT) scan
b) Administer intravenous imipenem and urgently call the general surgeons
c) Administer intravenous benzylpenicillin and arrange a magnetic resonance imaging (MRI) scan

d) Administer intravenous gentamicin and metronidazole and arrange a CT scan
e) Administer intravenous benzylpenicillin and urgently call the general surgeons

Question 158

Following emergency surgery a patient remains ventilated on the critical care unit. He needs a low dose noradrenaline intravenous infusion and now requires renal replacement therapy. He is to be commenced on continuous venovenous haemodiafiltration (CVVHDF). Which of the following flow rates of the total effluent (the sum of the dialysate and ultrafiltrate) of CVVHDF is the lowest that can still be considered effective for optimum renal replacement therapy?

a) 10 mL/kg of body weight per hour
b) 20 mL/kg of body weight per hour
c) 30 mL/kg of body weight per hour
d) 40 mL/kg of body weight per hour
e) 50 mL/kg of body weight per hour

Question 159

Regarding the management of a patient who has had a subarachnoid haemorrhage, which one of the following statements is most correct?

a) Systolic blood pressure should be carefully controlled within narrow limits
b) Hypervolaemia, haemodilution and hypertension ('triple H' therapy) should be introduced if cerebral oedema is suspected
c) Following procedural aneurysm management, prophylactic anticonvulsants should be administered
d) After an aneurysm has been coiled, aspirin and heparin are administered
e) Nimodipine 60 mg i.v. four-hourly for 21 days is used as prophylaxis against cerebral vasospasm

Question 160

One complication at the time of insertion of surgical or percutaneous dilational tracheostomy is bleeding. The following are true of peritracheal anatomy except which one?

a) The left brachiocephalic vein crosses from left to right, anterior to the trachea
b) The inferior thyroid veins run in the tracheoesophageal groove but form an anterior plexus
c) About 50% of people will have a thyroid ima artery
d) The thyroid isthmus lies anterior to the trachea at the level of the second and third tracheal rings
e) The jugular venous arch lies anterior to the trachea superior to the manubrium

Question 161

Urgent attendance in the recovery room is required. A patient is hypoxic and has overt features of residual neuromuscular blockade. A dose of neostigmine metilsulfate and glycopyrronium bromide is administered and the patient recovers quickly. On reviewing the patient's anaesthetic and drug charts, which of the following is least likely to have prolonged the action of the vecuronium that had been given?

a) The presence of an intraoperative metabolic acidosis
b) The isoflurane used as the maintenance anaesthetic

c) The gentamicin given prior to induction
d) The lithium the patient has been on to treat his long-standing bipolar disorder
e) Serum potassium 6.1 mmol/L

Question 162

Regarding a patient with Stage 3 chronic kidney disease, which one of the following statements is true?

a) They should have their haemoglobin maintained at 11 to 12 g/dL using iron supplements with or without erythropoietin
b) They should have their kidney function assessed every three months
c) They could be diagnosed during a period of acute kidney disease
d) If newly diagnosed, they should have a renal biopsy
e) They may have an average glomerular filtration rate of 25 mL/min per 1.73 m²

Question 163

Regarding the Valsalva manoeuvre, which one of the following statements is true?

a) Phase I involves raised intrathoracic pressure being transmitted to the aorta causing a transient decrease in blood pressure
b) Using a Valsalva manoeuvre therapeutically to terminate a supraventricular tachycardia takes advantage of Phase III physiology
c) Diabetic autonomic neuropathy disrupts the usual phases seen, most commonly by an exaggerated late hypertension
d) The Valsalva ratio is normally greater than 3
e) Congestive cardiac failure results in a square wave response

Question 164

Following the death of a patient, referral to the coroner or their deputy is mandatory in a number of situations. In which of the following situations is referral not mandatory?

a) A 52-year-old patient who has died six days after a proven myocardial infarction who was awaiting trial while on remand in prison
b) A 75-year-old man who has died of a subarachnoid haemorrhage with a past medical history including a diagnosis of pneumoconiosis
c) A 75-year-old woman admitted from a residential home with a bronchopneumonia and a core temperature of 34 °C
d) A 60-year-old patient with known COPD who had been discharged well following surgery three weeks previously and is then readmitted with bronchopneumonia from which they die two days later
e) A 40-year-old man who has died following admission for treatment of a urinary tract infection contributed to by a paraplegia sustained following an assault 20 years previously

Question 165

In the following options, $T_{1/2}$ is the half-life of the anticoagulant they are currently taking and T_{max} is the time taken from administration to reaching full activity. If a patient is anticoagulated and needs to have an epidural catheter removed, the ideal time between stopping the last dose of anticoagulant and starting the next dose of anticoagulant is:

a) $(3 \times T_{1/2}) + (8 \text{ hours} + T_{max})$
b) $(3 \times T_{1/2}) + (4 \text{ hours} - T_{max})$

c) $(2 \times T_{1/2}) + (8 \text{ hours} - T_{max})$
d) $(3 \times T_{1/2}) + (4 \text{ hours} + T_{max})$
e) $(2 \times T_{1/2}) + (8 \text{ hours} + T_{max})$

Question 166

A 20-year-old soldier is complaining of phantom limb pain (PLP) six months following lower-limb amputation. Which one of the following is incorrect regarding his condition and possible treatment options?

a) If he had had an epidural inserted prior to amputation his chances of developing PLP would have been reduced
b) The use of mirror therapy has been shown to reduce PLP in both upper- and lower-limb amputations
c) The incidence of PLP has been shown to be as high as 80%
d) The pain in PLP tends to be constant rather than intermittent
e) The incidence of PLP in adults is independent of age, gender and level of amputation

Question 167

Regarding tetanus, the following statements are true except which one?

a) May be diagnosed with the aid of the spatula test with high sensitivity and specificity
b) A patient who has survived the disease does not require further tetanus vaccination
c) Cardiovascular instability is best treated in intensive care with deep sedation
d) Musculoskeletal symptoms are caused by disruption of inhibitory neurotransmitter release by central nerves
e) Autonomic dysfunction may be successfully treated with magnesium

Question 168

A 58-year-old Afro-Caribbean female presents with clinical and radiological features of ischaemic colitis. She does not speak English. She is clinically dehydrated, tachypnoeic and distressed. Her laboratory results are as follows: Hb 10.8 g/dL; WCC 18 x 10^{10}/L; Platelets 146 x 10^9/L; Urea 10.1 mmol/L; Creatinine 89 micromol/L; pH 7.32; $PaCO_2$ 3.4 kPa; PaO_2 8.8 kPa; Base excess -4.0 mmol/L; Lactate 2.4 mmol/L. Erect chest X-ray does not show gas under the diaphragm. The surgical team proposes an urgent laparotomy. Oxygen is applied and aggressive fluid resuscitation commenced. Which one of the following statements is the most appropriate action to take next?

a) Once fluid resuscitated, proceed to surgery
b) Provide analgesia and order more blood tests
c) Give urgent antibiotics, then proceed to surgery
d) Transfuse packed red blood cells to a target haematocrit of 0.4
e) Intubate and ventilate on the intensive care unit and observe initially

Question 169

Occurring with an incidence of 1 per 7000 operations, which one of the following is the commonest cause of peri-operative loss of vision in patients undergoing non-ocular surgery?

a) Cortical infarction
b) Retinal ischaemia
c) Corneal abrasion

d) Ischaemic optic neuropathy
e) Electromagnetic retinal injury

Question 170

Regarding risk factors for the development of pre-eclampsia, the following statements are true except which one?

a) Pre-eclampsia is more likely to develop in women whose mothers had pre-eclampsia than in women whose mothers did not
b) Pre-eclampsia is more likely to develop in the daughters-in-law of women with a history of pre-eclampsia than in other women
c) Women with pre-existing chronic hypertension are more likely to develop pre-eclampsia
d) Among nulliparous women, black women have twice the risk of developing pre-eclampsia compared to white women
e) Nulliparous women who smoke have a similar risk of developing pre-eclampsia to non-smokers

Question 171

You are asked to review a patient in the recovery room one hour after the end of an anaesthetic for manipulation of a forearm fracture. He is 43 years old, unkempt and is of no fixed abode. He has a past history of schizophrenia for which he is on 75 mg of chlorpromazine per day. He is a 20 cigarette a day smoker, drinks up to 100 units of alcohol a week and has previously taken intravenous heroin. He has been in hospital for 24 hours. He is anxious, sweating, hypertensive, tremulous and hyperreflexic. As you arrive at the bedside, he has a self-limiting tonic-clonic seizure for 30 seconds. None of these symptoms or signs were present before induction and he has no history of epilepsy.
    Which one of the following is the most likely explanation?

a) Alcohol withdrawal
b) Nicotine withdrawal
c) Heroin withdrawal
d) Emergence from anaesthesia
e) Side effects of excess chlorpromazine

Question 172

When washing hands, which one of the following hand parts is most commonly missed?

a) The thenar eminence
b) The lateral aspect of the index finger
c) The dorsum of the thumb
d) The hypothenar eminence
e) The knuckle at the base of the little finger

Question 173

A 39-year-old patient presents for day case surgery. Which of the following is least likely to indicate that this patient is at risk of postoperative nausea and vomiting (PONV)?

a) The operation is laparoscopic sterilisation
b) The patient is female

c) The patient is a non-smoker
d) The patient had nausea following a rhinoplasty three years ago
e) The patient suffers from 'car-sickness'

Question 174

Which of the following is not considered a risk factor for the development of ventilator-associated pneumonia?

a) The presence of an orogastric tube
b) Acute respiratory distress syndrome (ARDS)
c) An *in situ* percutaneous tracheostomy
d) Treatment with muscle relaxants
e) Age >60 years

Question 175

Regarding the provision of anaesthesia for ENT surgery, which one of the following statements is most correct?

a) For microlaryngoscopy, a microlaryngoscopy tube (cuffed oral endotracheal tube, ID 5 mm) must be used
b) For functional endoscopic sinus surgery, given the operation's proximity to the patient's eyes, the eyes must be taped and padded
c) Of the various lasers available, carbon dioxide lasers do have the capacity to ignite endotracheal tubes
d) In myringoplasty using an overlay graft, use of nitrous oxide as part of the inhaled gas mixture is actually likely to be beneficial
e) In parotidectomy, neuromuscular blockade is recommended because coughing can cause surgical field disruption and significant haemorrhage

Question 176

A pulmonary artery flotation catheter is being used to monitor a patient on the cardiac intensive care unit following cardiac surgery. Which one of the following variables best reflects left ventricular preload?

a) Pulmonary capillary wedge pressure
b) Left ventricular end-diastolic pressure
c) Left ventricular wall tension
d) Left ventricular end-diastolic volume
e) Mean pulmonary venous pressure

Question 177

A hypothetical new anaesthetic vapour, jabetone, is presented as 600 g in a bottle costing £74.67. It has an atomic weight of 120 and a minimum alveolar concentration (MAC) of 2%. At a fresh gas flow of 1 L/min with an agent concentration of 2%, which one of the following options is the cost per hour?

a) 15 p/hour
b) 20 p/hour
c) 40 p/hour
d) 80 p/hour
e) 220 p/hour

Question 178

Regarding the eponymous descriptions of anaesthetic breathing systems the following statements are true except which one?

a) A Lack is a co-axial Mapleson A
b) A Water's circuit is a Mapleson C
c) A Magill is a parallel Mapleson A
d) An Ayre's T-piece is a Mapleson E
e) A Bain is a co-axial Mapleson D

Question 179

The following signs of anaphylaxis detected under anaesthesia are matched with the correct frequency except which one?

a) Cardiovascular collapse 88%
b) Bronchospasm 36%
c) Cutaneous erythema 45%
d) Angioedema of the face 24%
e) Bradycardia 3%

Question 180

Regarding the applied pharmacokinetics of opioids, which one of the following statements is true?

a) When administered intrathecally or extradurally, diamorphine is less likely than morphine to produce a delayed respiratory depressant effect due to its high lipid solubility
b) Alfentanil has a quicker onset time than fentanyl because it is more lipid soluble
c) The duration of action of morphine is longer than fentanyl because it has a longer terminal elimination half-life
d) Morphine may demonstrate a secondary peak effect due to gastro-enteric recirculation
e) When compared to morphine at equipotent doses, alfentanil has a shorter duration because it is subject to a more rapid clearance than morphine

Question 181

Regarding neurophysiology in the healthy, supine, adult subject, the following statements are true except for which one?

a) Brain parenchyma occupies 85% of the available intracranial volume
b) Cerebral blood volume accounts for 5 to 8% of the available intracranial volume
c) Cerebrospinal fluid occupies 7 to 10% of the available intracranial volume
d) Cerebrospinal fluid is produced at a rate of 0.1 to 0.2 mL/min
e) Intracranial pressure is 10 to 23 cmH$_2$O

Question 182

A 55-year-old overweight male presents during the evening. He was brought in by ambulance from a restaurant at which he had been at a celebration and had consumed a larger than average quantity of food and a large amount of alcohol. On leaving the restaurant he had vomited a small amount, but continued to retch and complained of severe left-sided chest pain. He soon developed haematemesis and subcutaneous emphysema in his neck. Which one of the following statements is true?

a) Admiral Boerhaave was famously a victim of this syndrome when it was originally described
b) The mechanism described is the commonest aetiology of the resulting surgical pathology
c) Mackler's triad, suggestive of the diagnosis, is the combination of dysphagia, epigastric pain and melaena
d) Management here should be with two large-bore thoracostomy tubes and observation on ITU, although thoracotomy is a possibility
e) Time from onset of symptoms until treatment is a major determinant of mortality with the two variables being directly related

Question 183

A 93-year-old man presents for reduction and repair of a large inguinal hernia that has made buttoning up his trousers uncomfortable. He is a lifelong non-smoker and still works two mornings a week in his son's bookshop. He wears a hearing aid and has had a previous haemorrhoidectomy, which was followed by postoperative vomiting. He has a thin, weak left arm, which he rarely uses following a brachial plexus injury in a tram accident at the age of 22. According to the American Society of Anesthesiologists (ASA) criteria, which of the following would be his correct ASA score?

a) I
b) I E
c) II
d) II E
e) III

Question 184

In morbidly obese patients which one of the following is the most reliable predictor of difficult intubation?

a) Height
b) Body mass index
c) Mallampati score
d) Neck circumference
e) Thyromental distance

Question 185

The following are recognised causes of the syndrome of inappropriate antidiuretic hormone secretion, except for which one?

a) Prone positioning
b) Positive-pressure ventilation
c) Subarachnoid haemorrhage
d) Pain
e) MDMA or 'Ecstasy' ingestion

Question 186

The five clinical risk factors that contribute to increased cardiac risk during major non-cardiac surgery, as proposed by Lee in 1999 and incorporated into the *ACC/AHA 2007 Guidelines on Perioperative Cardiovascular Evaluation*, are listed below. Indicate which one is incorrect.

a) History of ischaemic heart disease
b) History of pulmonary disease

c) History of cerebrovascular disease
d) Preoperative treatment with insulin
e) Preoperative serum creatinine >177 micromol/L

Question 187

Hospitals are required to invite patients, who are undergoing certain operations, to undertake a number of questionnaires designed to look at patient-reported outcome measures (PROMs) related to that specific operation. Which of the following is not one of these operations?

a) Elective hip replacement
b) Laparoscopic cholecystectomy
c) Groin herniorrhaphy
d) Varicose vein surgery
e) Elective knee replacement

Question 188

Regarding carbon monoxide poisoning, the following statements are true except which one?

a) Carbon monoxide shifts the oxyhaemoglobin dissociation curve to the left
b) The main route of carbon monoxide excretion is pulmonary
c) Observable tissue hypoxia is greater than would be expected from the reduction in oxygen delivery alone
d) Arterial carboxyhaemoglobin (COHb) percentage at the time of admission does not grade the severity of the injury
e) COHb of >30% should prompt consideration of hyperbaric oxygen therapy

Question 189

A 28-year-old woman has a retained placenta following uneventful vaginal delivery of her baby at term. She requires manual removal of the placenta for which subarachnoid anaesthesia is provided and the placenta is delivered. On arrival in the recovery room she suddenly becomes confused, agitated and clammy. She is noted to have a respiratory rate of 40 breaths/min, a heart rate of 50 bpm and a thready pulse volume. She then becomes unconscious. Her trachea is intubated and she is manually ventilated with 100% oxygen. Further examination reveals a blood pressure of 78/50 mmHg, SpO_2 of 88% and a loud murmur at the left sternal edge. She is unresponsive to painful stimuli despite no sedation, her pupils are small and gaze deviated to the right. Which one of the following is the most suitable action to take next?

a) Arrange a CT pulmonary angiogram
b) Insert a central venous catheter
c) Commence external cardiac massage
d) Place her in the left lateral position
e) Commence intravenous infusion of unfractionated heparin

Question 190

Regarding capnography, which one of the following statements is true?

a) Capnography is a sensitive marker of endobronchial intubation
b) Certain capnography traces are pathognomonic of particular equipment failures
c) $PaCO_2$ is always equal to or greater than $PETCO_2$
d) Pulmonary air embolism will decrease the magnitude of the Pa-ETCO$_2$ gradient
e) Capnography cannot be employed during high-frequency jet ventilation

Question 191

A 73-year-old, 68 kg male has a malignant intrathoracic tracheal stenosis. He needs a tracheal stent insertion on the thoracic surgery list for which your colleague is providing anaesthesia. The patient is considered at low risk of aspiration of gastric contents. He pre-oxygenates with the patient sitting up at 60°. He induces anaesthesia intravenously with 50 mcg of fentanyl and 80 mg of propofol, delivered very slowly until the patient is unresponsive and his eyelash reflex lost. His intention was to maintain spontaneous ventilation initially but on lying the patient supine and performing a chin lift he finds the patient coughs violently following which your colleague is unable to mask ventilate the patient. He performs direct laryngoscopy and finds a Cormack and Lehane Grade 4 view and is unable to intubate. He summons you to help and as you arrive the patient's SpO$_2$ is 82% and is showing no signs of regaining consciousness. In this 'can't intubate, can't ventilate' situation which one of the following is the most appropriate action?

a) Immediate cannula cricothyroidotomy and jet ventilation or tracheostomy by the surgeon, who is standing by
b) Insert a laryngeal mask airway and attempt to maintain ventilation and improve oxygenation
c) Give 100 mg suxamethonium intravenously to optimise the laryngoscopic view and intubate orally
d) Allow the patient to awaken from what was only a modest induction dose, and resume spontaneous ventilation sitting up
e) Give 100 mg of suxamethonium intravenously and request the surgeon perform rigid bronchoscopy

Question 192

Regarding botulinum toxin, the following statements are true except which one?

a) It is the most potent toxin found in nature
b) It produces non-competitive antagonism of post-synaptic acetylcholine receptors
c) It may cause a clinical condition in which the first parts of the body to be affected are often the cranial nerves
d) It is neutralised in canned food by heating the can to 121 °C for three minutes
e) It has been demonstrated to be successful in the management of anal fissure

Question 193

Transfusion of allogeneic donated bank blood exposes a patient to a number of risks. To reduce this risk, the patient's own erythrocytes may be re-transfused. The following statements are true of autologous blood transfusion except which one?

a) Acute normovolaemic haemodilution (ANH) is acceptable to some Jehovah's Witnesses
b) Preoperative autologous donation (PAD) negates the risk of transmission of infection
c) Postoperative cell salvage involves transfusing contents of wound drains once passed through an intrinsic filter in the reservoir – there is no further processing of transfusate
d) Cell salvage techniques may be used at caesarean section despite the presence of amniotic fluid
e) PAD involves collection of up to four units of blood over five weeks preoperatively with concurrent iron supplementation

Question 194

A ventilated patient is being monitored on the cardiac intensive care unit with a pulmonary artery flotation catheter. The values for some of the patient's parameters are as follows: Arterial blood pressure 115/70 mmHg; Pulmonary artery pressure 25/10 mmHg; Central venous pressure 10 mmHg; Pulmonary capillary wedge pressure 13 mmHg; Mean intrathoracic pressure 20 cmH$_2$0; Cardiac output 5 L/min. Measured in dyne.s.cm^{-5}, which one of the following options is his systemic vascular resistance?

a) 15
b) 18
c) 1080
d) 1200
e) 1680

Question 195

The following conditions are associated with digital clubbing except for which one?

a) Acromegaly
b) Pregnancy
c) Primary biliary cirrhosis
d) Infective endocarditis
e) Bronchitis

Question 196

In a patient known to be HIV positive, the following are all AIDS-defining clinical conditions except which one?

a) Invasive cervical cancer
b) Pneumocystis jiroveci pneumonia
c) Pulmonary tuberculosis
d) Salmonella septicaemia
e) Toxoplasmosis of the brain

Question 197

According to the Association of Anaesthetists of Great Britain and Ireland *Recommendations Regarding Monitoring* (4th edition, 2007) which one of the following statements is true?

a) Monitoring airway pressure is essential to the safe conduct of anaesthesia
b) A vapour analyser to detect volatile anaesthetic agents is mandatory
c) Monitoring must be maintained between theatre and the recovery area as for any other intra-hospital transfer
d) Under no circumstances should an anaesthetist leave an anaesthetised patient for whom they are responsible
e) In the recovery area clinical observations must be supplemented by electrocardiograph, pulse oximetry and non-invasive blood pressure measurement

Question 198

All the following drugs may prolong the QT interval on a patient's electrocardiograph, except which one?

a) Ketorolac
b) Haloperidol

c) Quinine
d) Tamoxifen
e) Ondansetron

Question 199

Which one of the following sites would lead to the greatest plasma concentration of local anaesthetic if the same dose of the same agent was administered to the same patient (on separate occasions)?

a) Intercostal
b) Interscalene
c) Caudal extradural
d) Tranversus abdominis plane
e) Deep cervical plexus

Question 200

Regarding cardiac pacing, which one of the following statements is true?

a) Epicardial pacing wires emerge directly through the anterior chest wall
b) VVI pacemakers deliver pacing stimulation regardless of the intrinsic activity of the heart
c) Biventricular pacemakers require insertion of the left ventricular lead via the systemic arterial vasculature
d) Unipolar diathermy during a surgical procedure is absolutely contraindicated
e) AOO pacemakers provide synchronous stimulation in cases of sinus bradycardia

Question 201

Regarding the use of spinal anaesthesia in the day case unit, the following statements are true except which one?

a) Muscle tone is preserved with a low dose spinal, which may necessitate adaptation of arthroscope insertion
b) Stage one recovery time is reduced with a subarachnoid block
c) In the UK, levobupivacaine 2.5 mg/mL is now licensed for intrathecal administration
d) 5 mg of bupivacaine plus 10 mcg fentanyl is adequate for a variety of lower limb day case procedures including knee arthroscopy
e) Time to readiness for discharge increases with dose of intrathecal bupivacaine but is not affected by its volume or concentration

Question 202

A 5-year-old is assessed on the children's ward prior to anaesthesia for tonsillectomy. Some topical local anaesthetic is prescribed to reduce the pain associated with subsequent cannulation. Regarding the available agents, which one of the following statements is true?

a) Application of amethocaine gel (Ametop) will make intravenous cannulation easier than application of a eutectic mixture of local anaesthetics (EMLA)
b) If the manufacturer's instructions are strictly followed there is no difference in the efficacy of Ametop compared with EMLA
c) Ametop reduces the pain associated with intravenous cannulation more than EMLA even when both have been applied for over 60 minutes
d) Ametop contains 2% amethocaine
e) A 5 g tube of EMLA will contain 150 mg of lidocaine and 150 mg of prilocaine

Question 203

The following conditions are associated with atlantoaxial instability except which one?

a) Rheumatoid arthritis
b) Neurofibromatosis
c) Hyperthyroidism
d) Down's syndrome
e) Ankylosing spondylitis

Question 204

Amiodarone is contraindicated in the following cardiac conduction disturbances or arrhythmias except which one?

a) The arrhythmias produced by digoxin toxicity
b) Wolff–Parkinson–White syndrome
c) Atrial fibrillation during thyrotoxicosis
d) Atrioventricular block
e) Torsades de pointes

Question 205

Regarding the practicalities of intrapleural chest drainage, the following statements are true except which one?

a) Obstructed inspiration can generate intrapleural pressures of negative 80 cmH$_2$O
b) Maintaining the collection chamber below the level of the patient promotes a pressure gradient with the higher pressure at the patient end
c) The connection tubing has a length of 1800 mm and 12 mm internal diameter thus an internal volume of around 0.2 L
d) The suction system applied to a chest drain must be high flow and low pressure to meet potential high fluid flow rates from the pleural cavity
e) Tubing must be at least 2 cm under the surface of the water to minimise resistance to expulsion while ensuring the volume above the tip is less than the volume of the tubing

Question 206

A 75-year-old male presents with a community-acquired pneumonia. He is oliguric and his admission blood biochemistry shows a creatinine level of 309 micromol/L with previously normal renal function. Which one of the following would be consistent with a diagnosis of acute tubular necrosis and not pre-renal uraemia?

a) Urinalysis shows hyaline casts
b) Specific gravity of 1.020
c) Osmolality 500 mOsm/kg
d) Fractional excretion of sodium 2%
e) Urinary sodium 20 mmol/L

Question 207

In a patient with asthma presenting with an exacerbation to the emergency department the following would be consistent with 'acute severe asthma' except which one?

a) PEF 50% of predicted
b) PaCO$_2$ 5.2 kPa

c) Heart rate 110 bpm
d) Respiratory rate 27 breaths per minute
e) Unable to complete sentences in one breath

Question 208

An 84 kg patient is listed for urgent surgery but gives a suspicious family history and you decide to treat him as if he were malignant hyperthermia susceptible. There are no target control infusion pumps available – just 100 mL bottles of 2% propofol and infusion pumps. You decide to use the original Bristol model for manual total intravenous anaesthesia. Consistent with the original work, the patient is premedicated with 20 mg oral temazepam. At induction he receives 250 mcg of fentanyl and 85 mg of propofol. Using the model mentioned, what volume of propofol will the patient receive in the following ten minutes?

a) 5.6 mL
b) 7.0 mL
c) 8.4 mL
d) 11.2 mL
e) 14.0 mL

Question 209

Which one of the following is least likely to reduce uterine tone?

a) Desflurane
b) Nifedipine
c) Diclofenac
d) Magnesium sulphate
e) Suxamethonium

Question 210

Pulmonary artery flotation catheters can be used to measure the following variables except which one?

a) Core temperature
b) Cardiac index
c) Mixed venous oxygen saturation
d) Pulmonary capillary wedge pressure
e) Mean pulmonary artery pressure

Question 211

Regarding the operation of a hydrogen electrode in order to measure pH, which one of the following statements is correct?

a) A special membrane is selectively permeable to H^+ ions
b) A calomel reference electrode describes a silver electrode in direct contact with silver chloride
c) The 'salt-bridge' is potassium chloride
d) A highly sensitive ammeter is required
e) A unit difference in pH will produce a voltage of 6 V

Question 212

A 26-year-old woman with a history of syncope requires spinal anaesthesia for lower segment caesarean section. The subarachnoid injection is performed with the patient sitting on the operating table, whereupon she is assisted in lying supine with a 15° left lateral tilt on the table. Four minutes later, the patient becomes drowsy and confused and her monitor shows a heart rate of 49 bpm and a non-invasive blood pressure of 78/ 35 mmHg. Rapid infusion of intravenous fluid is commenced, the left lateral tilt of the operating table is increased and an assistant manually displaces the gravid uterus. Given the mechanism of the evolving phenomenon, which ONE of the following agents should best treat this patient?

a) Ephedrine
b) Atropine
c) Glycopyrrolate
d) Phenylephrine
e) Adrenaline

Question 213

Which of the following would you find most surprising in a patient presenting to an intensive care unit with Guillain–Barré syndrome?

a) An elevated cerebrospinal fluid cell count
b) A recent history of a respiratory tract illness
c) Delayed F waves on nerve conduction studies
d) The presence of a bulbar palsy
e) No response to high dose oral corticosteroid therapy

Question 214

A 30-year-old obese male presents with an incarcerated femoral hernia. A rapid sequence induction of general anaesthesia is planned. He has a cannula *in situ* in his left antecubital fossa through which doses of thiopentone and suxamethonium are delivered and eventually the patient's trachea is intubated with a certain amount of difficulty, which is ascribed to the patient's body habitus. During the operation it is noticed that his fingers on the left hand are white and cold and that blood is pulsating up the tubing of the intravenous fluid-giving set. Which one of the following state-ments describes the most appropriate action to take next?

a) Remove cannula and commence immediate heparinisation via a new intravenous cannula
b) While under anaesthesia perform brachial plexus block
c) Infuse pressurised 0.9% saline through the existing cannula
d) Inject 10 mg of diluted papaverine into the existing cannula
e) Inject 10 mg of diluted bupivicaine into the existing cannula

Question 215

A patient's electrocardiogram is reviewed prior to surgery for suspected ischaemic bowel. The patient is unwell and it is noted they have a prolonged QT interval. Due to which of the following would you least expect this to be?

a) Beta blocker therapy
b) A history of breast carcinoma with known bone metastases
c) Jervell–Lange–Nielsen syndrome
d) A history of ischaemic heart disease with daily angina
e) Hypothermia

Question 216

An 18-year-old man with Marfan's syndrome requires anaesthesia for knee arthro-scopy and medial meniscal repair. He is tall, with very long arms and a thoracolumbar scoliosis. His father looks similar. Which of the following would be least likely to be noted in this patient?

a) An ejection systolic murmur radiating to the carotids
b) A pansystolic murmur loudest at the apex
c) High arched palate
d) Pectus excavatum
e) Needing to use glasses to see to sign the consent form

Question 217

While on-call for the obstetric unit you are urgently bleeped to a delivery room where a mother has delivered her baby. She is well but the baby has a heart rate of 90 bpm, cries weakly and flexes when stimulated, has poor muscle tone, blue hands and feet, but has a pink trunk. Which of the following is the correct Apgar score for this baby?

a) Six
b) Five
c) Four
d) Three
e) Two

Question 218

A 50-year-old woman presents to the pain clinic with a three-year history of low back pain with occasional radiation down the left leg. The severity and impact on her functional ability is increasing and her general practitioner feels he has explored all the options open to him. Careful history-taking eliminates the 'red flags' of chronic back pain. Which one of the following options is not a 'yellow flag' of chronic back pain?

a) A negative attitude that back pain is harmful or potentially severely disabling
b) Fear avoidance behaviour and reduced activity levels
c) An expectation that passive, rather than active, treatment will be beneficial
d) A comorbid psychiatric diagnosis or history of substance misuse
e) A tendency to depression, low morale and social withdrawal

Question 219

Regarding the properties of some local anaesthetics, with respect to levobupivacaine, which one of the following statements is correct?

a) It has the same potency as ropivacaine, and at equipotent doses has the same onset of action as racemic bupivacaine and the same duration of action as lidocaine
b) It has greater potency than lidocaine, and at equipotent doses has the same onset of action as racemic bupivacaine and the same duration of action as ropivacaine
c) It has greater potency than ropivacaine, and at equipotent doses has a slower onset of action than lidocaine and a longer duration of action than racemic bupivacaine
d) It has greater potency than racemic bupivacaine, and at equipotent doses has a slower onset of action than ropivacaine and a longer duration of action than lidocaine
e) It has greater potency than lidocaine, and at equipotent doses has a slower onset of action than ropivacaine and a longer duration of action than racemic bupivacaine

Question 220

The classical approach to the study of pharmacodynamics involves analysis of dose–response curves and application of various equations. Log(dose)–response curves can theoretically distinguish between competitive and non-competitive antagonists at a particular receptor. However, given that experiments are limited by dose ranges and responses that must be safe, data at the extremes are often incomplete. Via what transformation may 'mid-range' data be manipulated to reveal linear graphs that demonstrate whether an antagonist is competitive or non-competitive?

a) Gaussian distribution
b) Lineweaver–Burke plot
c) Bland–Altman plot
d) Michaelis–Menton equation
e) Conductance ratio application

Question 221

Regarding carbon dioxide transport, which one of the following statements is correct?

a) Between arterial and venous blood, the mechanism with the greatest proportional change in carbon dioxide carriage is the bicarbonate component
b) Dissolved carbon dioxide component contributes 0.0225 mL/dL/kPa to the carriage of the gas
c) Deoxygenated blood has greater carbon dioxide carrying capacity than oxygenated blood – the Bohr effect
d) Carbamino compounds are generated by the combination of carbon dioxide with blood proteins
e) Plotted with the same scales, the carbon dioxide dissociation curve is much shallower than the oxyhaemoglobin dissociation curve

Question 222

Which one of the following statements regarding cyanosis is true?

a) Central cyanosis is always a manifestation of hypoxaemia
b) Central cyanosis is always accompanied by a reduced arterial PaO_2
c) Central cyanosis is detectable at a concentration of arterial reduced haemoglobin of 2.5 g/dL
d) Peripheral cyanosis is detectable at a concentration of arterial reduced haemoglobin of 1.5 g/dL
e) Methaemoglobinaemia will cause a drop in arterial oxygen saturations without clinically apparent cyanosis

Question 223

Which one of the following would not be consistent with the initial neurohumoural response following major trauma in a previously well patient?

a) Serum cortisol concentration 1250 nanomol/L
b) An increase in serum tri-iodothyronine concentration
c) A release of arginine vasopressin from the posterior pituitary
d) A surge of interleucin-1 and interleucin-6
e) A small rise in glucagon secretion

Question 224

A 29-year-old male is involved in a road traffic collision on his motorbike. He suffers blunt trauma to his head, chest and abdomen. His Glasgow Coma Score (GCS) is 5 at the scene (abnormal flexion to pain). In the emergency department (ED), his GCS is 4 and his ventilation is inadequate. His cervical spine is already immobilised with a hard collar, sand bags and tape. His trachea is intubated by the ED registrar and mechanical ventilation commenced. Plain radiographs of the cervical spine, chest and pelvis are taken in ED. The cervical spine radiograph looks normal. The ED registrar escorts the patient to CT where the patient undergoes CT of head, chest and abdomen. Immediate surgery is not indicated so the ED registrar escorts the patient to the intensive care unit where the ICU trainee has been busy to this point. With respect to this patient's spinal clearance, which one of the following actions is most appropriate once the patient has been stabilised?

a) Return to the imaging department for thin-slice cervical spine CT
b) Leave hard collar in place, but elevate the head of the bed 30° because the patient's intracranial pressure must be minimised
c) Given a normal plain film of the c-spine, an MRI of the spine to identify unstable ligamentous injury should be arranged urgently
d) Arrange thoracolumbar spine plain X-rays
e) Remove hard collar to reduce sequelae of long-term immobilisation but continue to log-roll the patient

Question 225

A 36-year-old female patient presents to the pre-assessment clinic prior to undergoing surgery for removal of metalwork. Her full blood count shows haemoglobin 9 g/dL and mean cell volume 107.3 fL. Which of the following investigations or observations would be the least likely to be helpful in elucidating the cause of her macrocytic anaemia?

a) A positive β-HCG
b) A raised TSH and low T4
c) That the patient has end-stage renal failure and is on haemodialysis
d) A history of excess alcohol intake
e) Abnormal liver function tests

Paper D

Question 226

With regard to the monitoring of neuromuscular blockade, the following statements are true except which one?

a) An acceptable level of neuromuscular function for extubation is present if a patient has a train-of-four ratio of >0.90
b) The gold standard for accurately assessing train-of-four ratio is mechanomyography
c) Post-tetanic count is most useful for assessing deep neuromuscular blockade
d) The presence of a single twitch on train-of-four indicates a 90% reduction in muscle tone following electrical stimulation
e) At the wrist, the negative electrode should be placed proximally

Question 227

Regarding clonidine, which one of the following statements is correct?

a) Clonidine produces vasodilation and a compensatory tachycardia is observed
b) Clonidine is an agonist at α_1 and α_2 adrenoreceptors
c) Reduction of minimum alveolar concentration (MAC) of volatile anaesthetic agents is limited to 20%
d) With higher therapeutic doses, respiratory depression is observed
e) Clonidine may increase small bowel motility and cause diarrhoea

Question 228

It is suspected that a patient on an intensive care unit has become delirious following recent surgery for a perforated diverticular abscess and consequent peritonitis. Which of the following statements regarding their management is incorrect?

a) The CAM-ICU screening tool may be a valuable aid to diagnosis in this situation
b) Drugs with central antimuscarinic or dopaminergic activity should be avoided wherever possible in critically ill patients with or at risk of delirium
c) Once the diagnosis has been established treatment with haloperidol is useful
d) Benzodiazepines should, generally, be avoided in the management of patients with delirium
e) Opioids, noradrenaline and corticosteroids all reduce rapid eye movement (REM) sleep, which contributes to an increased risk of delirium

Question 229

Which of the following is not associated with a significantly raised serum troponin I?

a) Elective DC cardioversion
b) Meningococcal septicaemia
c) Subarachnoid haemorrhage
d) Acute renal failure
e) Pulmonary embolus

Question 230

Regarding positioning a patient prone under anaesthesia, which one of the following statements is true?

a) In one configuration, shoulder and abdominal rolls allow adequate chest excursion
b) The pleural pressure gradient is considerably increased when prone, compared with supine
c) When optimally positioned, the prone patient will virtually always have an increased cardiac index
d) One of the few advantages of partial inferior vena cava obstruction is reduced blood loss during lumbar spinal surgery
e) Pancreatitis is a recognised complication of positioning patients prone for scoliosis surgery

Question 231

A patient with known brittle asthma is admitted with a serious acute exacerbation. They have a respiratory rate of 30 with saturations of 93% on 15 L/min of oxygen via a non-rebreathing mask. In the management of this patient, which of the following treatments is the least likely to be of benefit?

a) Regular oral prednisolone
b) Heliox
c) A single dose of intravenous magnesium sulphate
d) Intravenous aminophylline
e) Nebulised ipratropium bromide

Question 232

Which of the following is not a question asked during the 'Time out' section of the WHO Surgical Safety Checklist?

a) Has the sterility of the instruments been confirmed?
b) Have all team members introduced themselves by name and role?
c) Has antibiotic prophylaxis been given within the last 60 minutes?
d) Does the patient have a known allergy?
e) Is essential imaging displayed?

Question 233

In order to achieve topical analgesia and vasoconstriction of the nasal mucosa prior to surgery, Moffett's solution is sometimes used. According to the original description, which one of the following describes the constituents of Moffett's solution?

a) 1 mL 10% cocaine, 2 mL 8.4% sodium bicarbonate, 1 mL 1:1000 adrenaline
b) 2 mL 8% cocaine, 2 mL 1% sodium bicarbonate, 1 mL 1:1000 adrenaline

c) 2 mL 10% cocaine, 2 mL 8.4% sodium bicarbonate, 1 mL 1:1000 adrenaline
d) 1 mL 8% cocaine, 2 mL 8.4% sodium bicarbonate, 2 mL 1:10 000 adrenaline
e) 2 mL 10% cocaine, 1 mL 8.4% sodium bicarbonate, 2 mL 1:1000 adrenaline

Question 234

The laboratory diagnosis of malignant hyperthermia involves exposure of a muscle biopsy of standardised dimensions to various chemicals while being electrically stimulated. Which one of the following chemicals is used with the greatest quantity in these tests?

a) Ryanodine
b) Caffeine
c) Enflurane
d) Dantrolene
e) Suxamethonium

Question 235

Regarding intravenous fluid administration with 0.9% saline solution to an adult surgical patient, the following statements are true except which one?

a) May produce abdominal discomfort
b) May reduce glomerular filtration rate principally due to the sodium load affecting the renin–angiotensin system
c) Involves infusing a solution with a higher calculated osmolality compared to plasma
d) Every litre infused provides 1½ times the guideline daily allowance for dietary salt (NaCl) intake
e) Will produce a greater immediate rise in chloride concentration than sodium concentration

Question 236

Prior to elective surgery a 47-year-old female patient wants to discuss the risk of awareness under anaesthesia. This is her first anaesthetic and she is American Society of Anesthesiologists (ASA) grade I. The following statements are true except which one?

a) A risk of awareness of 1 to 2 per 1000 general anaesthetics should be quoted to her
b) If she were ASA grade III her chance of awareness would be higher
c) If she were male her chance of awareness would be higher
d) If she were older, but still ASA grade I, her chance of awareness would be similar
e) Roughly 5% of patients will dream while under general anaesthesia

Question 237

Regarding clinical practice relevant to the potential transmission of Creutzfeldt–Jacob disease (CJD) the following statements are true except which one?

a) For tonsillectomy surgeons routinely use traceable re-usable instruments
b) Use of disposable laryngoscope blades for tonsil and adenoid surgery is strongly recommended
c) In a known case of CJD, high-infectivity tissues are brain, spinal cord and posterior eye
d) In the UK, in order to reduce the risk of transmission of variant CJD a donor may not give blood if they have received a blood transfusion since 1 January 1990
e) If a laryngeal mask airway is used for tonsillectomy, it must be disposable

Question 238

A 70-year-old man is admitted to the intensive care unit with severe sepsis needing multiorgan support. Blood cultures have come back positive for Gram-negative bacilli. Which of the following is least likely to be the infecting organism?

a) *Neisseria meningitidis*
b) *Klebsiella pneumoniae*
c) *Pseudomonas aeruginosa*
d) *Escherichia coli*
e) *Enterobacter cloacae*

Question 239

Anaesthesia is provided for a 23-year-old, ASA grade I male undergoing an elective orthopaedic procedure. The airway is managed with a Laryngeal Mask Airway ProSeal™ (LMA ProSeal™). Shortly after entering theatre, the patient coughs and a small volume of gastric contents is noticed in the drain tube of the LMA ProSeal™. Of the following sequences of actions, which one would be most appropriate?

a) Place the patient in the left lateral position; remove the LMA ProSeal™ and wake the patient up
b) Keep the patient supine; remove the LMA ProSeal™; give suxamethonium with cricoid pressure applied by a trained assistant; intubate the trachea and perform endobronchial suction prior to insufflations of the lungs
c) Place the patient in the left lateral position; remove the LMA ProSeal™; give suxamethonium with cricoid pressure applied by a trained assistant; intubate the trachea and perform endobronchial suction prior to insufflations of the lungs
d) Deepen your anaesthetic and observe the patient for any problems while cautiously proceeding with surgery
e) Suction down the drain tube with an endobronchial suction catheter, suction around the back of the oropharynx and proceed if there is no obvious gastric content contamination

Question 240

A 42-year-old male is diagnosed with Guillain–Barré syndrome of a severe nature requiring mechanical ventilation. Early in his intensive care unit admission, a percutaneous tracheostomy is sited and his sedation is ceased. Twelve hours after this procedure you are called to his bedside. The patient is agitated and cyanosed. The flange of the tracheostomy tube is 3 cm proud of the front of his neck. His pulse oximeter shows arterial oxygen saturation of 82%. The ventilator alarm is sounding indicating high airway pressures and low minute volume. Insertion of a suction catheter into the tracheostomy tube meets with resistance immediately beyond the tube.

Which one of the following is the most appropriate action?

a) Manually ventilate with 100% oxygen via the tracheostomy tube
b) Remove existing tracheostomy tube and reinsert one of a smaller size
c) Induce anaesthesia and perform orotracheal intubation
d) Insert an Aintree exchange catheter into the stoma and insufflate oxygen
e) Cover the stoma and perform facial mask ventilation

Question 241

Regarding ankylosing spondylitis, which one of the following statements is correct?

a) Disease prevalence in men and women is approximately the same
b) In over 90% of cases the patient is positive for the type I HLA antigen, HLA-B37

c) A presenting feature of the condition is reduced range of movement of the cervical spine

d) The anaesthetic technique of choice, where suited to the proposed operation, is central neuraxial anaesthesia

e) Providing the cervical spine has a normal range of movement, patients with ankylosing spondylitis do not pose challenges to intubation greater than normal controls

Question 242

When compared to mean plasma values, which one of the following statements regarding mean cerebrospinal fluid (CSF) values is true?

a) CSF potassium concentration is 2.9 mmol/L when plasma is 4.6 mmol/L
b) CSF protein concentration is approximately one fifth of the plasma value
c) CSF glucose concentration is slightly less than plasma glucose concentration
d) The pH of CSF is marginally alkaline
e) The partial pressure of carbon dioxide is lower in CSF than in plasma

Question 243

The following are considered therapeutic options for the treatment of trigeminal neuralgia except which one?

a) Stereotactic radiosurgery
b) Percutaneous radiofrequency thermoablation
c) Topical capsaicin
d) Oral lamotrigine
e) Microvascular decompression

Question 244

A patient with severe pancreatitis and CT-proven pancreatic necrosis becomes pyrexial, tachycardic and hypotensive two days after admission. Regarding the use of serum procalcitonin (PCT) as a marker of sepsis, which of the following statements is true?

a) PCT is less sensitive than CRP in the diagnosis of severe sepsis
b) PCT is less specific than CRP in the diagnosis of severe sepsis
c) PCT is undetectable in the bloodstream in the absence of sepsis
d) PCT has a bloodstream half-life of approximately six hours
e) For severe bacterial infection to be likely, the serum PCT level is greater than 20 ng/mL

Question 245

Of the following definitions regarding pain, which one is correct?

a) Allodynia: increased response to spontaneous or evoked pain
b) Hyperalgesia: stimulus and response mode are the same but response is exaggerated
c) Hyperpathia: intermittent, repetitive spontaneous pain sensation
d) Neuralgia: pain caused by primary lesion or dysfunction of the nervous system
e) Causalgia: properly known as complex regional pain syndrome type I

Question 246

A 68-year-old male patient with a history of well controlled hypertension, stable angina and hypercholesterolaemia is scheduled for lumbar microdiscectomy as the second case on the following morning's operating list. He normally takes simvastatin, losartan, bisoprolol, bendroflumethiazide and nicorandil. In addition, the aspirin he normally takes was stopped nine days previously. On your preoperative visit the evening before, the ward nurse asks you which drugs to give and which to omit between now and his anaesthetic, tomorrow morning.

Which of the following combinations is most appropriate?

a) Give the bisoprolol, the bendroflumethiazide and the nicorandil. Omit the simvastatin and the losartan

b) Give the nicorandil. Omit the bisoprolol, the bendroflumethiazide, the simvastatin and the losartan

c) Give the simvastatin, the bisoprolol and the nicorandil. Omit the bendroflumethiazide and the losartan

d) Give the losartan, the bisoprolol, the bendroflumethiazide and the nicorandil. Omit the simvastatin

e) Give all the drugs

Question 247

A patient has been admitted with suspected community-acquired pneumonia and has been referred to critical care outreach by the medical team for consideration of ventilatory support. A CURB65 score is completed. The following variables score one point except for which one?

a) Mental test score 7/10
b) Urea 9 mmol/L
c) Age 73 years
d) Diastolic blood pressure 55 mmHg
e) Respiratory rate 25 breaths per minute

Question 248

Which one of the following statements regarding volatile anaesthesia is correct?

a) End tidal agent monitoring on most anaesthetic machines allows display of minimum alveolar concentration (MAC) for the patient
b) The MAC of desflurane is 6%
c) The oil:gas solubility coefficient of halothane is among the lowest of the volatile anaesthetic agents
d) Female gender decreases MAC
e) Hyponatraemia decreases MAC

Question 249

The following are unwanted effects of suxamethonium except which one?

a) Masseter spasm
b) Tachycardia
c) Hyperkalaemia
d) Malignant hyperpyrexia
e) Prolonged muscle relaxation

Question 250

Concerning the presentation and treatment of a patient with suspected gas embolism the following statements are true except which one?

a) The reason hyperbaric therapy reduces the volume of a gas bubble is because volume is inversely proportional to pressure at a constant temperature, which is explained by Boyle's law
b) The reason hyperbaric oxygen therapy also reduces the size of the gas bubble is due to the alteration of diffusion gradients of both nitrogen and oxygen
c) The commonest reason for a paradoxical gas embolus is due to the presence of a patent foramen ovale that occurs in upto 30% of the adult population
d) The 'mill wheel murmur' sometimes heard over the praecordium is due to blood and air mixing within the left ventricle
e) A patient in the 'deckchair' position is at increased risk of gas embolism

Question 251

A 6-week-old term infant presents for surgery to treat hypertrophic pyloric stenosis (HPS). Which of the following statements regarding this child and its treatment is least correct?

a) Both acid and alkaline urine occur
b) Attempts by the surgeon to take the patient straight to theatre should be resisted until attempts have been made to correct the biochemical abnormalities
c) If the infant has acid urine they are likely to have a significant potassium deficit
d) The infant is more likely to be female than male and to have a parent who also had HPS
e) In HPS, potassium and hydrogen ion excretion by the kidneys is designed to maintain a normal pH

Question 252

Regarding Lee's revised cardiac risk index, which one of the following would score one point?

a) Serum creatinine 120 micromol/L
b) Open hemicolectomy
c) On insulin sliding scale to manage hyperkalaemia
d) Poorly controlled hypertension
e) Hypercholesterolaemia

Question 253

A patient presents to your chronic pain clinic with a two-month history of severe pain in the right forearm. Of the following features, which is least consistent with a diagnosis of a complex regional pain syndrome type I?

a) Pain that is in an ulnar nerve distribution
b) A history of a fractured ulna occurring 24 months previously that required reduction and immobilisation
c) Worsening of the pain when the arm is placed in a dependent position
d) Loss of hair on the right forearm but preservation of hair on the left forearm
e) The presence of a tremor in the right arm

Question 254

Regarding the administration of intravenous infusions to children, the following statements are correct except which one?

a) Sodium chloride 0.45% + glucose 2.5% may be safely administered to the majority of children

b) Sodium chloride 0.18% + glucose 4% should not be available in areas that treat children
c) Sodium chloride 0.45% + glucose 5% is hyperosmolar with respect to plasma and hypotonic with reference to the cell membrane
d) Ongoing losses may be replaced by, for example, compound sodium lactate solution
e) Severe acute hyponatraemia is defined as a decrease in plasma sodium from normal to less than 130 mmol/L in less than 24 hours

Question 255

Regarding paediatric surgical conditions, the following statements are true except which one?

a) The commonest type of tracheo-oesophageal fistula is oesophageal atresia with a distal fistula
b) Pyloric stenosis classically presents with bilious projectile vomiting at six weeks of age
c) Gastroschisis involves a defect in the anterior abdominal wall, usually on the right
d) In >50% of cases of intussusception, the patient is less than one year of age
e) Inguinal hernias are almost exclusively of the indirect type

Question 256

Regarding the management of acute pancreatitis, which one of the following has been most universally abandoned?

a) Maintaining the patient nil-by-mouth
b) Use of pethidine, rather than morphine, for analgesia
c) Administration of prophylactic antibiotics
d) Laparotomy
e) Early computerised tomography

Question 257

Following emergency surgery for a ruptured abdominal aortic aneurysm a 76-year-old patient is on noradrenaline 0.35 mcg/kg/min. They remain hypotensive (80/35) with a decreased urine output despite being warmed since returning from theatre (34.5 °C to 37.1 °C) and having received 500 mL of intravenous colloid. An oesophageal Doppler probe is inserted, which gives a corrected flow time (FT$_C$) of 290 ms (normal range = 330 to 360 ms) and a peak velocity (PV) of 40 cm/s (normal range = 50 to 80 cm/s). Which of the following represents the most appropriate immediate management plan?

a) Cautious introduction of low dose dobutamine with the aim to slowly escalate the dose
b) Fluid challenge with boluses of 250 mL of Gelofusine® titrated to response
c) Aim to slowly reduce noradrenaline dose and give fluid challenges based on response
d) Further, cautious escalation of noradrenaline dose
e) Introduce nitrate infusion combined with cautious fluid challenges

Question 258

A patient with alcohol dependency was found unconscious in the community and transferred to the emergency department in your hospital. His admission temperature is 32 °C. Which one of the following list is the most immediate threat to his outcome?

a) This severe hypothermia will result in malignant arrhythmias
b) Hypokalaemia causing myocardial depression
c) Acidaemia
d) Progressive reduction in ionised calcium with reduction in pH
e) Spontaneous central apnoea

Question 259

A patient is admitted to the intensive care unit with a reduced GCS and a serum sodium of 120 mmol/L. Which of the following potential causes of this hyponatraemia is most likely to result in a decreased extracellular fluid compartment volume?

a) Pancreatitis
b) Bronchopneumonia
c) Severe cirrhosis
d) Congestive cardiac failure
e) Nephrotic syndrome

Question 260

During their preoperative assessment, a patient volunteers the information that they are allergic to a number of fruit and vegetables. Which of the following would be the least likely to be associated with a potential latex allergy?

a) Avocado
b) Strawberry
c) Kiwifruit
d) Banana
e) Cauliflower

Question 261

With regard to central venous catheters (CVCs), which one of the following statements is true?

a) Approximately one third of all hospital-acquired bloodstream infections are CVC related
b) *Staphylococcus aureus* is the commonest organism implicated in CVC infection
c) Both CVCs that are externally coated and CVCs that are internally AND externally coated with antimicrobial substances significantly lower the risk of CVC-related infection
d) The administration of antibiotics at the time of CVC insertion is recommended as it reduces the risk of CVC-related bloodstream infection
e) 1% chlorhexidine in 70% isopropyl alcohol should be used to clean the skin at the site of the CVC

Question 262

Twenty-four hours after a road traffic accident and prolonged extraction a 27-year-old woman is found to have a creatine kinase (CK) of 57 000 units/L. You suspect rhabdomyolysis. Which of the following does not support your diagnosis?

a) Raised troponin I (TnI)
b) Urine microscopy showing red blood cells
c) Myoglobinuria
d) Urine dipstick positive for blood
e) Hypocalcaemia

Question 263

Regarding a patient presenting with myasthenia gravis (MG), the following statements are true except which one?

a) MG is an autoimmune condition in which IgG autoantibodies interact with acetylcholine receptors at the neuromuscular junction
b) MG is most common in young men and older women
c) Reflexes in a patient with MG are normal
d) There is no association with malignant disease
e) Diagnosis of MG is, in part, made by assessment of the response to administration of a reversible acetylcholinesterase inhibitor

Question 264

For satisfactory progression of surgery involving transposition and shortening of muscles of the eye, it may be preferable to use a non-depolarising muscle relaxant for which one of the following reasons?

a) Depth of anaesthesia can interfere with the forced duction test
b) Bell's phenomenon interferes with the position of the eye and thus surgical field
c) The incidence of the occulocardiac reflex is diminished with muscle relaxation
d) The incidence of postoperative nausea and vomiting is diminished if muscle relaxation has been used
e) Postoperative pain scores are reduced if muscles have been relaxed during traction or manipulation

Question 265

Eight weeks post-partum, a 30-year-old woman requires an emergency appendicectomy. She is currently breastfeeding and wishes to continue as soon as possible after her operation. Which one of the following drugs should be avoided to allow her to return safely to breastfeeding in the shortest possible time?

a) Oxycodone
b) Atracurium
c) Propofol
d) Suxamethonium
e) Diclofenac sodium

Question 266

A patient needs transferring from one hospital to another. He is ventilated with a minute volume of 14 L/min. The journey will take 90 minutes in total. Assume he is transferred with an FiO_2 of 1.0 on a 100% efficient ventilator that uses a minute volume's worth of oxygen every minute. You want to carry enough oxygen to last for twice the anticipated journey time. Which of the following oxygen volumes (in cylinders) is the nearest to the ideal calculated amount?

a) 1C + 1D + 1E + 1F
b) 2F
c) 2E + 5C
d) 1F + 3E
e) 5D + 1E

Question 267

Regarding Down's syndrome (DS), the following statements are true except for which one?

a) The commonest cardiac abnormality in a patient with DS is an atrial septal defect
b) There is an increased incidence of subglottic and tracheal stenosis in DS patients
c) The incidence of non-haematological solid tumours is lower in DS patients than in a matched non-DS population
d) Patients with DS have a higher incidence of hypothyroidism than the normal population
e) The incidence of Alzheimer's dementia is increased in patients with DS

Question 268

Regarding skewness and kurtosis, which one of the following statements is true?

a) With negatively skewed data, the mean > median > mode
b) Positive kurtosis indicates a tall peaked distribution with shorter tails than a normal distribution
c) The standard normal distribution has a kurtosis of zero
d) Power transformations may not be applied to positively skewed data
e) When compared to other transformers, logarithmic transformation has least impact on skew

Question 269

A previously healthy 68-year-old female presents with an acute abdomen with clinical and radiological features of small bowel obstruction. The general surgeons propose an urgent laparotomy. She reports she has had one previous anaesthetic – 12 years ago for a hysterectomy – and considers that she had no problems with the anaesthetic. A rapid sequence induction is performed with thiopentone and suxamethonium, and a peripheral nerve stimulator is used to establish return of neuromuscular function. Unexpectedly it is 40 minutes post-induction that one twitch is first detected on a train-of-four stimulation. Having excluded other causes, which one of the following is the most likely pseudocholinesterase genotype she carries?

a) $E_1^s E_1^u$
b) $E_1^a E_1^a$
c) $E_1^u E_1^a$
d) $E_1^f E_1^a$
e) $E_1^s E_1^s$

Question 270

Patients with chronic renal failure tend to have a coagulopathy prompting careful consideration of the use of regional anaesthetic techniques. Which one of the following tests is most likely to demonstrate the presence of a coagulopathy in a patient with end-stage renal failure?

a) Platelet count
b) Prothrombin time
c) Activated partial thromboplastin time
d) Serum fibrinogen concentration
e) Bleeding time

Question 271

On rising from the supine to the erect position and remaining still, the following physiological responses would be expected except which one?

a) 20% decrease in cerebral blood flow
b) A rise in venous pressure at the foot to 90 mmHg
c) 40% fall in stroke volume
d) An increase in plasma concentration of renin and aldosterone
e) Minimal change in cardiac output

Question 272

Which one of the following statements regarding anticoagulant agents is correct?

a) Low molecular weight heparins have a greater ability to inhibit thrombin than to inhibit Factor Xa
b) Fondaparinux is contraindicated for thromboprophylaxis in major joint replacement surgery
c) Unfractionated heparin inhibits platelet activation by fibrin and also binds reversibly to antithrombin III
d) Neuraxial blockade is acceptable 12 hours after ceasing an infusion of abciximab (ReoPro®)
e) In heparin-induced thrombocytopenia, danaparoid (a heparinoid) should be avoided as an alternative agent

Question 273

A 37-year-old female accidentally transected her dominant hand radial artery on a broken wine glass while washing-up at midnight after an evening of alcohol excess. It is now 09.00 hours and she has been transferred to the regional plastic surgery unit for urgent surgery. She describes herself as fit and well apart from having one of the worst hangovers she can ever remember suffering. Compared to normal values, all of the following are likely to be found except which one?

a) A low total body glutathione level
b) A low plasma magnesium level
c) A low level of the neurotransmitter glutamine in the brain
d) A high plasma acetaldehyde level
e) A low gastric pH

Question 274

Regarding the options for facilitating dental procedures in children, which one of the following statements is true?

a) A general anaesthetic may be used in a community setting if administered by a consultant paediatric anaesthetist
b) Orthodontic extraction of sound permanent pre-molar teeth in a healthy child rarely justifies a general anaesthetic
c) Conscious sedation or behavioural techniques (including hypnosis) should not be attempted in a child
d) Physical, emotional or learning impairment is not a justification for general anaesthesia in circumstances that do not otherwise justify general anaesthesia
e) The primary objective of comprehensive treatment planning is to ensure that follow-up general anaesthetic procedures are of minimal duration

Question 275

A 77-year-old female was admitted three days ago with diabetic hyperosmolar non-ketotic acidosis (HONK). This had been treated appropriately. The patient now requires urgent assessment because her heart rate of 160 beats per minute has triggered the medical early warning score system. The patient is found to be drowsy, spontaneously breathing oxygen via a facemask with a respiratory rate of 24 breaths per minute and an SpO_2 of 91%. She has some basal crepitations on chest auscultation. Her blood pressure is 92/50 mmHg – less than her recorded baseline of 154/88 mmHg. Her arterial blood gases show pH 7.35 and glucose 14 mmol/L. Her ECG shows a heart rate of 160 beats per minute, QRS duration of 160 ms and occasional capture and fusion beats.

Which one of the following is the highest priority action to take?

a) Adjust her intravenous sliding scale insulin to address recurrence of her metabolic disorder
b) Initiate infusion of intravenous amiodarone – 300 mg over one hour
c) Arrange for synchronised DC cardioversion
d) Introduce continuous positive airway pressure non-invasive ventilation
e) If vagal manoeuvres fail, try incremental boluses of adenosine intravenously

Question 276

A 55-year-old man requires elective formation of a vascular access graft to allow commencement of renal replacement therapy. His chest radiograph is reviewed. This shows an enlarged heart with a cardiac/thoracic diameter ratio of 0.65. Which of the following investigations would demonstrate the risk factor most commonly associated with this abnormal chest X-ray finding in this patient group?

a) Thyroid function tests
b) Coronary angiogram
c) Echocardiogram
d) 24-hour ambulatory blood pressure monitor and access to previous blood pressure measurements
e) A full blood count and access to copies of previous full blood counts

Question 277

Regarding the content of intravenous fluids, the following statements are correct except which one?

a) 1000 mL of Gelofusine® contains 60 mmol of chloride ions
b) 200 mL of sodium bicarbonate 8.4% contains approximately 200 mmol of sodium ions
c) 500 mL of 20% mannitol contains approximately 100 g of mannitol
d) 500 mL of 6% hydroxyethyl starch (Voluven®) contains approximately 77 mmol of sodium ions and 77 mmol of chloride ions
e) 500 mL of 10% hydroxyethyl starch contains approximately 77 mmol of sodium ions and 77 mmol of chloride ions

Question 278

Regarding intraoperative monitoring of the electrocardiogram, which one of the following statements is true?

a) Lead II is most sensitive for detecting ischaemia
b) The CM_5 configuration requires four wires/electrodes
c) The CH_5 configuration involves sticking an electrode on the patient's head

d) To achieve alternative monitoring configurations once the leads are arranged appropriately, lead III is selected on the monitor display
e) Intraoperative manipulation of electrode placement and lead display selection is not recommended

Question 279

A patient presents for surgery during which blood loss of more than 1000 mL is anticipated. The theatre team suggests using intra-operative cell salvage (ICS). Regarding the use of ICS the following statements are correct except which one?

a) If the scheduled surgery is radical prostatectomy for carcinoma of the prostate then ICS should be avoided
b) If the patient is presenting for surgery to control a significant post-partum haemorrhage then ICS can be used safely
c) If the rinse fluid from the swabs is not collected, usable yield is limited to 50 to 70% of total blood loss
d) The vast majority of Jehovah's Witnesses will agree to the use of blood obtained via ICS
e) The cost of the consumables for ICS in one case is approximately equal to the cost of one unit of transfused packed red cells

Question 280

Regarding levosimendan, which one of the following statements is true?

a) It elevates intracellular calcium concentration
b) It decreases afterload but not preload
c) It binds to troponin T thus increasing the force of myocardial contractility
d) It works throughout the cardiac cycle
e) It has an effect on adenosine triphosphate (ATP) sensitive potassium channels

Question 281

Concerning severe infection with malaria, the following statements are true except for which one?

a) The commonest laboratory finding in severe malaria is thrombocytopenia
b) Females contracting severe malaria have a higher mortality rate than males
c) A thin smear is more sensitive than a thick smear in the diagnosis of *Plasmodium falciparum* malaria
d) Only female mosquitoes are capable of haematophagy (drinking blood)
e) 'Blackwater fever' is usually not associated with acute renal failure

Question 282

Regarding the standard error of the mean (SEM), the following statements are true except which one?

a) Calculation of the SEM is the product of the standard deviation and the reciprocal of the square root of the sample size
b) The SEM can be regarded as a measure of spread of multiple means about the mean-of-means
c) The SEM is necessary for calculating the 95% confidence intervals
d) The SEM gives a better representation of spread of actual sample data than standard deviation
e) The SEM gives an impression of how precisely a sample mean corresponds to the true population mean

Question 283

Two patients have been admitted with acute coronary syndrome and require escalation of therapy. However, there is currently only one critical care bed available. In assigning priority for admission, which of the following, considered in isolation of other factors, is least likely to contribute to the patient being at high risk of a further cardiac ischaemic event?

a) That the patient had taken regular aspirin in the seven days leading up to hospital admission
b) That the patient had a serum creatinine of 220 micromol/L on admission to hospital
c) That the patient had a sinus tachycardia of 120 bpm on admission to hospital
d) That the patient is a hypertensive smoker
e) That the patient is 70 years old

Question 284

In the calculation of a P-POSSUM score, which of the following physiological parameters is not used?

a) Systolic BP
b) White cell count
c) Serum creatinine
d) Serum sodium
e) Glasgow Coma Score

Question 285

Which one of the following statements is not a criterion of the abbreviated mental test?

a) Name of hospital
b) Recognition of two people (e.g. a doctor and a nurse)
c) Name a pencil and a watch
d) Recall an address
e) Name of monarch

Question 286

Regarding the practicalities of one-lung ventilation, which one of the following statements is true?

a) During one-lung ventilation the clamp must be placed on the patient side of the universal connector of the unventilated lung and the catheter mount to that side must be open to air
b) A left-facing double lumen tube does not allow one-lung ventilation of the right lung
c) Size of double lumen endotracheal tubes can be estimated by considering patient weight
d) The depth of insertion of a double lumen endotracheal tube in an adult male is commonly 29 cm
e) At least 2 mL of air should be put in the bronchial cuff to prevent pendelluft ventilation

Question 287

A 73-year-old patient requires emergency laparotomy. During their preoperative assessment they are noticed to have a collapsing pulse. Which of the following conditions is least likely to be the cause of this finding?

a) An undiagnosed patent ductus arteriosus
b) Hyperthyroidism
c) Mixed aortic valve disease
d) Haemoglobin 8.2 g/dL
e) Temperature 38.5 °C

Question 288

An intravenous drug abuser has been brought into the emergency department (ED) in cardiac arrest secondary to ventricular fibrillation resistant to DC cardioversion. Assistance from the intensive care team is sought. The patient has had his trachea intubated, without drugs, by the paramedics; however, they and the ED physicians have been unable to secure intravenous access. The following drugs may be given via the intratracheal route except which one?

a) Adrenaline
b) Lidocaine
c) Amiodarone
d) Naloxone
e) Atropine

Question 289

A sick septic patient is admitted to the intensive care unit (ICU) and at day two, the following drugs can be found on his drug chart. Which of them is statistically most likely to cause him harm during his stay on the ICU?

a) Noradrenaline
b) Morphine
c) Gentamicin
d) Propofol
e) Insulin

Question 290

Regarding awake carotid endarterectomy, which one of the following statements is true?

a) Superficial and deep cervical plexus blocks are necessary for regional anaesthesia in the awake patient undergoing carotid endarterectomy
b) It is common to use an intermittent bolus sedation technique during clamping of the carotid
c) One advantage of the awake technique is that it obviates the need for a shunt
d) Agitation is common and should prompt reassurance of the patient
e) Chronic obstructive pulmonary disease may be a relative contraindication to the awake technique

Question 291

Eight months following a road traffic accident in which a 30-year-old man sustained a spinal cord injury, the same patient presents for surgery to treat a urethral stricture. Regarding potential autonomic dysreflexia (AD), the following statements are true EXCEPT which one?

a) A blood pressure of 120/80 mmHg would be inconsistent with a diagnosis of AD
b) Injuries below the sixth thoracic vertebra (T6) and incomplete spinal cord lesions are less likely to lead to AD than lesions above T6 and complete spinal cord lesions

c) Signs include flushed, sweaty skin above the level of the lesion and cool, pale skin below this level
d) Both tachycardia and bradycardia are commonly seen during an episode of AD
e) The most common triggers for episodes of AD are stimulation of the lower urinary tract or bowel distension secondary to faecal impaction

Question 292

Regarding neonatal physiology, which one of the following statements is true?

a) A neonate has low levels of endorphins compared to adults
b) A neonate has mature neuromuscular junctions by two weeks of age
c) A neonate has reversed direction of flow of CSF compared to adults
d) A neonate has blunted parasympathetic reflexes
e) A neonate has poor sympathetic response to bleeding

Question 293

Regarding osmolality, the following statements are true except which one?

a) Raoult's law applies to one of the colligative properties of solutions
b) Plasma osmotic pressure is approximately 7 atmospheres
c) One mole of a substance dissolved in one kilogram of solvent will produce a freezing point depression of 1.86 °C
d) Plasma osmolality may be estimated from a patient's urea and electrolytes, and their blood glucose
e) An osmolality gap may be observed following transurethral resection of the prostate

Question 294

Regarding acid–base management during cardiopulmonary bypass, which one of the following statements is true?

a) The solubility of carbon dioxide decreases as the temperature decreases
b) The 'alpha' of alpha-stat pH management refers to the alpha-globin subunit of haemoglobin
c) On cardiopulmonary bypass without correction, as the temperature falls, the pH of the blood falls
d) In alpha-stat management, carbon dioxide must be added to the bypass circuit
e) In pH-stat management, the arterial blood gas values are corrected for the temperature the patient was when they were taken

Question 295

A 35-year-old woman is admitted confused and vomiting to the emergency department following ingestion of a quantity of unknown tablets. The critical care team is called because of the following blood gas result:

pH 7.55; pO_2 19.02 kPa; pCO_2 2.53 kPa; HCO_3^- 18 mmol/L

Of the following drugs, which has most likely been ingested?

a) Paracetamol
b) Dothiepin
c) Aspirin
d) 3,4-methylenedioxymethamphetamine (MDMA)
e) Cocaine

Question 296

A 50-year-old lady has undergone emergency splenectomy following a road traffic accident. Regarding her follow-up care the following statements are correct except which one?

a) She should receive pneumococcal vaccination against *Streptococcus pneumoniae* approximately two weeks after her splenectomy
b) If not previously immunised she should be vaccinated with *Haemophilus influenzae* type B
c) Influenza vaccination is recommended for her on a yearly basis
d) She should be immunised against *Neisseria meningitidis*
e) She should receive ongoing prophylactic antibiotics to reduce the chance of serious infection with *Staphylococcus*

Question 297

A patient aspirates their stomach contents on emergence from anaesthesia while lying supine. They receive mechanical ventilation on ICU and are successfully weaned and extubated but still need supplementary oxygen. At day 12, they develop raised inflammatory markers, a temperature of 39.5 °C and evidence of pulmonary abscesses on their plain chest radiograph. Which one of the following is the most likely site of their abscess?

a) Superior segment of the right lower lobe
b) Superior segment of the lingular
c) Superior segment of the left lower lobe
d) Posterior basal segment of the right lower lobe
e) Lateral segment of the right middle lobe

Question 298

The following features would place a patient at risk of postoperative urinary retention except which one?

a) Male gender
b) 500 mL intravenous infusion of Hartmann's solution during knee arthroscopy
c) Previous history of severe bradycardia under anaesthesia
d) Open reduction and mesh repair of inguinal hernia
e) Intravenous midazolam sedation in recovery

Question 299

A patient has been accepted for non-heart beating organ donation (NHBD). Which of the following organs cannot be successfully transplanted if the patient dies 90 minutes after withdrawal of active treatment?

a) Heart valves
b) Corneas
c) Liver
d) Skin
e) Kidneys

Question 300

A 67-year-old, 75 kg woman requires anaesthesia for a total knee replacement. Her admission blood results are reviewed. Some of them are as follows: urea 15.1 mmol/L; creatinine 77 micromol/L; haemoglobin 8 g/dL.

Which of the following represents the least likely cause?

a) Regular non-steroidal use over the past six months
b) Chronic renal failure secondary to hypertension and non-insulin dependent diabetes mellitus
c) That she is on medication for treatment of cardiac failure
d) That she has been taking prednisolone, 20 mg daily, for the last six months
e) A history of alcohol excess, known hepatic cirrhosis and oesophageal varices on endoscopy

Answers

Paper A

1	b	26	a	51	d
2	c	27	a	52	b
3	b	28	e	53	d
4	b	29	b	54	c
5	e	30	a	55	e
6	c	31	a	56	e
7	b	32	a	57	d
8	d	33	d	58	c
9	e	34	c	59	c
10	a	35	c	60	b
11	c	36	d	61	e
12	e	37	a	62	e
13	a	38	b	63	c
14	d	39	e	64	a
15	a	40	d	65	b
16	d	41	c	66	d
17	a	42	c	67	b
18	c	43	d	68	c
19	c	44	d	69	d
20	c	45	e	70	b
21	e	46	e	71	d
22	b	47	d	72	c
23	e	48	d	73	b
24	b	49	a	74	c
25	a	50	c	75	c

Paper B

76	c	101	a	126	e
77	b	102	e	127	c
78	a	103	a	128	e
79	b	104	e	129	c
80	e	105	a	130	b
81	c	106	b	131	c
82	a	107	a	132	e
83	e	108	e	133	e
84	e	109	a	134	c
85	b	110	d	135	a
86	a	111	c	136	a
87	b	112	e	137	e
88	d	113	e	138	c
89	c	114	d	139	b
90	a	115	c	140	b
91	e	116	a	141	e
92	a	117	c	142	b
93	e	118	c	143	e
94	c	119	b	144	d
95	e	120	d	145	c
96	d	121	e	146	b
97	d	122	b	147	d
98	d	123	c	148	a
99	e	124	d	149	d
100	b	125	c	150	c

Paper C

151	d		176	c	201	c
152	d		177	d	202	c
153	d		178	c	203	c
154	a		179	e	204	b
155	c		180	a	205	e
156	b		181	d	206	d
157	b		182	e	207	b
158	b		183	a	208	b
159	d		184	d	209	e
160	c		185	a	210	b
161	e		186	b	211	c
162	a		187	b	212	a
163	e		188	e	213	a
164	d		189	d	214	c
165	c		190	e	215	b
166	d		191	e	216	a
167	b		192	b	217	b
168	b		193	b	218	d
169	d		194	d	219	b
170	e		195	e	220	b
171	a		196	c	221	d
172	c		197	a	222	a
173	a		198	a	223	b
174	a		199	a	224	a
175	c		200	a	225	e

Paper D

226	e	251	d	276	d		
227	b	252	b	277	a		
228	a	253	a	278	c		
229	a	254	e	279	a		
230	e	255	b	280	e		
231	b	256	a	281	c		
232	d	257	c	282	d		
233	b	258	c	283	d		
234	b	259	a	284	c		
235	b	260	e	285	c		
236	c	261	a	286	d		
237	b	262	b	287	c		
238	a	263	b	288	c		
239	b	264	a	289	a		
240	c	265	a	290	e		
241	a	266	a	291	a		
242	a	267	a	292	e		
243	c	268	c	293	c		
244	c	269	c	294	e		
245	b	270	e	295	c		
246	c	271	e	296	e		
247	e	272	c	297	a		
248	e	273	c	298	b		
249	b	274	b	299	c		
250	d	275	c	300	b		

Explanations

Paper A

Question 1: Albumin

Regarding albumin, the following statements are true EXCEPT which one?

a) Albumin is a negative acute phase protein
b) A common cause of hypoalbuminaemia is starvation or malnutrition
c) In health the liver produces approximately 10 g per day of albumin
d) The circulation half-life of albumin is approximately 18 days
e) The majority of total body albumin is found in the extravascular compartment

Answer: b

Explanation

Albumin is a single polypeptide of 585 amino acids and molecular weight 66kDa produced by the liver. Its molecular weight is variably quoted between 66 and 69kDa, which seems to be related to the degree of glycosylation. It is negatively charged and very soluble, and performs a number of crucial physiological roles. It is the most abundant plasma protein, responsible for maintenance of colloid oncotic pressure and transport, via protein-binding, of drugs, bilirubin, thyroid hormones, calcium ions and more. Despite its domination of plasma proteins, only 40% of total body albumin is intravascular. The rest is in the interstitial compartment having been filtered from the intravascular compartment (the transcapillary escape rate is 5% per hour) and slowly returned to the circulation via the thoracic duct. It performs similar roles in the interstitium, including exerting an oncotic pressure (consider Starling forces). However, although the interstitial albumin content is greater, the volume in which it resides is significantly greater such that resultant oncotic pressure is low and the gradient is maintained. It is a common misconception that serum albumin concentration is a marker of nutritional status and that it falls in starvation. It is correct that albumin is not stored in the liver so levels do reflect synthetic activity but during starvation with normal liver function, albumin will be maintained at the expense of proteolysis elsewhere. Albumin is not catabolised during starvation. It is common, however, that malnutrition accompanies disease states that are associated with hypoalbuminaemia. The causes of low albumin states are categorised into decreased synthesis (liver dysfunction), increased loss (e.g. renal dysfunction), redistribution (i.e. capillary leak) and very rarely increased catabolism. Acute and chronic inflammatory states provoke elements of each of these. Also albumin is referred to as a negative acute phase reactant as its manufacture is diminished as part of the inflammatory process.

Question 2: Sugammadex

Which of the following statements regarding sugammadex is TRUE?

a) It is a modified α-cyclodextrin
b) The drug forms complexes with steroidal neuromuscular blocking drugs with a ratio of 1:2
c) Following sugammadex administration to reverse rocuronium-induced neuromuscular blockade the measured total plasma rocuronium concentration will rise
d) The majority of the drug is metabolised and excreted by the kidneys
e) Sugammadex exerts its effect by binding with rocuronium at the neuromuscular junction

Answer: c

Explanation

Sugammadex is a modified γ-cyclodextrin of which there are three types (α, β and γ) all of which are doughnut shaped, have a hydrophobic, lipophilic cavity and a hydrophilic exterior. To create sugammadex, γ-cyclodextrin has been modified by the addition of eight side-chains to extend the cavity and negatively charged carboxyl groups to increase binding affinity. This has created a molecule that is able to bind with the steroidal neuromuscular blocking drugs (rocuronium > vecuronium > pancuronium). Sugammadex forms tight 1:1 complexes with these drugs in plasma, resulting in movement of neuromuscular blocker away from the neuromuscular junction into the plasma down a concentration gradient. Sugammadex has no effect on acetylcholinesterase or any receptor system in the body. The majority of sugammadex is excreted unchanged in the urine. For complete reversal of neuromuscular blockade to take place sugammadex need only reduce post-synaptic receptor occupancy from 100% to 70%. Several dose-finding studies have been carried out and suggested doses range between 2.0 to 4.0 mg/kg following reappearance of the second train-of-four twitch after administration of rocuronium. There is also emerging evidence that sugammadex, at a dose of 16 mg/kg, can promptly reverse high-dose rocuronium (1.0–1.2 mg/kg). This may lead to the intriguing possibility of rocuronium challenging the place of suxamethonium as the muscle relaxant of choice in rapid sequence induction.

Reference

Naguib M. Sugammadex: another milestone in clinical neuromuscular pharmacology. *Anesth Analg* 2007; **104**(3): 575–81.

Question 3: Pulmonary vasoconstriction

Pulmonary vasoconstriction may be caused by

a) Hypothermia
b) Smoking 'Crack' cocaine
c) Volatile anaesthetic agents
d) Calcium channel blockers
e) Positive end expiratory pressure

Answer: b

Explanation

'Crack' or free-base cocaine is a Class A illicit drug, which is used widely in the 'hard' drug taking community. In 2001, in the USA, 4.7% of young adults admitted to having used 'Crack' cocaine. Due to the illegal nature of the drug, 'Crack' has not been the subject of formal randomised controlled trials. There is a substantial body of case reports and good animal-model work to suggest that smoking 'Crack' puts a patient at risk of developing pulmonary vasoconstriction. All the other options here are known to inhibit pulmonary vasoconstriction.

Question 4: Central neuraxial block producing neurological injury

Regarding central neuraxial blocks, which one of the following is MOST likely to cause permanent neurological injury?

a) An epidural sited for obstetric indications
b) An epidural sited for adult general surgical indications
c) An epidural sited for paediatric general surgical indications
d) A spinal sited rather than an epidural
e) An epidural sited for chronic pain indications

Answer: b

Explanation
In 2009, the 'NAP3' study was published on the website of the Royal College of Anaesthetists. It is an impressive body of work that has given a numerator and denominator for injury following central neuraxial blocks (CNB). To ascertain the denominator they estimated the total number of CNB performed in a year by looking at a two-week snapshot. All of the units using epidurals in the UK returned information for the snapshot and a denominator figure of just over 700 000 CNBs per year was found. Potential cases of permanent neurological injury following CNB were reported and reviewed to determine the likelihood of the injury being due to the CNB. This allowed the reporters to attach an optimistic figure (in which only the highly likely to be due to the CNB were included) and a pessimistic figure (in which some of the more tenuous associations between CNB and injury were included). The findings showed that the risk was generally lower than people had previously thought. Epidurals caused more harm than spinals (6.1 vs. 2.2 cases per 100 000 for the 'pessimistic' interpretation) and the highest risk group for epidurals was in adult general peri-operative care. This was probably due to the high incidence of sicker patients having thoracic epidurals on a background of pharmacological or pathological derangement of their clotting cascade.

Reference
Royal College of Anaesthetists. Major complications of central neuraxial block in the United Kingdom. Report and findings of the 3rd National Audit Project of the Royal College of Anaesthetists. London: RCA, 2009. Online at www.rcoa.ac.uk/docs/NAP3_web-large.pdf (Accessed 30 October 2009)

Question 5: Nasogastric tube placement

A nasogastric tube is sited in a patient ventilated on the critical care unit. Which one of the following is considered the MOST ACCURATE way of confirming correct positioning?

a) Measurement of the aspirate using pH indicator strips
b) Auscultation of air insufflated through the nasogastric tube (the 'whoosh' test)
c) Testing the acidity/alkalinity of aspirate from the nasogastric tube using litmus paper
d) Observing the appearance of the aspirate from the nasogastric tube
e) Chest radiograph

Answer: e

Explanation

There have been a number of safety alerts involving the misplacement of nasogastric tubes. The only two recommended methods for confirming correct nasogastric tube placement are chest radiography and the use of pH indicator strips or paper. No other methods including the other three options listed in the question are considered safe. The most accurate method for confirming correct tube placement is accurately reported chest radiography. However, there have been multiple reports of X-rays being mis-interpreted and minimising X-ray exposure is also important, particularly in the critically ill patient. pH testing may be influenced by co-administration of medication that could elevate the pH level of gastric contents, e.g. antacids, H_2 antagonists and proton pump inhibitors. There are no known reports of pulmonary aspirates with a pH of less than 5.5 so this is a useful cut-off point. If the pH is greater than this then one should wait an hour then re-check, as the commonest reason for a higher pH is the presence in the stomach of enteral feed. The gold standard is radiography. In addition to following insertion, nasogastric tube position should be re-checked before administration of feed, at least once daily during continuous feed, following episodes of vomiting, retching or coughing and if there has been any evidence of tube displacement.

Reference

National Patient Safety Agency. Reducing the harm caused by misplaced nasogastric feeding tubes. Patient safety alert 05. NPSA, 21 February 2005. Online at www.npsa. nhs.uk (Accessed 30 October 2009)

Question 6: Prevention of infective endocarditis

Which of the following patient groups is NOT thought to be at increased risk of infective endocarditis and therefore does NOT require prophylaxis against infective endocarditis when undergoing an interventional procedure?

a) Moderate mitral regurgitation
b) A patient with a history of previous endocarditis but a structurally normal heart
c) Isolated atrial septal defect
d) Hypertrophic cardiomyopathy
e) Pulmonary stenosis

Answer: c

Explanation

Infective endocarditis (IE) is a rare condition with significant morbidity and mortality. Until relatively recently, in an attempt to prevent this disease, at-risk patients were given antibiotic prophylaxis before dental and certain non-dental interventional pro-cedures. This status quo was challenged for a number of reasons including the lack of efficacy of antibiotic prophylaxis regimes, the lack of association between episodes of IE and prior interventional procedures, and the prevalence of bacteraemias arising from everyday activities such as brushing teeth. As a result, in 2008 the National Institute for Health and Clinical Excellence (NICE) produced new guidelines on the prevention of IE. These guidelines identified patients at risk of IE. This included those with valve replacement, acquired valvular heart disease with stenosis or regurgitation, structural congenital heart disease (including surgically corrected or palliated structural condi-tions but excluding isolated atrial septal defects, fully repaired ventricular septal defects, fully repaired patent ductus arteriosus and closure devices that are considered to have epithelialised), hypertrophic cardiomyopathy or a previous episode of IE. The guidelines also stated that prophylaxis against IE should not, routinely, be offered to people undergoing dental procedures and those undergoing non-dental procedures at the following sites: upper and lower gastrointestinal (GI) tract, genitourinary (GU) tract (including childbirth) and the upper and lower respiratory tract unless they fall into the 'at-risk' group for IE. The antibiotic given to an 'at-risk' patient receiving antimicrobial therapy because they are undergoing a GI or GU procedure at a site where there is suspected infection should be broad enough to include those organisms known to cause IE.

Reference

NICE Clinical Guideline 64. Prophylaxis against infective endocarditis: antimicrobial prophylaxis against infective endocarditis in adults and children undergoing interventional procedures. London: NICE, 2008. Online at www.nice.org.uk/nicemedia/pdf/CG64NICEguidance.pdf (Accessed 30 October 2009)

Question 7: Crises in myasthenia gravis

A 40-year-old woman known to have myasthenia gravis presents to the emergency department with severe global weakness. She is pale, sweaty and cyanosed. Her partner explains that she was diagnosed some time ago and she is, to the best of his knowledge, compliant with her oral pyridostigmine therapy. She is a smoker and has been coughing more than usual recently. He has been worried about her low mood in past months. In order to distinguish between an excess or inadequacy of her myasthenia treatment, which one of the following features is likely to be the MOST HELPFUL?

a) Rapid onset of ventilatory failure
b) Response to dose of cholinesterase inhibitor
c) Flaccid muscle paralysis
d) Presence of bronchospasm
e) Loss of deep tendon reflexes

Answer: b

Explanation

Distinguishing myasthenic crisis from cholinergic crisis is difficult because the two conditions share many clinical features. A myasthenic crisis may be precipitated by non-compliance with medications, concurrent infection or any physiological insult, but the condition naturally varies in severity and it is expected that cholinesterase inhibitor therapy will have to be regularly adjusted. A cholinergic crisis is caused by relative overdosage of cholinesterase inhibitor medication causing acetylcholine excess and stimulation at nicotinic and muscarinic receptors in the locomotor and autonomic nervous systems. This produces a syndrome similar to organophosphate poisoning. Both may present with rapid onset flaccid paralysis. A curiosity of myasthenia gravis and cholinergic crisis is that deep tendon reflexes are preserved. Bronchospasm is a described feature of cholinergic crisis but may equally be present in myasthenic crisis, as inability to cough causes retained secretions and airway irritation. Both may cause sweating and cyanosis via ventilatory failure. Cholinergic crisis is associated with the SLUDGE syndrome (salivation, lacrimation, urinary incontinence, diarrhoea, gastrointestinal hypermotility and emesis) but is not consistently present and does not distinguish from myasthenic crisis. Despite the fact that one of these emergencies is caused by an excess of cholinesterase inhibitor, the conditions are differentiated by administration of intravenous edrophonium at escalating doses (1 mg, 3 mg, 5 mg). Myasthenic crisis will show transient improvement whereas in cholinergic crisis the SLUDGE syndrome, bradycardia or very rarely asystole may be precipitated. This is only acceptable as a diagnostic tool as the half-life of edrophonium is short. Atropine should be immediately available to administer, if required. The arrangement of this test should not distract from appropriate airway and ventilatory management with a small dose of non-depolarising muscle relaxant, if necessary, to facilitate endotracheal intubation.

Question 8: Tricyclic antidepressant poisoning

Which of the following is NOT a recognised cause of the toxic effects of tricyclic antidepressant drugs taken in overdose?

a) Inhibition of noradrenaline reuptake at nerve terminals
b) A myocardial membrane stabilising effect
c) An anticholinergic action
d) Indirect activation of $GABA_A$ receptors
e) Direct alpha adrenergic action

Answer: d

Explanation

Tricyclic antidepressant drugs are among the most commonly ingested substances in self-poisoning along with benzodiazepines, paracetamol and alcohol. They are rapidly absorbed from the GI tract, are highly protein bound, have a large volume of distribution and therefore have a long elimination half-life. The toxic effects are mediated in four main ways, direct alpha adrenergic blockade, an anticholinergic action, a membrane stabilising effect on the myocardium and inhibition of noradrenaline reuptake at nerve terminals. The clinical features of overdose may be divided into effects on the cardiovascular system, central nervous system (mainly sedative but also proconvulsant) and anticholinergic effects. The latter effects are common and include pyrexia, urinary retention, absent bowel sounds and dilated pupils. Sinus tachycardia and hypotension are the commonest cardiovascular effects but the major toxic effect is related to the slowing of depolarisation of the cardiac action potential by sodium current inhibition. Treatment following overdose is, in the main, supportive. Specific treatments include alkalinisation with intravenous sodium bicarbonate. This works by reducing the pharmacologically active unbound proportion of the drug by raising pH. Anti-arrhythmic treatment should be avoided where possible but there may be a role for magnesium in the treatment of ventricular arrhythmias. Tricyclic-specific antibody fragments have been developed but their use is limited by cost and the potential renal toxicity due to the large dose required.

Reference

Kerr GW, McGuffie AC, Wilkie S. Tricyclic antidepressant overdose: a review. *Emerg Med J* 2001; **18**(4) 236–41.

Question 9: Tourniquet use for limb surgery

Regarding the use of tourniquets in the theatre environment, the following statements are true EXCEPT which one?

a) Exsanguination and tourniquet inflation is associated with immediate rise in central venous pressure, arterial blood pressure and heart rate
b) After two hours' inflation time, a significant decrease in core temperature can be expected on deflation of the tourniquet
c) Pre-inflation, ketamine 0.25 mg/kg intravenously can prevent the hypertensive response to tourniquets
d) When using a double-cuff tourniquet for intravenous regional anaesthesia the proximal cuff is the first to be used

e) If the continuous tourniquet inflation time exceeds two hours, the ischaemic cell damage and lesions associated with acidosis are irreversible

Answer: e

Explanation

The use of a tourniquet for prevention of haemorrhage during limb surgery requires a pneumatic cuff of width at least half the diameter of the limb. The limb is exsanguinated and the cuff inflated to 50 mmHg greater than the systolic blood pressure for the upper limb or 100 mmHg greater than the systolic blood pressure for the lower limb. Exsanguination causes an autotransfusion of blood volume to the central compartment with consequent increase in central venous pressure, heart rate and blood pressure. This is exacerbated by the acute increase in systemic vascular resistance. The temperature of the ischaemic limb drops and metabolites accumulate in it. It is the release of these metabolites, and cold to the circulation, which causes the physiological changes seen on deflation. After about one hour of cuff inflation, characteristic resistant hypertension is seen. This may be avoided with pre-inflation ketamine as described or regional anaesthesia. An arbitrary inflation duration limit of two hours is often applied but some centres use in excess of this and at two hours' duration, cell lesions secondary to local acidosis are reversible. During intravenous regional anaesthesia the proximal cuff is inflated first before the local anaesthetic is injected in order that the site of the distal cuff is rendered insensate before the distal cuff is inflated such that tourniquet pain is avoided.

Reference

Malanjum L, Fischer B. Procedures under tourniquet. *Anaes Intens Care* 2009; **10**(1): 14–17.

Question 10: Blood sampling

You are called to the resuscitation room where an unwell, 34-year-old man is undergoing assessment. You agree to take the venous blood sample for investigations. The bottles and syringes required are all listed below. Select the sample that you would draw and fill THIRD.

a) Standard gold-topped sample bottle containing gel activator (SST) for urea and electrolytes
b) Standard grey-topped sample bottle containing fluoride oxalate for glucose
c) Standard blue-topped sample bottle containing citrate coagulation screen
d) Standard purple-topped sample bottle containing EDTA for full blood count
e) Blood culture bottles

Answer: a

Explanation

Typically, a blood culture sample would be drawn and filled first. This is to reduce the chance of bacterial contamination during sampling. Following that, the clotting screen in the citrate bottle should be filled next as the minimum amount of time for the blood to be out of contact with the circulation is ideal. This also reduces the risk of contamination with coagulants or anticoagulants in other bottles. Next comes the gold-topped SST bottle. If this is filled after the purple-topped bottle, EDTA contamination can interfere with biochemistry analysis. Finally the grey-topped oxalate bottle is filled. SST tubes used to appear higher up in the order of draw but have dropped down as they are now considered additive tubes, containing silica particles to promote clotting.

Reference
Advice available online at www.bd.com/vacutainer/pdfs/plus_plastic_tubes_
wallchart_orderofdraw_VS5729.pdf (Accessed 30 November 2009)

Question 11: Respiratory examination

A 55-year-old male smoker presents with lethargy, cough and intermittent chest pains. He requires assessment because of progressive respiratory failure. On examination he has a central trachea and reduced chest expansion. On the right he has a dull percussion note, easily audible breath sounds and whispering pectoriloquy. On the left his breath sounds seem less audible but there are no added sounds and vocal resonance is normal. Which of the following is the MOST likely diagnosis?

a) Right pleural effusion
b) Left pneumothorax
c) Right pneumonic consolidation
d) Left lobar collapse with patent major bronchi
e) Right bronchial proximal obstructing lesion

Answer: c

Explanation
Unilateral differences in breath sounds may represent a reduction in breath sounds in one hemithorax or an increase in audibility on the contralateral side. Bronchial breathing, as caused by increased sound transmission through a consolidated lobe, might be overlooked in favour of describing reduced breath sounds on the contralateral side. The examination is consistent with a right-sided pneumonia although crepitations were not mentioned in this case. A right-sided collapsed lobe with patent major bronchi may give virtually identical examination findings. This is intuitive, as in both cases tissues have been rendered more solid and conductive to sound. With a pleural effusion, the accumulated liquid fails to transmit sound – breath sounds and vocal resonance are reduced and the percussion note is stony dull. Similar findings might be seen where there is lobar collapse with an obstructed main bronchus as there is no air flow into the collapsed lobe. A pneumothorax will produce a hyperresonant percussion note as well as reduced breath sounds and vocal resonance with no added sounds.

Reference
Crompton G. The respiratory system. In: Munro J, Campbell I (eds) *Macleod's Clinical Examination*, 10th edn. Edinburgh: Churchill Livingstone, 2000; pp.117–44.

Question 12: Meta-analysis

Regarding meta-analysis, which one of the following statements is TRUE?

a) Is analagous to a systematic review
b) The size of a 'blob' in a 'blobbogram' reflects the degree of significance found in the individual study
c) If the centre line is crossed by the confidence interval of the combined result, there is no association between the variables
d) The 'x' axis of the results graph is usually expressed as relative risk
e) The funnel plot helps to identify selection bias

Answer: e

Explanation

Meta-analysis continues to suffer from criticism but remains a cornerstone of evidence-based medicine. As such, a good working knowledge of how meta-analysis works is essential. Systematic review is a rigorous technique for examining the medical literature. It usually starts with asking a question; working out which database(s) to examine; performing a search; selecting and then reviewing the best evidence; and synthesising an answer to the question with a level of recommendation. Meta-analysis is a statistical technique for combining the results of small trials to provide power through strength of numbers allowing questions to be answered. All meta-analyses start with a systematic review, but not all systematic reviews involve meta-analysis. The size of the 'blob' in a 'blobbogram' indicates the weighting towards the overall analysis that has been assigned to an individual study. It has nothing to do with the findings in the individual study, just the study's contribution to the meta-analysis. If the centre line is crossed by the confidence interval of the combined result, there may still be an association but the meta-analysis has failed to demonstrate it. The 'x' axis is usually either the odds ratio or favours treatment/favours control. Typically in meta-analysis, selection bias involves the study team missing small studies with negative findings as these are often less likely to be published. Big studies will tend to sit closer to the true mean, whereas smaller studies will spread out further from the mean in both directions. A funnel plot involves the studies plotted with decreasing size up the 'y' axis and demonstrated effect on the 'x' axis. They will show asymmetry at the broader part of the funnel if such a selection bias exists.

Reference

Crombie IK, Davies HTO. What is meta-analysis? 2nd edn. What is . . . ? series. Hayward Medical Communications, 2009. Online at www.medicine.ox.ac.uk/bandolier/painres/download/whatis/Meta-An.pdf (Accessed 30 October 2009)

Question 13: Postoperative thoracic surgery

Negative pressure may be applied to the chest drainage tube of the affected hemithorax in the following circumstances EXCEPT which one?

a) Post-pneumonectomy
b) Known bronchopleural fistula
c) Known haemothorax
d) Known empyema
e) Post-oesophagectomy

Answer: a

Explanation

Chest drainage tubes are sited intra-operatively or elsewhere to allow egress of fluid (such as air, blood, pus or effusion) from the intrapleural space. Often the pressure gradient between intrapleural space and atmospheric pressure are adequate to encourage outward flow. In cases where the gradient is insufficient, suction may be applied to the chest tube. Unlike 'wall-suction', chest tube suction is low-pressure (10 to $20\,cmH_2O$), high-flow suction. If a chest drain has been used for a pneumothorax and high-pressure, low-flow suction is applied (incorrectly), the rate of volume evacuation may not be sufficient thus allowing accumulation in the chest and potentially a tension pneumothorax. With bronchopleural fistula (BPF) there is no doubt that suction evacuation of the cavity may encourage further air leakage across the BPF causing increased volume of 'wasted ventilation'. It is recommended that if it is necessary in cases of BPF, suction should be maintained at the minimum effective level. The options quoted have caused controversy with respect to whether application of suction is appropriate. In cases of haemothorax, with potentially ongoing haemorrhage, might suction encourage bleeding? This is not thought to be the case. The role of chest tube suction with pleural infection is not agreed but it is not contraindicated. Following pneumonectomy the operative side fills with serous fluid. Although a chest tube is sited, it is usually left clamped and *must not* have negative pressure applied to it as doing this will evacuate the serous fluid, potentially disrupting the stump and shifting the mediastinum enough to produce a similar effect to a tension pneumothorax. Post-oesophagectomy the use of facemask non-invasive ventilation is contraindicated as it could cause anastomotic strain/leak.

Question 14: Acute phase proteins

The following are direct or indirect measurements of acute phase proteins EXCEPT which one?

a) C-reactive protein
b) Plasma viscosity
c) Haptoglobin
d) Rheumatoid factor
e) Erythrocyte sedimentation rate

Answer: d

Explanation

C-reactive protein (CRP) and haptoglobin are acute phase proteins. These are proteins whose levels fluctuate in response to tissue injury. C-reactive protein is elevated in a wide range of inflammatory diseases such as infections, connective tissue diseases and neoplasias. C-reactive protein was so called, when it was discovered, because it reacted with the C polysaccharide of *Streptococcus pneumoniae*. Haptoglobin is elevated in haemolysis, but also in many inflammatory processes. Erythrocyte sedimentation rate (ESR) measures how quickly red cells fall through a column of blood and as such is an indirect test of acute phase proteins. ESR has a number of factors, such as gender and haematocrit, that influence the value generated by the test. It is, however, cheap, quick and easy to perform but is fairly non-specific with regard to the type of inflammatory process detected. Plasma viscosity is also an indirect test of acute phase proteins with results that mirror ESR. It is not, however, affected by haematocrit and is therefore more reliable than ESR. Rheumatoid factor (RhF) is an autoantibody, found in about 75% of people known to have rheumatoid arthritis. It is also elevated in a number of other autoimmune diseases such as Sjögren's syndrome. The level of RhF may give some indication of severity of the rheumatoid arthritis but is not predictive of an acute inflammatory flare-up.

Question 15: Warfarin therapy

A patient has a CT-confirmed retroperitoneal haemorrhage. He is on warfarin for atrial fibrillation. His international normalised ratio (INR) is usually stable between two and three. It is now eight, and this may be explained by the recent commencement of a new drug. Of the following drugs, which is the LEAST LIKELY to be responsible for the derangement?

a) Clopidogrel
b) Paracetamol
c) Amiodarone
d) Fluconazole
e) Metronidazole

Answer: a

Explanation

Warfarin inhibits the effective synthesis of biologically active forms of the vitamin K-dependent clotting factors: II, VII, IX and X, as well as the regulatory factors: protein C, protein S and protein Z. The precursors of these factors require carboxylation of their glutamic acid residues to allow the coagulation factors to bind to phospholipid surfaces. This carboxylation is linked to oxidation of vitamin K to form vitamin K epoxide, which is in turn recycled back to the reduced form by the enzyme vitamin K epoxide reductase (VKOR). Warfarin inhibits VKOR thereby diminishing available vitamin K stores and inhibiting production of functioning coagulation factors. Most clinically relevant drug interactions with warfarin involve drugs from only a few classes and occur by only a handful of mechanisms. Drugs that impair platelet function (e.g. acetylsalicylic acid, clopidogrel and interestingly some selective serotonin reuptake inhibitors) increase the risk of bleeding in patients on warfarin but without raising the INR, hence option (a) is incorrect. The effect of NSAIDs on the gastric mucosa is another important cause of increased bleeding risk in a warfarinised patient with an INR within therapeutic range. Many antibiotics enhance the effects of warfarin by either reducing vitamin K levels by altering the intestinal microflora or by directly inhibiting hepatic warfarin metabolism. Commercially produced warfarin exists as a racemic mixture of two isomers, the S-isomer of which is five times more active and is metabolised by the cytochrome P450 isoenzyme 2C9. Drugs reducing the activity of this enzyme, e.g. antifungals, fluoxetine, metronidazole and amiodarone, will therefore lead to elevated warfarin levels and raised INR. The other major drug interaction of warfarin is with paracetamol. Research evidence suggests that N-acetyl (P)-benzoquinoneimine (the highly reactive paracetamol metabolite that causes hepatocellular injury in paracetamol overdose) inhibits vitamin K-dependent carboxylase thus interrupting the vitamin K cycle and augmenting the clinical effect of warfarin. For reasons that are unclear, some patients may experience a rapid rise in INR following standard doses of paracetamol.

Reference

Juurlink D. Drug interactions with warfarin: what clinicians need to know. *Can Med Assoc J* 2007; **177**(4): 369–71.

Question 16: Postoperative complications of trauma surgery

A horse rider falls at a jump and sustains a closed head injury without impairment of consciousness at any stage and a femoral shaft fracture, which is internally fixated with an intramedullary nail soon after admission. At 48 hours post-injury she becomes confused, tachypnoeic, hypoxaemic and pyrexial (38.2 °C). An atypical rash is also noted. Which one of the following statements is MOST APPROPRIATE?

a) Immediately alert the orthopaedic surgeons
b) Based on these features, anticoagulation is indicated
c) Transfusion of packed red cells is indicated
d) A chest X-ray will contribute to resolving the situation
e) An urgent CT head scan is highest priority

Answer: d

Explanation

The question is written to give rise to suspicion of fat embolism syndrome. Remember, however, that this is rare, and sensible exclusion of common, treatable diagnoses is required. The characteristic rash is present in less than half of cases of fat embolism syndrome and this diagnosis is less treatable than other differentials. Although the patient's orthopaedic team should be kept up to date, they will have little to contribute currently. There is no mention as to the presence or absence of blunt chest trauma during the accident, but at 48 hours a lower respiratory tract infection is a possibility, as might be a slowly worsening pneumothorax. Immediate introduction of supportive care and a prompt portable chest X-ray (and other basic investigations) will help work towards a solution.

Red cell transfusion would be indicated for haemorrhage, or sometimes fat embolism, but further investigation would be required in advance of this. Pulmonary embolism is a possibility but again anticoagulation should not be initiated based on these features. The history and chronology of the head injury prompts a low suspicion of primary intracranial pathology, but the possibility of a secondary bleed must be borne in mind. Beware any option that suggests that the 'highest priority' is anything other than applying oxygen and instigating resuscitation measures.

Reference
Gupta A, Reilly C. Fat embolism. *Contin Educ Anaesth Crit Care Pain* 2007; **7**(5): 148–51.

Question 17: Monoamine oxidase inhibitors

A 54-year-old male requires emergency laparotomy. He has long-standing depression and is taking a monoamine oxidase inhibitor. Which one of the following monoamine oxidase inhibitors is LEAST LIKELY to cause incident during conduct of general anaesthesia?

a) Moclobemide
b) Phenelzine
c) Isocarboxazid
d) Tranylcypromine
e) Iproniazid

Answer: a

Explanation
The popularity of monoamine oxidase inhibitors (MAOIs) for the treatment of depressive disorders, obsessive syndromes and chronic back pain rose in the 1970s and 1980s but has subsequently declined due to the emergence of superior medications with more favourable side-effect profiles. Nevertheless, patients still taking these medications will be encountered and awareness of the potential interactions should be maintained. Amine neurotransmitters and neurohumoural messengers are metabolised by monoamine oxidase (MAO) and catechol-O-methyl transferase (COMT). Inhibition of MAO causes indiscriminate increase in concentration of amines in the central nervous system and elsewhere. Co-administration with agents that rely on MAO for their metabolism (e.g. indirectly acting sympathomimetics, ephedrine) or agents that also increase concentration of amines (notably pethidine, which blocks neuronal reuptake of serotonin) can produce dramatic clinical syndromes. The type I reaction is excitatory and involves hypertension, hyperpyrexia, convulsions, coma and can be fatal. The type II reaction is depressive, producing respiratory depression, hypotension and coma essentially resembling opioid overdose. Iproniazid was the prototype MAOI, originally introduced in the 1950s as a treatment for tuberculosis for which its efficacy was limited. Tranylcypromine is the most hazardous as it possesses stimulant activity independent of its enzyme inhibition properties. Moclobemide is a selective reversible inhibitor of monoamine oxidase-A, thus is devoid of many of the side-effects and interactions of its historical counterparts. Unlike the older agents, which form covalent bonds with the enzyme, moclobemide's action is reversible spontaneously with a half-life of two to four hours. It may be continued peri-operatively but pethidine and indirectly acting

sympathomimetics should still be avoided. Carefully titrated morphine would be the opioid of choice where regional anaesthesia cannot be employed.

Question 18: Management of pulmonary embolism

You are asked to see a 65-year-old patient on the ICU who had been admitted 24 hours previously following emergency laparotomy for a bleeding duodenal ulcer. He had been extubated 24 hours previously. His haematology, coagulation and biochemistry profiles are normal and he was on 30% oxygen but has suddenly become very short of breath with some pleuritic central chest pain. He is cardiovascularly stable. You suspect a possible pulmonary embolism (PE) and start him on high-flow oxygen. Which of the following statements represents your BEST immediate management plan?

a) 12-lead electrocardiogram (ECG), blood for cardiac troponin, computerised tomography pulmonary angiogram (CTPA) and therapeutic dose unfractionated heparin if the CTPA shows a significant PE
b) 12-lead ECG, CTPA and thrombolytic therapy if the CTPA shows a significant PE
c) 12-lead ECG, CTPA and therapeutic dose unfractionated heparin if the CTPA shows a significant PE
d) CTPA and therapeutic dose enoxaparin sodium if the CTPA shows a significant PE
e) 12-lead ECG, D-dimer and if both are normal no further immediate interventions

Answer: c

Explanation
There is a great deal of information in this question that takes some sifting through. Option (a) is incorrect because cardiac troponin taken at the onset of chest pain is of little prognostic significance, particularly in a patient who has been critically ill. Option (e) is incorrect because a combination of a negative 12-lead ECG and D-dimer is not sensitive enough to exclude a diagnosis of PE. Option (d) can be discounted because an ECG should be done to exclude any obvious ST elevation or other evidence of myocardial ischaemia, and it would be unwise to start a low molecular weight heparin rather than unfractionated heparin in a patient on critical care following recent surgery, due to the risk of bleeding. Of note the often-quoted, classic 'S1, Q3, T3' pattern seen on an ECG in pulmonary embolus is extremely uncommon. This leaves Options (b) and (c). A 2006 *Cochrane Review* showed that, based on the limited available evidence, it was unclear whether thrombolytic therapy was better than heparin for pulmonary embolism. The reviewers felt that more double-blind randomised controlled trials, with subgroup analysis of patients presenting with haemodynamically stable acute pulmonary embolism compared to those patients with a haemodynamic unstable condition, were required. In addition, thrombolytic therapy in a patient who has recently undergone laparotomy for a bleeding duodenal ulcer may be potentially hazardous.

Reference
Dong BR, Hao Q, Yue J, Wu T, Liu GJ. Thrombolytic therapy for pulmonary embolism. *Cochrane Database of Systematic Reviews* 2009, 3. CD004437. Summary online at www.cochrane.org/reviews/en/ab004437.html (Accessed 30 October 2009)

Question 19: Electrical safety

Regarding electrical equipment designed to optimise patient safety, which one of the following statements is TRUE?

a) Under single fault conditions, type I, CF equipment should have a leakage current in the order of 5mA
b) Type BF equipment is safe because the patient circuit is earthed

c) To promote patient safety a theatre suite should have an uninterruptible power supply (UPS)

d) Class III equipment is defined as that which operates at 'safety extra-low voltage' of less than 12V

e) A current-operated earth-leakage circuit breaker relies on an unacceptable current causing disintegration of a fuse that then breaks the circuit

Answer: c

Explanation

A patient's safety may be jeopardised by a lack of electricity as well as an excess of it. UPS ensure continued operation of safety-critical equipment in the event of a mains power failure. Rather frustratingly for the purposes of exams, values for allowable leakage currents vary according to source. However, the order of magnitude is incorrect in Option (a) – any device potentially forming a direct electrical link with the heart and thus with the potential to cause microshock, should have leakage currents in the order of microA, not mA. The 'F' of type BF equipment indicates a floating circuit – one in which there is no electrical contact with any other circuit or earth. The only current that flows in it is induced by a step-down transformer. Safety extra-low voltage (SELV) is less than 24V. A current-operated earth-leakage circuit breaker (COELCB) incorporates equal coils of live and neutral wires inducing a self-cancelling magnetic field. In the presence of an unacceptable current the magnetic fields no longer match: one dominates and operates a solenoid that breaks the circuit.

Question 20: Heart murmurs

A 57-year-old woman is listed for elective abdominal surgery. She has a history of rheumatoid arthritis. On auscultation of her praecordium, a murmur is detected. Regarding this patient, the following statements are true EXCEPT for which one?

a) If this murmur is related to a left-sided valve abnormality it will be heard louder in expiration than inspiration

b) The most likely murmurs would be an apical pansystolic murmur radiating to the axilla or a diastolic murmur heard best at the left sternal edge

c) If this murmur was secondary to aortic stenosis then a grade one sounding murmur is of less significance than a grade five sounding murmur

d) If this murmur was secondary to mitral regurgitation, a quiet first heart sound would be not altogether unsurprising

e) Atrial fibrillation would prompt suspicion of a mitral source of the murmur

Answer: c

Explanation

The usual heart sounds S1 and S2 are due to closure of the mitral and tricuspid valves and the aortic and pulmonary valves respectively. Extra heart sounds S3 and S4 may be normal (e.g. heard in athletes and young children) or abnormal, as in congestive cardiac failure. Mitral regurgitation will therefore give a quiet S1. The audibility of murmurs is graded from one to six – the higher the number, the louder the murmur. A patient with aortic stenosis and a failing left ventricle will have a quieter murmur than a similar degree of stenosis with a vigorous ventricle, so beware the quiet but significant aortic stenosis! Rheumatoid arthritis is associated with both mitral and aortic regurgitation, as is ankylosing spondylitis. Atrial fibrillation (AF) is most commonly associated with mitral valve lesions, and the breathlessness associated with mitral stenosis often worsens considerably with the onset of AF. In general, diastolic murmurs are always pathological, mixed valve disease is common, and the valve lesion you don't want to miss as an anaesthetist is tight aortic stenosis. In general, murmurs related to left-sided valve abnormalities will be heard louder in expiration than inspiration, and vice versa for murmurs related to right-sided valve lesions. This is because inspiration leads to increased venous return causing an increased blood volume in the right side of the heart. This increased volume restricts the amount of blood entering the left side of the heart, hence why left-sided murmurs are then quieter. The opposite is true for expiration due to the reduced venous return that is seen.

Question 21: Colloids

Regarding colloid preparations for intravenous infusion, which one of the following statements is CORRECT?

a) Gelofusine® consists of urea-linked gelatin component molecules
b) Regarding pentastarches, the 'pent' refers to 50% esterification with succinyl groups
c) Dextran 70 and 110 interfere with platelet aggregation and have an anticoagulant action, whereas Dextran 40 does not
d) Gelatin used for medical colloids is derived from exposing collagen from sheep bones to a strong alkali then boiling water
e) Hetastarch contains molecules with mean molecular weight of 450 kDa

Answer: e

Explanation
A colloid is a suspension of molecules of a particular size in another continuous medium. It is someway between a true suspension and a true solution because although the added molecules are not dissolved in the carrier liquid, they will not settle out of it under the action of gravity. The suspended particles will not traverse a semi-permeable membrane, which is the rationale for their use as a plasma substitute in hypovolaemia as the infused volume will remain in the intravascular compartment (or at least it will not be distributed over larger fluid compartments as quickly as crystalloid solutions). Aside from blood component therapy there are three main categories of colloid solutions: gelatin preparations, hydroxyethyl starches and dextrans. Gelatin is a collagen-like substance manufactured by boiling cattle bones (thermal degradation) following alkali treatment (although it may be derived from boiling up most animal connective tissues). The gelatin molecules are then urea-linked to form the colloid particles in Haemaccel® or succinylated for use in Gelofusine®. They have average molecular weights of 35 and 40 kDa respectively. Hydroxyethyl starches are glucose backbones with hydroxyethyl esterification to different extents, which lends them their name. Hetastarches have 70% substitution, hexastarches 60%, pentastarches 50% and tetrastarches 40% hydroxyethyl substitution. They have mean molecular weights of 450, 250, 200 and 130 kDa respectively. Haes-steril® is a pentastarch while Voluven® is a tetrastarch. Dextrans are polysaccharides derived from the action of the bacterium *Leuconostoc mesenteroides* on sucrose. They are presented in preparations of average molecular weights 40, 70 and 110 kDa, hence their names. They all interfere with platelet aggregation and have at least the potential to interfere with blood crossmatching. Each of the colloid preparations has different intravascular residence time, metabolism/excretion rate and rate of immune-mediated adverse reactions, as well as lists of other advantages and disadvantages.

Question 22: Korotkoff sounds

During an emergency in the hospital you are evacuated with an anaesthetised patient into the hospital car park. You want to measure the patient's blood pressure and are handed a stethoscope and a sphygmomanometer. What sounds on auscultation would you use to identify the systolic and diastolic blood pressure?

a) The peak of the first Korotkoff sound and the muffling of the fourth Korotkoff sound
b) The start of the first Korotkoff sound and the start of the fifth Korotkoff sound

c) The start of the first Korotkoff sound and the muffling of the fourth Korotkoff sound
d) The peak of the first Korotkoff sound and the peak of the fifth Korotkoff sound
e) The start of the first Korotkoff sound and the peak of the fifth Korotkoff sound

Answer: b

Explanation

In these days of non-invasive blood pressure monitoring with machines, the older skills of measuring blood pressure in a way that uses no electricity may seem irrelevant. Equipment malfunction, power failure, or remote anaesthesia are circumstances where the technique is still necessary thus knowledge of it is core. Judging by recent short answer questions set for the Final FRCA, the College shares this opinion.

The five Korotkoff sounds are heard as the sphygmomanometer cuff is deflated from a pressure above systolic. The first sound is the snapping sound first heard, the second is quieter murmurs, the third is a snapping sound, the fourth is thumping or muting of the sound and the fifth is the onset of silence. Traditionally systolic pressure has been measured at the onset of the first sound and diastolic has been at the last audible point of the fourth sound (muffling). Since 2000, there has been a change over to using the start of the fifth Korotkoff sound as diastolic pressure as this was thought to be more reproducible between different operators as it was a quantitative assessment rather than a qualitative one. Some have argued that, sometimes, the fourth sound never disappears. The cause for this is thought to usually be excessive pressure on the head of the stethoscope, and a lighter touch is recommended.

Question 23: Drug infusion rate

You are told to draw up a new inotrope for infusion to be administered to an 80 kg patient. The drug comes as an ampoule containing 200 mg in 20 mL. You are instructed to draw the whole ampoule up with water for injection to make a final volume of 50 mL. You only have a basic syringe driver that runs in mL/h. The product information recommends starting the infusion at 20 mcg/kg/min. How many mL/h would you set the syringe driver to?

a) 9.6 mL/h
b) 12.0 mL/h
c) 16.7 mL/h
d) 18.0 mL/h
e) 24.0 mL/h

Answer: e

Explanation

200 mg in 50 mL gives a concentration of 4 mg/mL or 4000 mcg/mL.
1 mL/h would be 50 mcg/kg/h or 50/60ths mcg/kg/min.
The required rate is therefore $20 \div 50/60 = 120/5 = 24$ mL/h

Question 24: Lung volumes

Of the following techniques, which one may be used to measure residual volume?

a) Carbon monoxide dilution
b) Total body plethysmography
c) Bohr's method
d) Pendelluft analysis
e) Wet spirometry

Answer: b

Explanation

Total body plethysmography involves sitting the subject in a closed box while they make a series of respiratory efforts against an open and closed valve. Collection of measurable pressure and volume changes with the application of Boyle's law allows the derivation of functional residual capacity and subsequently residual volume. Other methods include helium dilution (carbon monoxide is involved in determining diffusion capacity), and single- and multiple-breath nitrogen washout analysis. The former is Fowler's method and can be used to determine anatomical dead space and closing capacity as well. The multiple-breath nitrogen washout technique is also used in studies of uniformity of ventilation. Bohr's method is used to measure physiological dead space. Wet spirometry can measure every volume of gas that may pass the subject's lips but cannot deduce what volume remains in the subject's lungs at the end of a maximal expiration. Pendelluft is the phenomenon where gross mismatching of compliance in different lung regions (classically caused by a flail chest but also occurring in acute respiratory distress syndrome) causes gas transfer between lung regions during the respiratory cycle, rather than in and out of the trachea.

Question 25: Cardiotocograph

Listed below are five descriptions of a cardiotocograph trace. With regards to signs of foetal distress, which one of the following is the SECOND most concerning trace?

a) Heart rate 90 beats/min, late decelerations, variability 5 beats/min
b) Heart rate 145 beats/min, early decelerations, variability 25 beats/min
c) Heart rate 40 beats/min, no decelerations, variability 2 beats/min
d) Heart rate 160 beats/min, variable decelerations, variability 30 beats/min
e) Heart rate 100 beats/min, early decelerations, variability 20 beats/min

Answer: a

Explanation

A healthy cardiotocograph (CTG) has foetal heart rate in the range of 110 to 150 beats/min; decelerations of the heart rate only occur early with respect to uterine contractions, and variability is in the range of 5 to 25 beats/min.

Bradycardia between 100 and 110 is suspicious, and below 100 is almost always pathological. If sustained, this is a sign of foetal distress and the foetus should be delivered. Tachycardia in the range of 150 to 170 beats/min is suspicious. Over 170 is likely to be pathological, usually indicating problems such as foetal infection or distress. Early decelerations are worst at the peak of uterine contraction, are caused by foetal head compression and are usually benign. Variable decelerations occur after the peak of contraction, but their timing is erratic. They may be a sign of umbilical artery obstruction. Late decelerations are worst after the peak of contraction and may be a sign of foetal hypoxia. Sustained reduction of variability, especially in combination with sinister decelerations, would be indicative of foetal distress. In the question, the traces would rank (c), (a), (e), (d), (b) with (c) the most sinister. Option (c) describes an arresting bradycardia; (a) is a pathological bradycardia; (e) is a suspicious bradycardia; (d) is a borderline tachycardia and (b) is normal.

Question 26: Transfusion immunology

A 25-year-old female presents with significant haemorrhage secondary to a ruptured ectopic pregnancy. Which blood component transfusion practice is MOST LIKELY to cause harm?

a) Transfusion of A +ve packed red cells to an AB −ve recipient
b) Transfusion of A −ve packed red cells to an AB +ve recipient

c) Transfusion of AB +ve fresh frozen plasma to AB –ve recipient
d) Transfusion of B +ve cryoprecipitate to an O –ve recipient
e) Transfusion of AB –ve platelets to an O +ve recipient

Answer: a

Explanation
The issues here are ABO compatibility and rhesus D compatibility requirements of various blood components and awareness of the risk of rhesus D isoimmunisation in a Rh –ve woman of childbearing age. Cryoprecipitate need not be ABO or Rh compatible. Fresh frozen plasma (FFP) must be ABO compatible but Rh compatibility is not considered. Platelets should ideally be ABO and Rh identical, or at least compatible. However, there is only a very low risk of any sort of reaction. If matching is not possible due to scarce resources, ABO incompatible platelets are acceptable (with some exceptions), but with the potential for reduced efficacy. In terms of red cells, the AB +ve patient is the universal recipient and can be transfused any type if cross-matched, identical-type red cells are not available. Type AB recipients may receive type A red cells as the small amount of anti-B antibodies from the donor seldom causes a problem. Haemolytic disease of the newborn occurs where maternal Anti-Rh-D antibodies (produced in response to a previous sensitisation event in a Rh –ve mother) cross the placenta and destroy foetal Rh +ve cells. The resultant foetal anaemia can have disastrous consequences. This is why it is crucial that Rh –ve women are not transfused Rh +ve components – red cells clearly carrying the greatest risk. We are accustomed to using O –ve blood in an emergency but in fact for males over 16 or females beyond childbearing, use of O +ve blood in an emergency is acceptable and indeed written into the transfusion practice guidelines in some US centres.

References
McClelland DBL (ed) *Handbook of Transfusion Medicine*, 4th edn. UK Blood Transfusion and Tissue Transplantation Services. London: TSO, 1997. Online at www.transfusion guidelines.org.uk (Accessed 30 October 2009)
Serious Hazards of Transfusion (SHOT) website. Online at www.shotuk.org (Accessed 30 October 2009)
Serious Adverse Blood Reactions and Events (SABRE) webpage. Online at www.mhra. gov.uk (Accessed 30 October 2009)

Question 27: Malignant carcinoid syndrome

Regarding malignant carcinoid syndrome, the following statements are true EXCEPT which one?

a) Malignant carcinoid syndrome occurs in around 50% of those patients with a carcinoid tumour
b) Fibrosis of heart valves is more commonly seen on the right side of the heart than the left
c) Carcinoid tumours can produce insulin
d) For a patient to have malignant carcinoid syndrome they are likely to have liver metastases
e) Carcinoid tumours originating in the appendix are likely to be benign

Answer: a

Explanation
The term carcinoid can be applied to all tumours of the diffuse endocrine system. Carcinoid tumours may produce a wide variety of vasoactive substances, polypeptides and amines including histamine, somatostatin, 5-hydroxytryptamine and very rarely

insulin. Malignant carcinoid syndrome (MCS) is the constellation of symptoms typically exhibited by patients where the vasoactive substances they produce bypass and hence are not broken down by the liver. This circumstance usually arises in those patients with metastatic liver deposits, but is not exclusively limited to it (e.g. bronchial carcinoid tumours). MCS occurs in around 15% of patients with a carcinoid tumour. Patients with MCS can present a significant anaesthetic challenge. Their clinical presentation mainly depends on the site(s) of the tumour(s) and the substance(s) they secrete. Flushing, diarrhoea and bronchospasm are the commonest presenting features. Greater than 90% of carcinoid tumours originate from the distal ileum of appendix. Those originating from outside the gut have the highest incidence of MCS. Patients with MCS tend to have right-sided heart problems including tricuspid and pulmonary valve lesions and right-sided heart failure, as the vasoactive substances are metabolised by the lungs so tend not to reach the left side of the heart.

Question 28: Asthma in pregnancy

Regarding asthma in pregnancy, which one of the following statements is TRUE?

a) Asthma attacks in brittle asthmatics are more common during labour than at any other stage of the pregnancy
b) Theophyllines are contraindicated for treating asthmatics in pregnancy
c) Oral steroid therapy should be avoided in gravid patients with acute severe asthma
d) Intravenous magnesium sulphate should not be administered to an asthmatic in labour
e) Uncontrolled asthma is associated with pre-eclampsia

Answer: e

Explanation
One third of asthmatic patients will experience an improvement in their symptoms during pregnancy, one third will suffer a worsening and one third notice no change. In those that deteriorate, the peak severity is between weeks 24 and 36 after which symptoms improve with attacks being very unusual in labour because of endogenous steroid production. No adverse outcomes have been demonstrated with the use of inhaled β_2 agonists, inhaled steroids, theophyllines or magnesium during pregnancy. Oral steroids do not have convincing evidence of harm and the British Thoracic Society concludes that the detriment to mother and foetus by not adequately treating acute severe asthma outweighs the potential, unproven risk of systemic steroids in pregnancy. Uncontrolled asthma during pregnancy is associated with hyperemesis, hypertension, pre-eclampsia, premature delivery and low birthweight babies. Emphasis is therefore on maintaining good control with the patient's pre-pregnancy medications, regular clinical review and rapid treatment of acute severe asthma with drug therapy as for the non-pregnant patient.

Reference
British Thoracic Society/Scottish Intercollediate Guidlelines Network. *101 British Guideline on the Management of Asthma: a National Clinical Guideline.* NHS QIS, May 2008, revised June 2009. Online at www.sign.ac.uk/pdf/sign101.pdf (Accessed 30 October 2009)

Question 29: Acid–base physiology

A lactic acidosis will be accompanied by a normal anion gap in the presence of which one of the following circumstances?

a) Concurrent diabetic ketoacidosis
b) Hypoalbuminaemia

c) Lithium poisoning
d) Intractable vomiting
e) Hypoaldosteronism

Answer: b

Explanation

The anion gap describes the apparent discrepancy between the summed concentrations of the anions and cations that are commonly measured in the plasma. It is relevant when considering the origin of a metabolic acidosis. It is, of course, an artefact of measurement as laws of electrochemical neutrality dictate that the summed concentrations of the anions and cations must be equal. It is the 'unmeasured' anions that account for the gap. Commonly measured anions are Cl^-, HCO_3^- and PO_4^- while commonly measured cations are K^+, Na^+, Mg^{2+} and Ca^{2+}. There are typically more unmeasured anions, and around 80% of these are the negatively charged molecule, albumin. Others include sulphate (SO_4^{2-}), bromide (Br^-), and other plasma proteins. Unmeasured cations consist of some normal plasma proteins and notably the paraproteins found in multiple myeloma. Although strictly one should sum all the cations measurable and compare to the sum of all the measurable anions, the anion gap is simplified to $Na^+ - (HCO_3^- + Cl^-)$ with a reference range of 8 to 12mEq/L. Renal physicians often include potassium (K^+) in the calculation, thus their range is a little higher. If acid is added to plasma, it will be buffered by HCO_3^- whose concentration will fall. If the acid added is hydrochloric acid (H^+Cl^-) then the corresponding rise in Cl^- concentration will render the anion gap unchanged. However, any other acid will decrease the HCO_3^- level while adding unmeasured anions to the plasma and the anion gap will increase. Typical examples of this include ketoacids, lactic acid, urea, aspirin, ethylene glycol, methanol and ethanol. If HCO_3^- is lost from the plasma (e.g. diarrhoea, renal tubular acidosis, hypoaldosteronism) and endogenous or exogenous Cl^- restores electroneutrality then the anion gap is normal and a hyperchloraemic acidosis has developed. Given that albumin accounts for the large majority of 'unmeasured' anions, its significant influence on the anion gap should not be overlooked. A fall in serum albumin concentration will cause a corresponding drop in the anion gap, such that a hypoalbuminaemic patient with even a severe lactic acidosis may have a normal anion gap.

Question 30: Number needed to treat (NNT)

Regarding the calculation of number needed to treat (NNT), which one of the following formulae is used?

a) 1/absolute risk reduction
b) 1/the odds ratio
c) The odds ratio/absolute risk reduction
d) Relative risk reduction/absolute risk reduction
e) 1/relative risk reduction

Answer: a

Explanation

The number needed to treat (NNT) is the reciprocal of the absolute risk reduction expressed as a decimal. For example, if a new agent reduces the risk of postoperative vomiting from 25% to 15%, the absolute risk reduction is 10%, or 0.1. In 100 patients, the 75 not suffering from vomiting and the 25 who were initially suffering would all have to have the treatment to stop 10 from vomiting. You would treat 100 to stop 10 vomiting, or 10 to stop 1 vomiting; NNT is 10 or 1/0.1.

'Number needed to treat' is bandied around regularly when doctors discuss papers, it is loosely understood and a simple statistical concept that is easy to define.

Reference

McQuay HJ, Moore RA. Using numerical results from systematic reviews in clinical practice. *Ann Intern Med* 1997; **126**(9): 712–20. Online at www.medicine.ox.ac.uk/bandolier/booth/painpag/NNTstuff/numeric.htm (Accessed 30 October 2009)

Question 31: Hyperchloraemic acidoses

Based on their associated biochemical derangements, which one of the following surgical pathologies is the odd one out?

a) Pyloric stenosis
b) Enteric fistula
c) Ureterosigmoidostomy
d) Toxic megacolon
e) Villous adenoma of the rectum

Answer: a

Explanation

Pyloric stenosis is associated with a hypochloraemic metabolic alkalosis. Enteric fistulas, ureterosigmoidostomies, severe diarrhoea (e.g. that caused by inflammatory bowel disease flare) and villous adenomas are all responsible for hyperchloraemic acidoses. In pyloric stenosis, persistent vomiting with loss of stomach contents rich in hydrochloric acid causes the alkalaemia and hypochloraemia. Potassium ions are lost at the kidneys in favour of preserving hydrogen ions to correct the alkalosis. This, as well as potassium ion loss in the vomitus, means hypokalaemia is also a problem. Hypernatraemia may be present if the patient is very dehydrated but hyponatraemia may also be seen. In health, the acidic stomach contents are usually rendered neutral soon after arrival in the duodenum by the abundant bicarbonate ions secreted by the pancreas, biliary system and duodenum. These bicarbonate ions are effectively reabsorbed in the jejunum so minimal bicarbonate is ultimately lost in the faeces. Any diarrhoeal state where this process is jeopardised results in bicarbonate loss. Alternatively if bowel contents, biliary or pancreatic juices are externally drained, bypassing reabsorption, a similar consequence ensues. Villous adenomas secrete bicarbonate-rich mucus. Renal chloride retention, resulting in hyperchloraemia, is a compensatory response to the bicarbonate loss.

Question 32: Paediatric postoperative pain

The FLACC scale is a commonly used tool for assessing pain in a population who may not be able to verbalise postoperative pain or discomfort. Which one of the following statements is CORRECT?

a) The tool is applicable to the age range: two months to seven years
b) The 'A' in FLACC stands for 'Arms'
c) The maximum score, indicating the worst possible pain, is 15
d) A child who is kicking with their legs drawn up would score 1 for legs
e) The nature of the child's crying has no impact on the score

Answer: a

Explanation

The tool scores from zero to two points each for five parameters: face, legs, activity, cry and consolability. The sum of these gives the final score – a score of ten being the maximum, indicating the worst pain. As described, the tool is validated for children between two months and seven years of age. The scale has not been validated for children with developmental delay. This is a behavioural tool as opposed to one that relies upon patient participation. A child who is kicking and drawing their legs up scores a maximum 2 points for legs. With respect to the nature of crying: moans or whimpers score 1, whereas steady screaming scores 2. In the literature the tool has been compared with other paediatric behavioural pain assessment tools: CHEOPS (Children's Hospital of Eastern Ontario pain scale), OPS (Objective pain scale), TPPPS (Toddler-pre-school postoperative pain scale). The Wong & Baker FACES scale and visual analogue scales are patient-reporting tools.

Reference
Merkel SI, Voepel-Lewis T, Shayevitz JR, Malviya S. The FLACC: a behavioral scale for scoring postoperative pain in young children. *Pedatr Nurs* 1997; **23**(3): 293–7.

Question 33: Physiology of pregnancy

Regarding normal physiological changes in a healthy pregnancy, which one of the following changes would NOT be consistent with expected changes?

a) 10% increase in heart rate by 12 weeks gestation
b) 20% increase in stroke volume by 12 weeks gestation
c) 20% increase in red cell volume by 28 weeks gestation
d) 20% increase in anatomical dead space by 28 weeks gestation
e) 50% increase in glomerular filtration rate by 12 weeks gestation

Answer: d

Explanation
Virtually every organ system exhibits physiological change during pregnancy to compensate for the increased demands of sustaining the mother and growing foetus and in preparation for the enormous physiological challenge of parturition. Causing some frustration to candidates is that authoritative sources occasionally differ in their account of some of the variations. An example of this is the calibre, volume and resistance of large conducting airways. Some argue that capillary engorgement and oedema reduce calibre whereas others propose that prostaglandin-mediated smooth muscle relaxation causes dilation of conducting airways resulting in a marked reduction in resistance and an increase in anatomical dead space by up to 45% at the third trimester. Either way, Option (d) stands out as incorrect when compared to the correctness of the other four options. The 20% increase in red cell volume is tempered by the 50% increase in plasma volume in the same period giving rise to the 'physiological anaemia of pregnancy'. Total blood volume increases by 40%. Other changes are not listed here but it aids recall if they are categorised into cardiovascular, respiratory, gastrointestinal (and hepatic), renal, haematological (including volumes), neurological and those other changes secondary to the placenta as an endocrine organ.

Reference
Power I, Kam P. Maternal and neonatal physiology. In: *Principles of Physiology for the Anaesthetist*. London: Arnold, 2001; pp. 345–52.

Question 34: Heat loss

You are providing general anaesthesia to a 47-year-old patient having an open hemi-colectomy. You have been infusing all fluids through a fluid warmer but notice that the patient's temperature has dropped to 35 °C. The patient will be losing MOST heat by which one of the following processes?

a) Conduction into the patient's general surroundings
b) Convection with the room air

c) Radiation to the patient's general surroundings
d) Evaporation from wound and skin
e) Respiratory losses from conduction, convection and evaporation

Answer: c

Explanation

Radiation is responsible for about 40% of the initial heat loss from an anaesthetised patient. Convection into the operating room air accounts for another 30%. Evaporative losses from the wound contribute another 15%, with respiratory losses and general conduction only responsible for the small remaining heat loss. All of this may be further complicated by factors such as infusing-room-temperature fluids or fridge-temperature blood. The allocation of resources to combat peri-operative cooling should be considered with these figures in mind.

Reference

NICE Guideline CG65. Online at www.nice.org.uk/Guidance/CG65 (Accessed 30 November 2009)

Question 35: Antimicrobials

Which one of the following statements regarding antimicrobials is TRUE?

a) Carbapenems are not β-lactam antibacterial drugs
b) Action against Gram-negative bacteria was superior with the earlier generations of cephalosporins but Gram-positive cover has been sequentially improved
c) Fluoroquinolones include norfloxacin, ofloxacin and lomefloxacin
d) Tazocin® is the trade name for the generic antimicrobial tazobactam
e) Aminoglycoside antibacterial drugs include gentamicin, netilmicin, vancomycin and tobramycin

Answer: c

Explanation

β-lactam antibacterial drugs may be subdivided into four groups: penicillins, cephalosporins, carbapenems and monobactams. Each of these four may be further subclassified. Cephalosporins maintain good Gram-positive action, and with each successive generation Gram-negative cover is improved. Tazocin® is the trade name for the combination preparation piperacillin (a broad spectrum agent with anti-pseudomonal action) with tazobactam (a β-lactamase inhibitor with no intrinsic antimicrobial activity of its own). Vancomycin is a glycopeptide antibacterial agent. It is synergistic with aminoglycosides. Ciprofloxacin is the most commonly encountered fluoroquinolone but the others do have their specific indications.

Question 36: 12-lead electrocardiogram

Regarding misplacement of limb leads prior to recording a 12-lead electrocardiogram, the following misplacements would mimic the stated condition EXCEPT which one?

a) Left-arm electrode and right-arm electrode switch – dextrocardia
b) Right-leg electrode and right-arm electrode switch – pericardial effusion
c) Left-arm electrode and left-leg electrode switch – inferior myocardial infarction
d) Right-leg electrode and left-leg electrode switch – true posterior myocardial infarction
e) Clockwise rotated limb leads (with right leg correctly sited) – extra-nodal atrial rhythm

Answer: d

Explanation

When making a diagnosis from any investigation, recognition of an artefact is as important as identification of a pathology. A 12-lead electrocardiogram (ECG) uses ten wires and electrodes: six chest leads plus four limb leads (the right leg of which is the ground or indifferent electrode). As the display of this electrical activity uses a positive deflection to represent current in the direction of that electrode and from which territory of pathology is deduced, it is easy to see why lead misplacement can cause misleading changes. In this question the false statement is recognisable without knowledge of the correctness of the others. True posterior myocardial infarctions provoke 'mirror' changes in the anterior chest leads (V_1-V_3) and do not (unless there is an inferior component) produce changes in the limb leads. For this reason limb lead misplacement and misleading changes in the limb leads could not lead to erroneous diagnosis of posterior myocardial infarction. It is intuitive why switching right- and left-arm leads would mimic dextrocardia as the heart axis would appear grossly deviated to the right. Switching the right-arm and right-leg electrode would involve putting the indifferent electrode at the main origin of activity so all complexes would be reduced in magnitude as seen in pericardial effusion. Switching left-arm and left-leg would produce Q waves in II, III and aV_f. If the indifferent electrode remains on the right leg, clockwise rotation of the limb leads would produce p-wave inversion, suggesting an extra-nodal origin of rhythm.

Reference

Vardan S, Vardan S, Mookherjee D, *et al*. Guidelines for the detection of ECG limb lead misplacements. *Resid Staff Physician* 2008; **54**(1). Online at www.residentandstaff. com/issues/2008-01.asp (Accessed 30 October 2009)

Question 37: Intraocular pressure and anaesthetic drugs

Regarding intraocular pressure and drugs used in anaesthesia, the following statements are true EXCEPT which one?

a) Intravenous midazolam reduces intraocular pressure
b) Metoclopramide causes an increase in intraocular pressure
c) Atracurium has no effect on intraocular pressure
d) Rocuronium reduces intraocular pressure
e) All intravenous induction agents reduce intraocular pressure, except ketamine

Answer: a

Explanation

The three agents commonly encountered in anaesthesia that raise intraocular pressure are ketamine, suxamethonium and metoclopramide. Oral benzodiazepines and intravenous midazolam have no effect, whereas intravenous diazepam reduces intraocular pressure. Atracurium has no effect on intraocular pressure while all other non-depolarising muscle relaxants reduce it. Opioids, volatile anaesthetic agents and induction agents (except ketamine) reduce intraocular pressure. Knowledge of these factors is of particular relevance to providing anaesthesia for ophthalmic surgery involving traumatic or surgical disruption of globe integrity where a rise in intraocular pressure may cause extrusion of globe contents and significant patient detriment.

Reference

Raw D, Mostafa S. Drugs and the eye. *Contin Educ Anaesth Crit Care Pain* 2001; **1**(6): 161–5.

Question 38: Thromboelastography

A 58-year-old male patient is recovering on the cardiac intensive care unit following first-time coronary bypass grafting. The surgeon is concerned that the drain output is greater than acceptable. You take a blood sample for thromboelastography. Which of the following findings would be consistent with a diagnosis of thrombocytopaenia?

a) A prolonged r time, an increased k time, a decreased alpha angle, a decreased MA
b) A normal r time, an increased k time, a normal alpha angle, an extremely decreased MA
c) A decreased r time, a decreased k time, an increased alpha angle, an increased MA
d) A normal r time, a normal k time, an increased alpha angle, a continuously decreasing MA
e) A prolonged r time, a normal k time, an increased alpha angle, a normal MA

Answer: b

Explanation

The thromboelastograph (TEG) measures how the shear elasticity of a blood sample changes as a clot is formed. Measurements of strength and stability give an idea whether the clot will do the job of haemostasis, and the kinetics of clot formation give a quantitative indication of whether the patient has sufficient factors for clot formation. Five parameters are measured by the basic TEG. The 'r' is the time from start of the test to initial fibrin formation. The 'k' is the time from beginning of clot formation until the amplitude reaches 20 mm, the 'alpha angle' is the angle between the middle of the TEG and a line drawn along the main body of the developing TEG trace. This represents the acceleration of the fibrin burst. The 'MA' is the maximum amplitude and represents how strong the clot is. The Ly30 is the amplitude 30 minutes after the MA. This represents how stable the clot is. Typically, in a patient with low platelets, the TEG would show a normal r time, an increased k time, a normal alpha angle, and an extremely decreased MA. A prolonged r time, an increased k time, a decreased alpha angle and a decreased MA is typical of blood clotting factor deficiency. A decreased r time, a decreased k time, an increased alpha angle and an increased MA is found in hypercoagulable states. A normal r time, a normal k time, an increased alpha angle and a continuously decreasing MA is found in thrombolysis. The final option given is not a typical pattern.

Reference

Curry A, Pierce T. Conventional and near-patient tests of coagulation. *Contin Educ Anaesth Crit Care Pain* 2007; **7**(2): 45–50.

Question 39: Neurophysiological monitoring

In an anaesthetised, intubated patient various neurophysiological monitors may be used. Of the following monitors, which one is LEAST LIKELY to be affected by a concurrent remifentanil infusion?

a) Auditory evoked potentials
b) Electroencephalography
c) Bispectral index
d) Spectral entropy
e) Somatosensory evoked potentials

Answer: e

Explanation

The search for a monitor with good sensitivity and specificity to measure the depth of an anaesthetic has been one of the great challenges in academic anaesthesia that has thwarted many great minds. The electroencephalograph (EEG), auditory evoked potentials (AEP), the bispectral index (BIS) and spectral entropy have all been proposed and used with varying degrees of success and adoption. The electroencephalograph was the first to be investigated. With increasing anaesthesia there is a reduction in the activity of the EEG, there is a shift from higher frequency signals to lower frequency and correlation between signals from different parts of the cortex becomes more random. The multiple leads, bulky equipment and complicated read-out stopped it from ever being a practical candidate for monitoring depth of anaesthesia. A number of commercial products employing BIS, AEPs or spectral entropy are currently available. Generally these involve a simplified set of electrodes attached to the patient connected to a small unit that measures electrical waveforms produced within the central nervous system. These are then analysed and usually reduced down to a linear dimensionless scale from 0 to 100 with the lower scores indicating deeper levels of anaesthesia. Bispectral index and entropy monitors use specific analysis of the EEG, and AEP interprets the EEG following an auditory stimulus. All of these four monitors have been the subject of studies demonstrating an alteration in reading when a remifentanil infusion is used. Somatosensory evoked potentials (SSEPs) have substantially taken the place of wake-up tests in spinal surgery and are adversely affected by volatile anaesthetics. As a result, target controlled anaesthesia with propofol, usually with supplementary remifentanil, tends to be the anaesthetic of choice when SSEPs are used.

Question 40: Non-respiratory functions of the lung

Which one of the following options is a function performed by the lung?

a) Conversion of angiotensinogen to angiotensin I
b) Secretion of immunoglobulin E into bronchial mucus
c) Uptake and metabolism of histamine
d) Deactivation of prostaglandin E_2
e) Manufacture of phosphatidylinositol biphosphate, the phospholipid component of surfactant

Answer: d

Explanation

The non-respiratory functions of the lung are numerous and should not be overlooked in favour of the more commonly questioned functions of gas exchange. Angiotensinogen is converted to angiotensin I in the plasma by renin produced by the juxtaglomerular apparatus of the kidney. Angiotensin I is virtually devoid of physiological action except as a precursor to angiotensin II. This conversion occurs in the lungs catalysed by angiotensin converting enzyme (ACE) located on pulmonary capillary endothelial cells. As angiotensin II is a significant vasoconstrictor (more potent than noradrenaline) it follows that ACE inhibitor drugs are effective antihypertensives. Angiotensin converting enzyme also inactivates almost all of the bradykinin in the lung. The accumulation of bradykinin in patients on ACE inhibitor therapy is responsible for the side effect of cough, as bradykinin is an irritant. The lung secretes immunoglobulin A into bronchial mucus as a component of defence against infection (cf. IgE component in asthma pathophysiology). 5-hydroxytryptamine (serotonin) is almost completely eliminated by passage through the lungs – it is taken up intact rather than metabolised. Noradrenaline is partially deactivated, whereas histamine and dopamine traverse the pulmonary circulation without decrement. Prostaglandin E_1, E_2 and $F_{2\alpha}$ are deactivated in the lung whereas prostaglandin A_2 and I_2 (prostacyclin) are not. Phosphatidylinositol biphosphate (PIP_2) is a component of G-protein second messenger systems. The active phospholipid in surfactant is dipalmitoyl phosphatidylcholine. Some other non-respiratory lung functions are: as a reservoir of blood; a filter of debris, platelet clumps and bubbles; storage of heparin in mast cells; arachidonic acid metabolism; and maintenance of the connective tissue architecture of the lung.

Question 41: Side effects of antihypertensives

The following antihypertensive agents are linked with well recognised side effects EXCEPT which one?

a) Lisinopril may cause angioedema
b) Metoprolol may cause impotence
c) Diltiazem may cause insulin resistance
d) Bendroflumethiazide may cause hyperuricaemia
e) Losartan may cause a dry cough

Answer: c

Explanation
A lot of development has gone into improving antihypertensives' side-effects profiles, as the pathology itself often exists without symptoms. A drug that makes a patient feel symptomatic is less likely to be a clinical and commercial success due to non-compliance. Mild side effects due to antihypertensives, such as headache and lethargy, are common. Lisinopril has been known to cause angioedema. This potentially life-threatening side effect occurs in about 0.1 to 0.2% of patients on lisinopril. All the beta-blockers may cause impotence. Lisinopril commonly produces a dry cough (97% of cases), and although this is much less common with losartan (18%) it may also trouble patients. Hyperuricaemia with thiazide use is well described.

Even though there have been a few isolated case reports linking diltiazem with insulin resistance, a clinical trial showed no effect on circulating glucose or insulin levels in patients on diltiazem, and another showed an improvement in insulin levels in insulin-resistant patients started on insulin. It would certainly not be identified as a recognised side effect.

Reference
Chan P, Tomlinson B, Huang TY, et al. Double-blind comparison of losartan, lisinopril, and metolazone in elderly hypertensive patients with previous angiotensin-converting enzyme inhibitor-induced cough. *J Clin Pharmacol* 1997; **37**(3): 253–7.

Question 42: Antiemetics

Regarding antiemetics, which one of the following statements is TRUE?

a) Dexamethasone has been shown to downregulate 5-HT_3 receptors in the chemoreceptor trigger zone
b) As an anticholinergic, glycopyrrolate has useful antiemetic properties
c) Cyclizine acts as an antiemetic by antagonism of muscarinic acetylcholine receptors
d) Ondansetron exerts antagonism at 5-HT_3 receptors only in the chemoreceptor trigger zone and the nucleus tractus solitarius
e) Nabilone is an antagonist at endogenous cannabinoid receptors

Answer: c

Explanation

The mechanism via which steroids prevent and treat nausea and vomiting remains unknown. They may act by reducing central and peripheral prostaglandin production, or via an anti-inflammatory process that may reduce stimulation from an operative site, or block 5-HT$_3$ production from the gut. Muscarinic acetylcholine receptors are found in the nucleus ambiguous, nucleus tractus solitarius and the dorsal motor nucleus of the vagus. Central receptors are also involved in the vestibular initiation of motion sickness. As all these target sites are within the blood–brain barrier only tertiary amine anticholinergics reduce nausea and vomiting. The quaternary ammonium compound glycopyrrolate does not cross the barrier and has no antiemetic properties. Cyclizine is an H$_1$-antagonist (antihistamine) and blocks centrally located H$_1$ receptors; however, a significant proportion of its antiemetic properties are due to an anticholinergic action. Ondansetron antagonises central and peripheral (mainly gut) 5-HT$_3$ receptors. Nabilone is a novel agent, which is an agonist at endogenous cannabinoid receptors – a mechanism not previously employed pharmaceutically. The pharmacology of antiemetics is best recalled by learning the physiological pathways, anatomical sites and neurotransmitters involved in the induction of vomiting then considering where each of these pathways may be interrupted with appropriate antagonists.

Reference

Forrest K, Simpson K. Physiology and pharmacology of nausea and vomiting. In: Hemmings J, Hopkins P (eds) *Foundations of Anesthesia: Basic Sciences for Clinical Practice*, 2nd edn. Philadelphia: Mosby-Elsevier, 2006; pp. 763–72.

Question 43: Heat moisture exchanger filter

A heat moisture exchanger incorporating a standard high efficiency particulate air (HEPA) filter has a pore size as small as or smaller than all of the following pathogens, EXCEPT which one?

a) *Mycobacterium tuberculosis*
b) *Staphylococcus aureus*
c) *Legionella pneumophilia*
d) *Mycoplasma pneumoniae*
e) *Pseudomonas aeruginosa*

Answer: d

Explanation

A standard HEPA filter is tested to ensure a 0.3 μm pore size. At this size, protection is not just about the sieve effect of the filter pore size as electrostatic attraction also has an important role. *Mycobacteria tuberculosis* are 0.2 to 0.4 μm wide and 2 to 4 μm in length. It is thought that a HEPA filter would still be protective against tuberculosis. *Staphylococcus aureus* are about 0.6 μm in diameter. *Legionella pneumophilia* are 0.5 to 1.0 μm wide and 1.0 to 3.0 μm long. *Mycoplasma pneumoniae* are the smallest known free-living organisms and can be as small as 0.15 μm. *Pseudomonas aeruginosa* are 1 μm by 3 μm in size.

Question 44: Narrow-complex tachycardia

A previously fit and well 52-year-old patient develops a regular narrow-complex tachycardia in recovery, but is otherwise stable with a blood pressure of 125/85 mmHg. You apply oxygen on high flow via a facemask, perform a 12-lead ECG and start carotid sinus massage, which fails to correct the tachycardia. You give adenosine 6 mg intravenously, which fails to alter the rhythm, followed by a further adenosine 12 mg intravenously, again with no improvement. What would you do next?

a) Give digoxin 500 mcg intravenously
b) Give amiodarone 300 mg loading dose intravenously
c) Give verapamil 2.5 mg intravenously over two minutes
d) Give adenosine 12 mg intravenously
e) Perform synchronised DC cardioversion

Answer: d

Explanation

The patient described is stable. The Resuscitation Council (UK) recommends an ECG during each manoeuvre. This is important as it may help to detect an underlying arrhythmia such as atrial flutter if the heart rate slows. Carotid sinus massage failed, so the next step would be to give adenosine as described. If this fails, you would try one more 12 mg dose of adenosine. If this fails, the verapamil should be given. Digoxin may be of use in a stable irregular narrow-complex tachycardia , and cardioversion may be required if the patient becomes unstable.

Reference

Nolan J. Peri-arrest arrhythmias. In: *Advanced Life Support*, 5th edn. London: Resuscitation Council (UK), 2005; pp. 59–67. Online at www.resus.org.uk/pages/ periarst.pdf (Accessed 30 October 2009)

Question 45: Hydrogen ion measurement

During arterial blood gas analysis, representation of quantity of hydrogen ions present in the sample may be displayed as pH, hydrogen ion concentration or both. The following statements are correct equivalences EXCEPT which one?

a) pH 7.6 = 25 nanomol/L
b) pH 7.4 = 40 nanomol/L
c) pH 7.3 = 50 nanomol/L
d) pH 7.2 = 63 nanomol/L
e) pH 7.0 = 114 nanomol/L

Answer: e

Explanation

This question might seem unreasonable but in fact tests recollection of the fact that pH is the negative logarithm to the base 10 of the hydrogen ion concentration. Where the pH is an integer it follows that the hydrogen ion concentration must be a multiple of ten (it is simply ten raised to the power of that integer (as a negative) i.e. pH 7 is 10^{-7} mol/L $= 100 \times 10^{-9}$ mol/L $= 100$ nanomol/L) so Option (e) is quite clearly incorrect. In fact a hydrogen ion concentration of 114 nanomol/L has a pH of 6.94. Just as a clinician might be challenged by working in a clinical area where mmHg are used instead of kPa for expressing gas tensions, an anaesthetist must be familiar with working in pH or nanomol/L as an expression of hydrogen ion concentration.

Question 46: Tissue donation

There are a number of absolute contraindications to tissue donations. These include the following circumstances EXCEPT for which one?

a) A patient with a family history of Creutzfeldt–Jacob disease (CJD)
b) A patient with Alzheimer's disease
c) A patient with multiple sclerosis

d) A patient who has had a previous transplant requiring immunosuppressive treatment even if that treatment was not being received at the time of death

e) Donation of corneas and sclera from a patient who has died with a proven diagnosis of metastatic carcinoma of the colon

Answer: e

Explanation

The criteria for tissue donation are different to those for organ donation and vary in terms of age and medical suitability depending on the tissue to be donated. There is no defined upper age limit for any tissue donation. Tissue can be retrieved up to 24 hours after death and up to 48 hours after death for heart valves. Tissues that can be donated include eyes for corneal and scleral donation, heart for heart-valve donation, bone, tendons, menisci and skin. There are a number of absolute contraindications for tissue donation. These include the following.

Patients who have ever:

- tested positive for HIV, hepatitis B, hepatitis C, human T cell lymphotrophic virus or syphilis or have high-risk behavioural factors for contracting these infections
- suffered from Creutzfeldt–Jacob disease or have a family history of CJD
- had a progressive neurological disease of unknown pathophysiology, e.g. multiple sclerosis, Alzheimer's disease, Parkinson's disease or motor neurone disease
- suffered from leucaemia, lymphoma or myeloma
- had a previous transplant requiring immunosuppressive treatment
- had a systemic malignancy (of note, patients with systemic malignancy can donate eye tissue).

Reference

The Intensive Care Society Working Group for Organ and Tissue Donation. Guidelines for adult organ and tissue donation. The Intensive Care Society, 2005. Online at www. ics.ac.uk (Accessed 30 October 2009)

Question 47: Cardiovascular autonomic reflexes

The following are eponymous cardiovascular reflexes EXCEPT which one?

a) Anrep effect: acute increase in afterload causes reduction in stroke volume then reflex restitution

b) Cushing's reflex: raised intracranial pressure causes hypertension and reflex bradycardia

c) Bainbridge reflex: an increase in venous pressure causes tachycardia

d) Bowman effect: as heart rate increases, contractility increases

e) Bezold–Jarish reflex: seen in myocardial ischaemia – stimulation of ventricular receptors cause bradycardia and hypotension

Answer: d

Explanation

The Bowditch effect is the increase in contractility associated with an acute increase in heart rate, provided the tachycardia is not excessive (thus inducing ischaemia).

The Bowman principle is from pharmacology and regards non-depolarising muscle relaxants. Less potent non-depolarising muscle relaxants must be given in larger doses in order to achieve the same maximal effect where sufficient acetylcholine receptors are occupied to prevent post-synaptic activation by endogenous acetylcholine. As larger doses are required, the peak plasma concentration and thus gradient to promote occupation of receptors is greater with these less potent relaxants. In summary, the onset time is shorter with less potent relaxants. Clinically this is exploited with rocuronium at high dose (0.9 mg/kg) producing flaccid paralysis in less than 60 seconds thus making it suitable for 'modified rapid sequence induction'. The other options are all genuine eponymous cardiovascular reflexes and may arise in SBAs or indeed vivas.

Question 48: Mixed venous oxygen saturations

Regarding mixed venous oxygen saturations, which one of the following statements is CORRECT?

a) In septic shock, SvO_2 is unlikely to be normal or supranormal
b) With a ventricular septal defect, a reduction in SvO_2 will be observed
c) If oxygen flux is fixed, elevated oxygen consumption results in increased SvO_2
d) If arterial oxygen saturation, haemoglobin and oxygen consumption are constant, SvO_2 varies directly with cardiac output
e) Cyanide toxicity causes a reduction in SvO_2

Answer: d

Explanation
True mixed venous oxygen saturations are those found in the pulmonary artery, measured with a pulmonary artery flotation catheter either by sampling the blood or fibreoptic oximetry incorporated into the device. The oxygen content of venous blood is a function of how much oxygen the body is using (oxygen consumption – $\dot{V}O_2$) balanced against how much oxygen it was supplied with (oxygen delivery – $\dot{D}O_2$). Oxygen flux is oxygen delivery per unit time (i.e. oxygen content of arterial blood x cardiac output). The law of mass action tells us essentially 'what goes in, must come out or have been used up'. This is the basis of Fick's law, which when applied here gives:

$$Q = \dot{V}O_2/(CaO_2 - CvO_2)$$

Now, ignoring the dissolved component, oxygen content of blood is $1.34 \times$ (Sats/100) $\times$ Hb

so, $CaO_2 = 1.34 \times$ (Sats/100) $\times SaO_2$ and $CvO_2 = 1.34 \times$ (Sats/100) $\times SvO_2$

If this is substituted into the Fick equation and rearranged we find:

$$SvO_2 = SaO_2 - 100VO_2/(1.34 \times Hb \times Q)$$

Thereby proving the statement in Option (d)
A VSD causes a left-to-right shunt, so oxygenated blood is contributed to that blood ultimately exiting the right side of the heart, thus SvO_2 is elevated. Cyanide toxicity causes reduced oxygen consumption via disruption of the cellular cytochrome oxidase system, so SvO_2 will rise. In septic shock it is not unusual to find elevated SvO_2 because of the direct cellular toxic effect of the physiological insult and response causing reduced tissue oxygen consumption. Despite this it is recommended that we aspire to maximal oxygen delivery in our goal-directed therapy in sepsis with targeted SvO_2 or $ScvO_2$ as a guide (65% or 70% respectively).

Question 49: Muscles of the larynx

Which one of the following options is a TRUE statement regarding the intrinsic muscles of the larynx?

a) The cricothyroids are the only muscles to tense the cords
b) The posterior cricoarytenoids, supplied by the recurrent laryngeal nerve, adduct the cords

c) Vocalis is supplied by the recurrent laryngeal nerve but is not considered an intrinsic muscle of the larynx
d) Thyrohyoid elevates the larynx
e) The internal laryngeal nerve supplies only one of these muscles

Answer: a

Explanation

There are six intrinsic muscles of the larynx (although they may be paired or subdivided). The first five are supplied by the recurrent laryngeal nerve, which is a branch of the tenth cranial nerve (the vagus): posterior cricoarytenoid, lateral cricoarytenoid, transverse arytenoid, thyroarytenoid and vocalis (of thyroarytenoid). The sixth intrinsic muscle is the cricothyroid and is supplied by the external laryngeal nerve, which is a branch of the superior laryngeal nerve, another branch of the vagus. The superior laryngeal nerve also branches to the internal laryngeal nerve, which supplies sensation to the laryngeal mucosa above the cords including the underside of the epiglottis. Above this, including the vallecula, sensation is from the glossopharyngeal nerve. Sensation below the cords is supplied by the recurrent laryngeal nerve. In terms of the action of each of the intrinsic muscles, they are as follows: posterior cricoarytenoid – abducts cords; lateral cricoarytenoid – adducts cords; transverse arytenoids – adducts cords; thyroarytenoids – relaxes cords; vocalis – adjusts cords; cricothyroid – tenses cords.

Sternohyoid (depresses larynx), thyrohyoid (elevates larynx) and the posterior constrictor of the pharynx are extrinsic muscles of the larynx.

Question 50: Anorexia nervosa

A 30-year-old woman presents for elective surgery. She is 170 cm tall, weighs 35 kg and has a long history of an eating disorder. The following statements about this patient are true EXCEPT for which one?

a) She is more likely to have mitral valve prolapse than a similar patient with a normal body mass index (BMI)
b) She is more likely to be bradypnoeic and bradycardic than a similar patient with a normal BMI
c) She is likely to be anaemic and leucopaenic
d) Her gastric emptying time is likely to be slower compared to a similar patient with a normal BMI
e) Common electrocardiogram (ECG) findings in this patient would include atrioventricular block, QT prolongation, ST segment depression and T-wave inversion

Answer: c

Explanation

The prevalence of anorexia in 15 to 30-year-old women in the UK is between 5 and 10%. Bulimia has a prevalence of 3 to 30% in the same population. The prevalence in males is approximately 1% for each condition. These conditions carry a significant morbidity and mortality due to the associated multiorgan dysfunction. Hypothermia is a routine finding as is sinus bradycardia, hypotension and bradypnoea, the latter as respiratory compensation for the metabolic alkalosis that occurs. ECG changes are seen in up to 80% of anorexia nervosa sufferers with atrioventricular block, QT prolongation, ST segment depression and T-wave inversion all being common. Mitral valve prolapse (probably due to a decrease in ventricular volume and mass) is more commonly seen in this population as are cardiac arrhythmias. The glomerular filtration rate in anorexic patients is reduced and proteinuria is seen in approximately two-thirds of these patients. Delayed gastric emptying is common as is thrombocytopaenia and leucopaenia. Surprisingly anaemia is an uncommon finding and if it does occur it is generally mild and secondary to bone marrow hypoplasia. Endocrine abnormalities are also common with elevated growth hormone and cortisol levels as well as impaired thermoregulation with resting core temperatures often less than 36.3 °C. Of interest, some patients suffering with anorexia nervosa report decreased pain sensitivity but this is probably linked with disturbances of thermoregulation rather than impaired nociception.

Reference
Seller CA, Ravalia A. Anaesthetic implications of anorexia nervosa. *Anaesthesia* 2003; 58(5): 437–43.

Question 51: APACHE II

Regarding the Acute Physiology and Chronic Health Evaluation II (APACHE II) scoring system, which one of the following statements is TRUE?

a) There are 15 physiological variables incorporated within the APACHE II scoring system
b) The maximum number of age points that can be assigned is ten
c) A similar patient will score fewer chronic health points if they are a non-operative critical care admission than if they are admitted following elective surgery
d) Points for the Glasgow Coma Score (GCS) are calculated by subtracting the actual GCS from 15
e) The scores for the physiological variables are obtained by recording the most abnormal variable in each category within the first 12 hours of admission to the critical care unit

Answer: d

Explanation
The APACHE II scoring system remains the most widely used intensive care scoring system, in part due to the slightly superior APACHE III scoring system's predictive equations being commercially protected. First described in 1985, APACHE II gives a score (maximum 71) that represents the summation of points awarded for 12 physio-logical variables, age and chronic health. The physiological variables examined are temperature, mean arterial pressure, heart rate, respiratory rate, oxygenation, arterial pH, serum sodium, serum potassium, serum creatinine, white cell count, GCS and haemocrit. The number of points awarded represents the most abnormal value for each physiological variable within the first 24 hours following intensive care unit admission. Ten of the physiological variables score a maximum of four points each. Creatinine scores a maximum of four or eight depending on whether the patient is in acute renal failure. The score for the GCS is calculated by subtracting the actual GCS from 15. If a patient leaves the intensive care unit and is then readmitted a new APACHE II score must be calculated. The maximum number of points scored for age is six if the patient is ≥75 years old. Chronic health points are awarded if the patient has a history of severe organ system insufficiency or is immunocompromised. The definitions of organ insuf-ficiency cover the cardiovascular, hepatic and renal systems. Five points are awarded if severe organ insufficiency or an immunocompromised state is present and the patient is admitted for a non-operative reason or following emergency surgery, and two points for elective postoperative patients.

Question 52: Cardiac tamponade

A 25-year-old man requires urgent assessment in the emergency department. Recently admitted following a fall of 20 m while climbing, he has suddenly become hypotensive (BP 55/30 mmHg), hypoxaemic (SpO_2 88% on 15 L/min O_2 via a non-rebreathe mask) and tachycardic (HR 160 bpm) having been cardiovascularly stable with good saturations on admission 60 minutes earlier. He has sustained multiple bilateral rib fractures, a sternal fracture, bilateral fractured scapulae and a mid-shaft femoral fracture but no pelvic fracture. Auscultation of his lung fields reveals bilateral air entry, his trachea is midline, his abdomen is soft and non-distended and there has been no response to administration of 3000 mL of crystalloid. Which of the following is the MOST LIKELY diagnosis to explain the sudden deterioration?

a) Blood loss secondary to multiple fractures
b) Cardiac tamponade
c) Severe, bilateral pulmonary contusions
d) Tension pneumothorax
e) Liver laceration

Answer: b

Explanation

This is a challenging case but, although rare, one should consider a traumatic cardiac tamponade as a possible cause especially in the presence of a fractured sternum. The classic triad (Beck's triad) of muffled heart sounds, elevated JVP and hypotension may be difficult signs to elicit in the emergency department so echocardiography may be invaluable in this situation. The other four options are all possibilities but elements of the history make them less likely. It would be unusual to have equal air entry and a midline trachea in a tension pneumothorax and one would expect some sort of response to fluid if multiple fractures were the cause, especially if the pelvis is intact. Significant intra-abdominal pathology would usually manifest some signs and significant bilateral pulmonary contusions would be unlikely to cause such profound hypotension so soon after injury.

Question 53: Stridor

Regarding aspects of acute stridor in children, which one of the following statements is CORRECT?

a) Respiratory syncytial virus (RSV) most commonly causes laryngotracheobronchitis
b) Because of the potential for complete airway obstruction, an intravenous cannula should be sited as a priority
c) Steroids no longer have a place in the treatment of croup
d) Once intubated, patients with a diagnosis of croup tend to have longer time to extubation than those with epiglottitis
e) A two day history of high fever and barking cough in a 4-year-old is typical for a diagnosis of croup

Answer: d

Explanation

This question focuses on just one cause of acute stridor in children (croup) although the candidate should be familiar with croup, epiglottitis, bacterial tracheitis and foreign body aspiration. The commonest cause of croup is parainfluenza virus. Although it may be caused by the respiratory syncytial virus (RSV), the commonest manifestation of RSV infection is bronchiolitis or pneumonia, not croup. It is accepted practice that disturbance or distress of the stridulous child should be avoided at the risk of precipitating complete airway obstruction. This includes postponing placement of an intravenous cannula until after stability has been achieved. The treatment of croup involves humidified oxygen, nebulised adrenaline and steroids. Heliox may be useful if high inspired concentrations of oxygen are not required. Time to extubation tends to be 48 hours with epiglottitis but if croup has been severe enough to warrant intubation, extubation may take up to ten days. A two day history of high fever and barking cough in a four-year-old is not typical. Although the onset and barking cough are usual, the patient is a little old for croup and a low-grade pyrexia is more common. A rapid onset, high grade fever in a very unwell 4-year-old with stridor is more consistent with epiglottitis.

Reference
Maloney E, Meakin G. Acute stridor in children. *Contin Educ Anaesth Crit Care Pain* 2007; **7**(6): 183–6.

Question 54: Gadolinium

Regarding the magnetic resonance imaging (MRI) contrast medium gadolinium, which one of the following statements is TRUE?

a) Gadolinium is usually administered as the soluble salt, gadolinium chloride
b) Unlike X-ray contrast media, gadolinium is safe to administer to patients with stage 3 chronic kidney disease
c) Gadolinium is paramagnetic in its Gd^{3+} state
d) The main role in MRI for gadolinium is to enhance the brightness of neural tissue
e) Gadolinium produces a similar incidence of severe allergic reactions compared to X-ray contrast media

Answer: c

Explanation
Gadolinium is a metal element of the lanthanide group, used in MRI scanning as a contrast agent. Gadolinium stays in intact blood vessels so will make the circulatory system, vascular organs or areas of active bleeding appear brighter. It is usually administered as a chelate with organic molecules such as diethylenetriaminepenta-acetic acid (DTPA). Gadolinium chloride, acetate or sulphate have low solubility at physiological pH and are toxic. Gadolinium is paramagnetic in its Gd^{3+} state and it is in this form that it is used in MRI. Gadolinium has a half-life of 30 to 90 minutes and is excreted through the kidneys. Severe side effects from gadolinium administration are extremely uncommon. There have been around 300 million administrations of gadolinium over the last 30 years. There have been about 200 reports of a skin condition called nephrogenic systemic fibrosis, mainly in patients with kidney disease following the use of gadolinium for MRI scanning. Gadolinium is not nephrotoxic to healthy patients but has been found to produce acute renal failure in 12% of patients with pre-existing stage 3 or 4 chronic kidney disease (glomerular filtration rate <60 mL/min/1.73 m²). The incidence of severe allergic reactions is low at 1 per 18 000 administrations compared to 1 per 1000 X-ray contrast administrations.

Reference
Ergün I, Keven K, Uruç I, *et al*. The safety of gadolinium in patients with stage 3 and 4 renal failure. *Nephrol Dial Transplant* 2006; **21**(3): 697–700.

Question 55: Burns fluid replacement

A 55-year-old, 75 kg male sustains 40% body surface area (BSA) burns in a house fire. Using the Parkland formula, in addition to maintenance fluids, the extra intravenous fluid he should receive in the first eight hours following injury is:

a) 3000 mL of crystalloid
b) 3000 mL of colloid
c) 750 mL colloid and 2250 mL of crystalloid
d) 4000 mL of crystalloid
e) 6000 mL of crystalloid

Answer: e

Explanation

The Parkland formula only involves crystalloid. It is simply $4\,\text{mL}/\text{kg} \times \%\text{BSA}$ over 24 hours. Half is given over eight hours, the rest over the next 16 hours. In this case $4 \times 75 \times 40 = 12\,000$ mL in 24 hours with 6000 mL in the first eight hours *following injury* (not following admission).

Hartmann's solution is favoured over 0.9% saline to avoid the hyperchloraemic metabolic acidosis associated with large volumes of saline. The Brook formula uses $0.5\,\text{mL}/\text{kg} \times \%\text{BSA}$ of colloid and $1.5\,\text{mL}/\text{kg} \times \%\text{BSA}$ of crystalloid in the first 24 hours, again half in eight hours and the rest over 16 (as for Option (c)). The Muir Barclay (Mount Vernon) formula uses colloid aliquots of $0.5\,\text{mL}/\text{kg} \times \%\text{BSA}$ over durations of four, four, four, six and six hours (as for Option (b)).

It should be remembered that these formulae are in addition to maintenance requirements and are a guide only. Fluid management in burns is based on frequent clinical assessment and measurements along with laboratory investigations (including four-hourly electrolytes, haematocrit, urine and plasma osmolality).

Question 56: Fentanyl and morphine

Regarding opioids, which one of the following statements is CORRECT?
  Compared to fentanyl, morphine has

a) A higher lipid solubility, a lower potency and a higher proportion bound to plasma protein
b) A lower lipid solubility, a higher potency and a higher proportion bound to plasma protein
c) A higher lipid solubility, a higher potency and a lower proportion bound to plasma protein
d) A lower lipid solubility, a lower potency and a higher proportion bound to plasma protein
e) A lower lipid solubility, a lower potency and a lower proportion bound to plasma protein

Answer: e

Explanation

Morphine and fentanyl are drugs commonly used in UK anaesthesia. A candidate at Final FRCA level should understand their pharmacology inside out. Fentanyl is more lipid soluble than morphine and therefore crosses the blood–brain barrier more easily. It is about 100 times more potent than morphine and is 80 to 95% plasma protein bound compared to 20 to 40% for morphine.

Question 57: Autonomic neuropathy

Regarding making the diagnosis of autonomic neuropathy, which one of the following statements is CORRECT?

a) Anhydrosis is the most common presenting symptom
b) A normal sinus arrhythmia involves mild elevation of heart rate during expiration and mild depression during inspiration
c) A Valsalva manoeuvre is of no use as a bedside test
d) During a sustained handgrip, a normal response would be an increase in diastolic blood pressure of >16 mmHg in the opposite arm
e) The patient's ability to perform mental arithmetic may aid diagnosis at the bedside

Answer: d

Explanation

Autonomic neuropathy describes a central or peripheral lesion of the autonomic nervous system, which results in dysfunction of its homeostatic function. Consequences for anaesthesia should not be underestimated as dramatic hypotension may be seen at induction of general anaesthesia or while establishing central neuraxial blockade. The patient may be at increased risk of aspiration of gastric contents and anaesthesia, surgery and recovery may provoke cardiac or respiratory arrest without prodrome. The causes may be considered in terms of their anatomical level: central or peripheral nervous system, primary or secondary. Diabetic and alcoholic neuropathies are two common causes and Guillian–Barré syndrome and porphyria are other diagnoses that the anaesthetist will remember; however, the list of described causes is extensive. The patient will most commonly present with orthostatic hypotension and may develop hypohydrosis. Bedside tests involve provoking the autonomic nervous system to respond to a predictable stressor. Lying–standing blood pressure measurement may provoke a drop of over 30 mmHg. Normal sinus arrhythmia (inspiration increases heart rate, expiration decreases it) and normal Valsalva response may be sought. In healthy subjects an increase in blood pressure will be seen caused by elevated sympathetic outflow associated with isometric exercise (sustained hand grip over three minutes), cold pressor test (immersion of hand in ice-cold water for 90 seconds) or mental arithmetic (serial 7 or 17 subtraction from a given figure). With respect to Option (e), it is not the patient's ability to perform mental arithmetic that aids diagnosis, more their haemodynamic response to performing the task.

Reference

Arbogast SD, Miles JD. Autonomic neuropathy. *eMedicine* 25 June 2009. Online at http://emedicine.medscape.com/article/1173756-overview (Accessed 30 October 2009)

Question 58: Preoperative airway assessment

A 45-year-old male presents for microlaryngoscopy following the development of a persistent hoarse voice. He mentions that when he had an appendicectomy age 12, the anaesthetist told him he had struggled to place his breathing tube. Which one of the following would MOST PREDICT a potential difficulty with tracheal intubation?

a) Thick beard and moustache
b) Maximal mouth opening of 4 cm
c) Sternomental distance of 12 cm
d) Patel's distance of 6.5 cm
e) Wilson score 1

Answer: c

Explanation

Each of the values is within normal range except the Savva (sternomental) distance, which below 12.5 cm indicates a potential difficulty with direct laryngoscopy and intubation. The critical Patel (thyromental) distance is 6 cm, where less than this may predict a challenging intubation. Delikan's test grades the extent of neck extension and of course Mallampati score indicates the extent of intraoral anatomy that can be seen from inspection through the open mouth. A Wilson score grades five different predictors of difficult intubation – a score of two or more indicating potential difficulty. A thick beard may pose a challenge to effective mask ventilation but is not a specific inhibition to intubation. Beware, however, those patients who have grown a beard to cosmetically compensate for a relatively small mandible, which might pose a challenge at laryngoscopy (a mandibular length of <9 cm predicts difficulty). It is important to distinguish a potentially difficult intubation from a difficult airway or difficult ventilation. Difficulty with one may be rescued or ameliorated by effectively addressing the other two. The anaesthetist must be vigilant to detect when two or three may be concurrently present in order to avert a potentially avoidable disaster.

Reference

Vaughan R. Predicting difficult airways. *Contin Educ Anaesth Crit Care Pain* 2001; **1**(2): 44–7.

Question 59: Peri-operative risks

In peri-operative care, which one of the following interventions reduces the risk of wound infections by 80%, the risk of requiring secondary surgery by 70% and the risk of pulmonary complications by 80%.

a) Screening for and treating MRSA colonisation
b) Avoiding inadvertent peri-operative hypothermia
c) Stopping smoking eight weeks pre-operatively
d) Intraoperative goal directed therapy
e) Preoperative safety briefing

Answer: c

Explanation

Much effort is put into many activities to improve outcome in surgery, but the single intervention that will produce the best returns for the above complications (and an additional raft of complications including stroke and myocardial infarction) is for the patient to stop smoking a good amount of time pre-operatively.

Reference

Møller AM, Kjellberg J, Pedersen T, Tønnesen H. Effect of preoperative smoking intervention on postoperative complications: a randomised clinical trial. *Lancet* 2002; **359**(9301): 114–17.

Question 60: Ketamine

A 78-year-old male with advanced dementia presents with a large incarcerated inguinal hernia. He is extremely confused, agitated and combative. He is being physically violent and despite his age and weighing only 60 kg he is requiring four theatre staff to prevent him from falling off the theatre table. He has already kicked one theatre support worker and attempts to secure venous access have failed, prompting further violent outbursts from the patient. It is your judgement that he requires a rapid sequence induction but that he currently poses a risk of harm to himself and others.

It is your intention to provide sedation sufficient to tolerate intravenous cannulation whereupon you will pre-oxygenate and perform an intravenous rapid sequence induction. You request ketamine, 100 mg/mL, which you plan to deliver intramuscularly. Which one of the following is the most suitable volume to administer?

a) 0.6 mL
b) 1.2 mL
c) 2.4 mL
d) 4.2 mL
e) 6.0 mL

Answer: b

Explanation

Ketamine is a versatile drug with numerous applications but is often avoided because of concerns over its psychomimetic side effects. It may be delivered by virtually any route, but in the UK is licensed for intravenous and intramuscular use. It has a wide dose range according to delivery route and intended degree of depression of conscious level. For induction of anaesthesia, an intravenous dose of 1 to 2 mg/kg is quoted but 0.5 mg/kg may often be adequate in an older patient. For intramuscular induction of anaesthesia, 4 to 10 mg/kg is suggested. Sedation dose needs to accommodate the clinical state of the patient and the nature of the procedure to be facilitated (in terms of likely stimulation). A dose of 0.2 to 0.5 mg/kg is sufficient intravenously or 2 to 4 mg/kg intramuscularly. In this case, the patient is unwell, poses a risk of aspiration and only needs to tolerate intravenous cannulation and pre-oxygenation. Inadvertent induction of anaesthesia is a possibility. For this reason, the lowest dose of the intramuscular range is selected: 2 mg/kg, 120 mg or 1.2 mL of a 10% preparation.

Question 61: Contrast-induced nephropathy

A 55-year-old man requires cerebral angiography and possible coiling of a large basilar aneurysm. He is diabetic with impaired renal function. Which of the following has been shown to reduce most the chances of the patient developing a contrast-induced nephropathy (CIN)?

a) An infusion of isotonic sodium bicarbonate commenced prior to contrast infusion
b) An N-acetylcysteine infusion commenced prior to contrast infusion
c) The use of the lowest dose of an iso-osmolar contrast medium possible
d) Commencement of an aminophylline infusion prior to contrast infusion
e) An infusion of 0.9% sodium chloride commenced prior to contrast infusion

Answer: e

Explanation

Contrast-induced nephropathy (CIN) is among the commonest causes of hospital-acquired acute renal failure. There are a number of factors variably associated with increased rates of CIN including diabetes, age over 75 years, peri-procedure volume depletion, heart failure, cirrhosis or nephrosis, hypertension, proteinuria, concomitant use of non-steroidal anti-inflammatory drugs, and intra-arterial injection of contrast medium. High doses of contrast medium also increase the likelihood of renal dysfunction. The risk of a decline in kidney function after the administration of contrast medium rises exponentially with the number of risk factors present. Contrast-induced nephropathy is usually transient, with serum creatinine levels peaking at three days after administration of the medium and returning to baseline within ten days. A decline in kidney function after the administration of a contrast medium is associated with a prolonged hospital stay, adverse cardiac events, and high mortality both in the hospital and in the long term. However, the association between these outcomes and the decline in function may be explained, at least in part, by coexisting conditions, the severity of the acute illness and other causes of acute kidney failure. The pathogenesis of CIN in humans is not clear, but is probably related to a combination of toxic injury to the renal tubules and ischaemic injury partly mediated by reactive oxygen species. A large number of treatments have been tried to reduce the incidence of CIN. Of these there is clear evidence for peri-procedure infusion of 0.9% saline solution and the use of the smallest dose possible of a low osmolality contrast medium. The evidence for N-acetylcysteine, isotonic sodium bicarbonate or aminophylline infusions is equivocal and further data is needed on the benefits of iso-osmolar contrast media.

Reference
Barrett BJ, Parfrey PS. Clinical practice. Preventing nephropathy induced by contrast medium. *N Engl J Med* 2006; **354**(4): 379–86.

Question 62: Signs of anaphylaxis

In severe anaphylaxis under anaesthesia, which of the following is MOST COMMONLY the first to be detected?

a) Flushing of the skin
b) Facial oedema
c) Desaturation
d) Difficulty in ventilating
e) Decrease in arterial pressure

Answer: e

Explanation
Decrease in arterial pressure is the first sign to be detected in 28% of cases, with difficulty in ventilating at 26%, flushing at 21%, desaturation at 3% and swelling at <3%.

Reference
Harper NJ, Dixon T, Dugué P, *et al*. Suspected anaphylactic reactions associated with anaesthesia. *Anaesthesia* 2009; **64**(7): 199–211. Online at www.aagbi.org/publications/guidelines/docs/anaphylaxis_2009.pdf (Accessed 30 October 2009)

Question 63: Physics of vaporisers

An Ohmeda Isotec 5 vaporiser filled correctly with isoflurane has a 1 L/min fresh gas flow delivered to it at sea level and 20 °C. The control dial is set such that the splitting ratio is 5%. What is the resulting concentration of isoflurane at the outlet of the vaporiser?

a) 0.8%
b) 1.6%
c) 2.4%
d) 3.2%
e) 5.0%

Answer: c

Explanation
There is a temptation to oversimplify calculations with respect to vaporisers. This can cause errors that are significant given the small concentrations of volatile agent that are

clinically useful. The saturated vapour pressure of isoflurane is 33.2kPa. Assuming an atmospheric pressure of 101.325kPa it can be seen that in the vaporising chamber, a saturated mixture of about one third isoflurane in carrier gas will be produced (recall Dalton's law of partial pressures). Amagat's law of partial volumes states that at a fixed temperature and pressure, the sum of the volumes of components of a gas mixture equals the total volume of that mixture (admittedly for ideal gases). Some texts incorrectly state that as 5% of the fresh gas flow (FGF) enters the vaporising chamber, which contains 33% isoflurane, then when this mixture rejoins the 95% that travelled through the bypass channel the resulting concentration is $0.05 \times 0.33 = 0.0165$ or 1.65%. This fails to acknowledge that the volume *leaving* the vaporising chamber is greater than the volume that *entered* the chamber as there has been volatile added to the gas with no increase in pressure. Consider the volumes in one minute. FGF 1000mL. Splitting ratio 5%. 50mL enters the chamber. This 50mL of carrier gas must also exit the chamber but a volume of pure isoflurane vapour has been added to it such that the exit gas proportion of isoflurane is one third (SVP/P_{atm} as previously established). It can be seen that 25mL of isoflurane has been added to the carrier gas ($25/(50 + 25)$ is one third). At the exit of the chamber the carrier gas (still 50mL) with added isoflurane (25mL) rejoins the 950mL of bypass carrier gas that now leaves at the vaporiser outlet. 25mL of isoflurane in 1025mL total volume is 2.4%.

Question 64: Clinical features of valvular heart disease

An 82-year-old female is awaiting a hip hemiarthroplasty having sustained a fractured neck of femur. She has mild dementia and is unable to relate her medical history. Her old notes are currently unavailable and as she has recently moved from out of the region her computer records are unhelpful. On examination she has a small volume, regular pulse. Her blood pressure is 136/72 mmHg and her JVP is not raised. She has an undisplaced, tapping apex beat. On auscultation, she has a short rumbling diastolic murmur audible all over the praecordium. Which one of the following is the MOST LIKELY valve lesion?

a) Mitral stenosis
b) Aortic regurgitation
c) Mixed aortic valve disease
d) Tricuspid stenosis
e) Pulmonary regurgitation

Answer: a

Explanation
This is most likely to be a mild form of mitral stenosis, as if the severity increased the features are so florid as to present no doubt as to the valve lesion in question. Each of these valve lesions may cause a diastolic murmur, so this case needs to be distinguished via its other clinical features. Mitral stenosis tends to be associated with atrial fibrillation, but in mild forms of the condition sinus rhythm is preserved. The small volume pulse and normal pulse pressure eliminates aortic regurgitation in which a wider pulse pressure and collapsing pulse is expected. Aortic stenosis in mixed aortic valve disease might give a small volume pulse as described, but then a systolic component to the murmur would be heard. The palpable first heart sound and 'opening snap' that gives the tapping apex beat is characteristic of mitral stenosis and not present in pulmonary valve regurgitation. Tricuspid stenosis shares many clinical features with mitral stenosis. If sinus rhythm is preserved, prominent jugular venous 'a' waves will be observed. It might be a contender for the answer here except that it is far less common than mitral stenosis so the 'most likely valve lesion' is still mitral stenosis.

Reference
Camm A. Cardiovascular disease. In: Kumar P, Clark M (eds) *Clinical Medicine*, 4th edn. Edinburgh: W.B.Saunders, 1998; pp. 700–10.

Question 65: Acute liver failure

Regarding acute liver failure, which one of the following statements is TRUE?

a) Subacute liver failure carries a better prognosis than hyperacute liver failure
b) Acute liver failure refers to 'jaundice to encephalopathy time' of one to four weeks
c) The commonest cause in the UK is infective hepatitis
d) Hyperglycaemia and hypokalaemia is the common metabolic derangement at presentation
e) Deliberate self-harm patients cannot be considered for liver transplantation

Answer: b

Explanation
Acute liver failure is the triad of jaundice, coagulopathy and encephalopathy developing in the context of an individual with previously normal liver function (in order to distinguish from acute or chronic liver failure or decompensated liver disease). The timings of acute liver failure refer to the time from onset of jaundice until the development of encephalopathy. In hyperacute, this is seven days; acute is one to four weeks; and subacute is five to twelve weeks. Subacute liver failure carries the worst prognosis. Around 70% of acute liver failure in the UK is secondary to paracetamol overdose with a much smaller proportion being caused by hepatitis. Worldwide, hepatitis B is the leading aetiology. At presentation the common metabolic derangements include hypoglycaemia, hypokalaemia and hypo- or hypernatraemia. As well as the classical triad mentioned, patients may present with failure of virtually every organ system, posing a significant challenge to the critical care practitioner. Patients are not excluded from liver transplantation on grounds of self-induced liver failure. The criteria for consideration for liver transplantation vary with whether the case is a paracetamol overdose or of other origin and include factors such as blood pH, prothrombin time, serum creatinine, grade of encephalopathy, serum bilirubin, age of the patient and chronology.

Question 66: Coronary artery blood flow

Regarding normal coronary artery blood flow, the following statements are true EXCEPT which one?

a) Total left coronary artery flow is initially decreased by tachycardia
b) At rest, right coronary artery blood flow is greater than left coronary artery blood flow at the beginning of systole
c) Flow in the left coronary artery at rest may be as high as 100 mL/min
d) Right coronary flow is at its lowest at the beginning of diastole
e) At rest, peak left coronary artery flow may be six times higher than peak right coronary artery flow

Answer: d

Explanation
In health, the development of a tachycardia will initially lead to a drop in left coronary artery flow, as the time in diastole during which flow normally occurs is reduced. In health, this is rapidly compensated for and flow matches any increase in demand. Left

coronary artery flow is very low during the whole of systole and may be absent at the beginning of systole. Right coronary flow is generally more even throughout the cardiac cycle, and despite being at its lowest rate in the cardiac cycle, is higher than left coronary flow at the beginning of systole. However, overall, right coronary flow is lower than left, and the peak left-sided flow at rest is around 100 mL/min, compared to 15 mL/min for the right side.

Question 67: Brachial plexus anatomy

Which one of the following statements regarding the anatomy of the brachial plexus is TRUE?

a) The median nerve derives contributions from spinal nerve roots C5 to C8
b) The upper, middle and lower trunks each have divisions that unite to form the posterior cord
c) The axillary and radial nerves are both derived from the lateral cord
d) The medial cutaneous nerves of the arm and forearm are branches of the ulnar nerve
e) The lateral cutaneous nerve of the forearm is a terminal branch of the radial nerve

Answer: b

Explanation

The candidate should be able to draw the brachial plexus and a quick sketch might aid the answering of this question. The median nerve is derived from spinal roots C5 to T1. The axillary and radial nerves are derived from the posterior cord. The medial cutaneous nerves of the arm and forearm are branches of the medial cord (as is the ulnar nerve). The lateral cutaneous nerve of the forearm is a branch of the musculocutaneous nerve. The radial nerve gives off the posterior cutaneous nerve of the forearm and the lower lateral cutaneous nerve of the arm.

Question 68: Oxygenation indices

Regarding oxygenation indices the following statements are correct EXCEPT for which one?

a) Calculating venous admixture requires a pulmonary artery flotation catheter
b) A PaO_2:FiO_2 ratio <26.6 kPa is a criterion for diagnosis of ARDS
c) P (A – a) O_2 is the respiratory index
d) Ideally an oxygenation index should not vary with changes in FiO_2
e) The alveolar gas equation is required for a number of oxygenation indices

Answer: c

Explanation

Maintaining a patient's oxygenation is high on an anaesthetist's list of priorities. It is reasonable to expect knowledge of the quantification of adequacy of oxygenation and gas exchange. It is also important to appreciate the limitations of each index in truly representing the performance of the lung. Venous admixture may be defined as 'that degree of true right-to-left shunt that would explain the observed difference in alveolar and arterial oxygen levels'. 'Levels' is used deliberately here because although the equation uses oxygen contents in its calculation, venous admixture can be used to quantify observed differences in tension, saturation or content. It is also widely regarded as the gold-standard oxygenation index, even if the source of deficient gas exchange is not primarily due to shunt. It does require true mixed venous blood content, which is found in the pulmonary artery. Central venous oxygen content may be substituted (with a correction factor) to give an approximation to the value.

$P (A - a) O_2$ is the alveolar-arterial oxygen difference and may be expected to be less than 2kPa in a young healthy individual but does increase with age. $(P (A - a) O_2) / PaO_2$ is the respiratory index and attempts to eliminate the variation of the index with FIO_2. These two indices and the PaO_2/PAO_2 ratio all rely on the assumptions of the alveolar gas equation.

The ideal oxygenation index should be a representation of the function of the lung and not be influenced by external factors that we may manipulate (like FIO_2). The index $PaO_2:FIO_2$ attempts to accommodate this. If inspired oxygen is manipulated, oxygen tension should change accordingly thus the index of oxygenation should remain constant.

Reference

Armstrong J, Guleria A, Girling K. Evaluation of gas exchange deficit in the critically ill. *Contin Educ Anaesth Crit Care Pain* 2007; **7**(4): 131–4.

Question 69: Peptic ulcer disease

Regarding the diagnosis and management of peptic ulcer disease, which one of the following statements is CORRECT?

a) In the UK, gastric ulcers are, overall, more common than duodenal ulcers
b) Alcohol consumption is an independent risk factor for peptic ulcer disease
c) Peptic ulcers, almost universally, present with pain as one of the clinical features
d) The presence of night-pain tends to suggest a duodenal rather than gastric ulcer
e) A perforated peptic ulcer necessitates urgent laparotomy

Answer: d

Explanation

One hundred years ago peptic ulcers were likely to be gastric and affect young female patients. More recently patients presenting with peptic ulcers (in the UK) are likely to be elderly, from lower socioeconomic groups and have a duodenal ulcer. Duodenal ulcers, especially in the elderly, can be completely painless and present with anaemia, upper gastrointestinal bleeding or perforation. Night-pain, as a presenting complaint, does tend to indicate a duodenal rather than gastric ulcer. The epigastric pain of both gastric and duodenal ulcers is relieved by eating or antacids thus these factors are not helpful in distinguishing the two. There is no proven link between alcohol consumption per se and peptic ulcers; in fact, ethanol may reduce the probability of developing duodenal ulcers. However, cirrhosis or chronic pancreatitis (often consequences of excessive drinking of alcohol) are associated with increased rates of peptic ulceration. The role of surgery in the management of perforated ulcers is unquestioned if peritonitis or pneumoperitoneum has developed; however, in the absence of these features, conservative management is an accepted strategy and not just in patients with high-risk comorbidity.

Question 70: Urinalysis

Regarding urinary chemical reagent dipstick testing, the following are true EXCEPT which one?

a) The presence of leucocytes with no nitrites is more common than the presence of nitrites with no leucocytes
b) Urine specific gravity measurements may need to be adjusted upwards if the urine is strongly acidic

c) If the stick is left with a coating of excess urine after dipping, errors are most likely to be found in the pH reading

d) Concurrent nephrotic syndrome may lead to overdiagnosing the syndrome of inappropriate antidiuretic hormone (SIADH) when analysing dipstick specific gravity

e) If the urine is allowed to stand for one hour, glucose testing may produce a false negative

Answer: b

Explanation

Nitrites are often found on urine dipsticks during infection as bacteria convert nitrates to nitrites. This is not the case for all bacteria, so the absence of nitrites does not equal the absence of bacteria. Specific gravity is in the range of 1.001 to 1.035 in health. Strongly acidic urine may raise the dipstick measurement of specific gravity so values may have to be adjusted downwards. If the stick is left with an excess of urine, errors are most likely to be seen on the pH recording as there may be run-off from the strongly acidic protein test pad. Dipstick measurement may read high specific gravity in the presence of ketones or protein in the urine. If the investigator is using dipsticks to aid with diagnosing SIADH, the proteinuria found in nephrotic syndrome may lead to a false positive diagnosis. If urine is allowed to stand, for any length of time, bacteria may use up any glucose for metabolism, rendering abnormally high glucose levels undetectable.

Question 71: Avoiding drugs

According to the product information leaflets, which one of the following statements is TRUE?

a) Albumin solution should not be used in patients with known egg allergy

b) The use of 20% Intralipid is safe in patients with a known peanut allergy

c) Gelofusine® may be unacceptable for the management of a Hindu patient

d) Propofol should not be used in patients with a known egg allergy

e) The use of hydroxyl ethyl starch solutions in patients with gluten-sensitive enteropathy should be avoided

Answer: d

Explanation

The aim of this question is to emphasise the point that propofol now explicitly states in its product information that it should be avoided in patients with a known egg allergy. Intralipid, which is very similar to the lipid emulsion used with propofol, is also not recommended in patients with a known soya or peanut allergy. This is despite containing no peanuts. Recommendations in guidelines from the European Commission now require products containing soya to be labelled as unsuitable for peanut allergy sufferers because of the high risk of cross-sensitivity. Albumin solution is sourced from human plasma and is different from the albumen of eggs, which may contain a number of ovalbumins. Gelofusine® is a bovine-sourced gelatin solution. Even though this may prove unacceptable to some members of the Hindu faith, this is not mentioned in Gelofusine's product information. Currently marketed hydroxyl ethyl starch solutions are made from either maize- or potato-sourced starch and so would be unlikely to create a problem in gluten-sensitive enteropathy, even if swallowed.

Question 72: *Clostridium difficile*

A patient on the intensive care unit develops offensive diarrhoea following treatment for ventilator-associated pneumonia. *Clostridium difficile* toxin has been detected in the stool. Which one of the following statements regarding *C. difficile* infection is TRUE?

a) Following initial treatment of *C. difficile* colitis recurrence is uncommon
b) Over 50% of adults carry *C. difficile* asymptomatically
c) The pathogenesis of *C. difficile* is secondary to the production of two types of exotoxin
d) Treatment with broad spectrum cephalosporins carries the highest risk of developing *C. difficile* colitis compared with treatment with other antibiotic types or groups
e) Non-toxin producing strains of *C. difficile* may cause pseudomembranous colitis

Answer: c

Explanation

C. difficile is a Gram-positive anaerobic bacillus, so named because originally it was a 'difficult' organism to isolate and culture. It is a normal commensal in up to 5% of the adult population and upto 50% of infants. In the latter, resistance to *C. difficile* colitis is thought to be secondary to the immaturity of an infant's enterocyte membrane toxin receptors. Hospitalised patients are at highest risk of *C. difficile* colitis because they often receive broad spectrum antibiotics in an environment where contamination with *C. difficile* spores is commonplace. These spores may survive for years in the environment. Broad spectrum cephalosporins and penicillins are the most commonly implicated antibiotics due to the number of prescriptions, but clindamycin is the most likely to cause *C. difficile* colitis. The pathogenic *C. difficile* organisms are those that produce toxins of which there are two: toxin A and toxin B. Outbreaks of *C. difficile* 027 are of particular concern because this particular strain produces much more of the toxins than most other types because a mutation has knocked out the gene that normally restricts toxin production. The colitis caused by the toxins may occur with or without pseudomembrane formation. Treatment is supportive along with discontinuation of any implicated antibiotics and commencement of metronidazole or vancomycin. Colonic resection is sometimes indicated in the most severe cases.

Reference

Kelly CP, LaMont JT. *Clostridium difficile* – more difficult than ever. *New Engl J Med* 2008; **359**(18):1932–40.

Question 73: Obstetric mortality

According to the CEMACH report (2003–5) published in 2007, which one of the following is TRUE?

a) The leading cause of indirect maternal death is psychiatric
b) There has been a significant rise in direct deaths due to amniotic fluid embolism
c) A third of the women who died from direct or indirect causes were overweight or obese
d) Thromboembolism is the second highest cause of direct maternal death
e) The time frame applied to late maternal death is >30 days and <1 year from the end of the pregnancy

Answer: b

Explanation

Direct maternal deaths are those resulting from conditions, complications or their management that are unique to pregnancy, occurring during the antenatal, intra-partum or post-partum period. Indirect maternal deaths are those resulting from previously existing disease or disease that develops during pregnancy, not due to direct obstetric causes, but which was aggravated by the physiological effects of pregnancy. Late maternal death is defined as the death of a woman from direct or indirect causes more than 42 days but less than one completed year after the end of the pregnancy.

The leading cause of indirect maternal death is cardiac. More than half of the women who died from direct or indirect causes were overweight or obese. Thromboembolism is the highest cause of direct maternal death. In the triennium mentioned there were six direct deaths due to anaesthesia and 31 direct and indirect deaths in which poor anaesthetic management contributed and lessons could be learned.

Reference

Lewis G (ed) The Confidential Enquiry into Maternal and Child Health (CEMACH). Saving Mothers' Lives: reviewing maternal deaths to make motherhood safer – 2003–2005. The Seventh Report on Confidential Enquiries into Maternal Deaths in the United Kingdom. London: CEMACH, 2007. Online at www.cmace.org.uk (Accessed 30 October 2009)

Question 74: Brain-stem testing

Regarding cranial nerve examination during testing for brain-stem death, the following cranial nerves are examined EXCEPT which one?

a) Cranial nerve VIII
b) Cranial nerve V
c) Cranial nerve XI
d) Cranial nerve IX
e) Cranial nerve X

Answer: c

Explanation

Although there is currently no formal definition of death in the United Kingdom, death may be defined as the irreversible loss of the capacity for consciousness, combined with the irreversible loss of the capacity to breathe. The irreversible cessation of brain-stem function will produce this clinical state. This therefore means that cessation of brain-stem function equates with the death of the individual and thus allows physicians to certify death in this situation. These definitions and the process involved in the certification of brain-stem death have recently been summarised (see reference below). Prior to brain-stem testing a number of preconditions must be satisfied. The patient's condition must be due to brain damage of known aetiology; they must be deeply comatose, unresponsive, apnoeic and be mechanically ventilated. There should be no evidence that this state is due to depressant drugs and their core temperature should be >34 °C at the time of testing. Any potential circulatory, metabolic or endocrine disturbances must have been excluded as the cause of continuation of the unconsciousness. Testing is done by two doctors registered for more than five years who are competent in carrying out the procedure. At least one should be a consultant. Testing should be undertaken by the doctors together and must be undertaken successfully and completely on two separate occasions. The test looks for the absence of brain-stem response, motor response and response to apnoea and consequent hyper-capnia. As part of this, the cranial nerves (whose nuclei are located in the brain stem) amenable to testing are II (pupillary response to light), V and VII (corneal reflex and response to painful stimuli), VIII (caloric testing) and IX and X (gag and cough reflex).

Reference
Academy of Medical Royal Colleges. A code of practice for the diagnosis and con-firmation of death. October 2008. Online at www.aomrc.org.uk/aomrc/admin/reports/docs/DofD-final.pdf (Accessed 30 October 2009)

Question 75: Implantable cardiac defibrillators

Regarding implantable cardiac defibrillators, which one of the following statements is TRUE?

a) An implantable defibrillator must be turned off before surgery involving diathermy
b) If the indifferent grounding pad is greater than 15 cm from the defibrillator, the risk from unipolar diathermy electrocautery is eliminated
c) An internal cardioversion shock of two joules will cause painful skeletal and diaphragmatic contraction in the awake patient
d) External cardiac pacing is contraindicated in the presence of implantable defibrillator leads
e) In approaching 90% of cases, a functioning implantable defibrillator will successfully terminate a malignant arrhythmia within 15 seconds

Answer: c

Explanation
An implantable cardiac defibrillator (ICD) consists of a pulse generator and leads embedded in the endocardium and responsible for detection of a malignant tachy-arrhythmia and delivery of the shock to terminate it. This function may be its only responsibility or it may complement other pacemaking functions. If the unit functions as a pacemaker as well, turning it off prior to surgery may result in reversion to the intrinsic bradyarrhythmia with deleterious consequences. Instead the unit should be reprogrammed to a safer, fixed VVI mode. If it functions solely as a defibrillator, it may be turned off pre-operatively. In this circumstance, pharmacological therapy and external pacing pads should be available for use in the event of malignant tachy-arrhythmia. External pads should be placed at least 10 cm from the pulse generator and leads. Unipolar electrocautery may be used but the indifferent pad should be as far as possible (at least 15 cm) from components of the implanted system. The surgeon should be advised to use low-energy, short bursts to minimise electromagnetic interference or induction. Alternatives such as bipolar or ligation techniques should be considered where possible. An internal shock of two joules will cause the symptoms described in the awake patient. For asynchronous defibrillation of ventricular fibrillation energies of 10 to 40 joules may be used. Implantable cardiac defibrillator batteries may contain 20 000 joules of energy. The efficacy of ICDs is higher than quoted in Option (e), approaching 100% in 5 to 15 seconds.

Reference
Bukhari A, Gars S, Mehta Y. Anaesthetic management of patients with implantable cardioverter defibrillator. *Ann Card Anaesth* 2005; 8(1): 61

Paper B

Question 76: Phenylephrine

Regarding the use of phenylephrine following central neuraxial block in obstetric anaesthesia, the following statements are true EXCEPT which one?

a) Continuous infusion produces fewer periods of hypotension than intermittent boluses
b) It results in less umbilical artery acidaemia than ephedrine
c) It produces less bradycardia compared to ephedrine
d) It produces less supraventricular tachycardia compared to ephedrine
e) It has not been shown to exhibit tachyphylaxis

Answer: c

Explanation
Following an inversion of what would have seemed heresy ten years ago, phenylephrine has become widely established as *the* drug for maintaining blood pressure following regional block in obstetric anaesthesia. This α_1 agonist gives smoothest blood pressure control as an infusion. Studies have shown that phenylephrine produces less acidosis on umbilical sampling, although there is conflicting evidence as to whether it produces less actual foetal acidosis. Phenylephrine produces less maternal supraventricular tachycardias but more bradycardias. There are some rare reports of tachyphylaxis outside of the obstetric literature.

Question 77: Refeeding syndrome

Refeeding syndrome can manifest with the following derangements EXCEPT which one?

a) Hypophosphataemia
b) Hyperkalaemia
c) Hypomagnesaemia
d) An increase in the minute volume and respiratory quotient
e) Increased extracellular fluid volume

Answer: b

Explanation
Refeeding syndrome occurs in patients after recommencement of feeding following a period of starvation, and this syndrome is not infrequently seen in the critically ill

patient. It may occur up to four days after either enteral or parenteral feed has been recommenced. During a period of starvation the secretion of insulin is decreased due to the reduced intake of carbohydrates and the switch to fat and protein catabolism. This results in intracellular depletion of electrolytes, in particular phosphate. This may be in spite of the maintenance of normal serum phosphate levels. Following the commencement of feeding, carbohydrate metabolism resumes and hence insulin production increases. This stimulates cellular uptake of electrolytes, which can lead to profound hypophosphataemia and hypokalaemia. The hypomagnesaemia is secondary to the phosphate depletion and is due to increased urinary excretion of magnesium. As phosphate is essential for ATP generation, hypophosphataemia can lead to a wide range of problems including rhabdomyolysis, cardiac and respiratory failure, leucocyte dysfunction, metabolic acidosis and arrhythmias. In addition, recommencement of carbohydrate metabolism will cause a sudden increase in CO_2 production and O_2 consumption, thus increasing both the respiratory quotient and minute volume. Awareness of the potential to develop refeeding syndrome is essential and the mainstays of treatment are aggressive electrolyte replacement and frequent monitoring of electrolyte levels.

Question 78: Disseminated intravascular coagulation

A 29-year-old multiparous woman suffers an antepartum haemorrhage secondary to placental abruption and in the course of the resuscitation and subsequent emergency caesarean section receives twelve units of packed red blood cells and four units of fresh frozen plasma. The following laboratory results would be expected in acute disseminated intravascular coagulation EXCEPT which one?

a) Reduced soluble fibrin
b) Moderate thrombocytopenia
c) Decreased factor VII levels
d) Gradual decrease in fibrinogen
e) Prolonged activated partial thromboplastin time

Answer: a

Explanation
Disseminated intravascular coagulation (DIC) is an acquired phenomenon whereby a precipitating event induces widespread and generalised activation of the blood clotting systems thereby producing a consumptive coagulopathy and fibrinous occlusions of the microvasculature. Precipitants are often inflammatory in nature and there is evidence that development of DIC is cytokine mediated. The pathophysiological phases are thrombin burst, anticoagulant suppression, fibrinolysis inhibition and inflammatory activation. The diagnosis is made from a combination of an at-risk patient with positive clinical features and compatible blood tests. There is not a specific test for DIC. Intravascular coagulation is largely due to activation of the intrinsic clotting pathway, but this does not translate to specificity of laboratory tests in acute DIC where virtually all tests relevant to coagulation may be deranged. As DIC involves massive fibrin production, elevated levels of soluble fibrin would be expected although most laboratories do not routinely test for this. Note that the intuitive decrease in fibrinogen is not always seen as fibrinogen is an acute phase protein released at times of heightened inflammation, so despite massive fibrin generation, fibrinogen may be slow to fall.

Reference
Becker JU, Wira CR. Disseminated intravascular coagulation: differential diagnoses and workup. *eMedicine* 10 September 2009. Online at http://emedicine.medscape. com/article/779097-diagnosis (Accessed 30 October 2009)

Question 79: Fluid management

Regarding peri-operative fluid management, which one of the following statements is MOST CORRECT?

a) In patients with acute kidney injury, potassium-containing balanced electrolyte solutions should be avoided
b) Higher molecular weight hydroxyethyl starch solutions should be avoided in severe sepsis
c) For patients with acute kidney injury, if free water is required 5% dextrose solution should be avoided
d) In patients without gastric emptying disorders, oral water is acceptable pre-operatively except in the last hour prior to induction of anaesthesia
e) Elderly patients are more likely to benefit from 4% dextrose/0.18% saline fluid as maintenance

Answer: b

Explanation

Hetastarch or pentastarch solutions with an average molecular weight >200kDa have been shown to increase the risk of precipitating renal failure in severe sepsis. Patients with acute kidney injury should have their fluid and electrolyte status regularly reviewed, therefore the use of balanced electrolyte solutions is not prohibited as its advantages over 0.9% saline are still present. If a free-water deficit is demonstrable then 0.18% saline or 5% dextrose should be used but with vigilance to avoid hyponatraemia. The risks of hyponatraemia in children is well publicised; however, the elderly are equally susceptible and hypotonic and/or hyposmolar intravenous infusions as maintenance should be avoided (4% dextrose/0.18% saline is hypotonic but isosmolar). There is high-grade evidence that fasting times for oral non-particulate clear fluids should not exceed two hours in order to reduce peri-operative complications. The GIFTASUP 2008 guidelines (see reference below) give a thorough summary.

Reference

Powell-Tuck J, Gosling P, Lobo DN, *et al*. British consensus guidelines on intravenous fluid therapy for adult surgical patients (GIFTASUP). 2008. Online at www.ics.ac.uk/icmprof/standards.asp?menuid=7 (Accessed 30 October 2009)

Question 80: Stopping smoking

After cessation of smoking 20 cigarettes a day for 20 years, which one of the following takes the LONGEST to show signs of significant improvement?

a) Small airway function
b) The negative inotropic effect of smoking
c) Excess sputum production
d) Polycythaemia
e) Risk of chest infection

Answer: e

Explanation

Stopping smoking 12 hours before surgery significantly reduces the level of carboxyhaemoglobin, increases oxygen carrying capacity of blood, and reduces the negative inotropic and arrhythmic effects of smoking. Stopping smoking for 12 to 24 hours will reduce elevated heart rate and blood pressure, and improve peripheral vasoconstriction. Stopping smoking for a week will improve raised blood viscosity and polycythaemia. Stopping smoking for one month improves small airway function, which continues to improve for a further six months. Stopping smoking for six weeks will produce gains in reducing excess sputum production, with a 50% reduction in the first two weeks. Stopping smoking for two months reduces the risk of postoperative chest infection with a risk approaching that of non-smokers if the patient stops for six months. The longer the period of abstinence, the less likely a wound complication.

Reference
Doctors and Tobacco. The Tobacco Control Resource Centre website. Online at www. tobacco-control.org/ (Accessed 30 October 2009)

Question 81: Somatosensory evoked potentials

In a patient having cortical somatosensory evoked potentials monitoring of spinal cord integrity during spinal surgery, the following may produce important inaccuracies EXCEPT which one?

a) Blood pressure variations
b) Temperature variations
c) Neuromuscular blocking drugs
d) Haemorrhage down to a haemoglobin of 5.5 g/dL
e) Maintenance of anaesthesia with sevoflurane

Answer: c

Explanation
Somatosensory evoked potentials (SSEPs) are monitored during spinal surgery and in many centres they have replaced wake-up testing during spinal surgery. The technique involves the analysis of recorded signals picked up by recording electrodes sited over the spine or scalp and caused by stimulating peripheral nerves. The signal may be affected by temperature variation and hypotension. Anaemia to a haematocrit of <15% may also affect SSEPs. The motor tracts are not monitored, so SSEPs are unaffected by neuromuscular blocking drugs and may actually be enhanced as muscle blockade decreases the 'noise' from muscle tissue. Volatile anaesthetic agents increase SSEP latency and decrease amplitude. SSEPs use usually involves an anaesthetic with target-controlled propofol infusion, which has little significant affect.

Reference
Boisseau N, Madany M, Staccini P, et al. Comparison of the effects of sevoflurane and propofol on cortical somatosensory evoked potentials. Brit J Anaesth 2002; **88**(6): 785–9.

Question 82: Preoperative anaemia

A 30-year-old Chinese woman who has been in the United Kingdom for the last year is scheduled to have a laparoscopic cholecystectomy. She has no significant past medical history other than rheumatoid arthritis for which she takes occasional analgesia only. She has been feeling tired over the last few months. Clinical examination is consistent with rheumatoid arthritis but otherwise unremarkable. She has a microcytic, hypo-chromic anaemia with a haemoglobin of 9.6 g/dL. Which of the following is LEAST LIKELY to be the cause?

a) HbH disease
b) Alpha-thalassaemia trait

c) Anaemia secondary to rheumatoid arthritis
d) Beta-thalassaemia minor
e) Anaemia secondary to menorrhagia

Answer: a

Explanation
The alpha-globin gene is located on chromosome 16, the beta globin gene on chromosome 11. The prevalence of beta- or alpha-thalassaemia is up to 15% in some parts of the world. Alpha-thalassaemia is found in populations in the Mediterranean, Africa, the Middle East and South East Asia. Beta-thalassaemia affects individuals in China, the Mediterranean, the Middle East and India. There are four subtypes of alpha-thalassaemia. These subtypes are characterised by the number of alpha-globin chain genes deleted (from one to four). The subtypes, from a single gene deletion through to the genes coding for all four alpha genes are named silent carrier, alpha-thalassaemia trait, HbH disease and hydrops foetalis respectively. The severity of symptoms is proportional to the number of genes deleted. Silent carriers are asymptomatic, alpha-thalassaemia trait sufferers are usually asymptomatic but they may be anaemic with a hypochromic-microcytic picture. Both these subtypes have a normal life expectancy, HbH disease is characterised by haemolytic anaemia with splenomegaly and bone changes, so it is very unlikely that a patient with HbH would have remained asymptomatic to the age of 30. Patients with hydrops foetalis are stillborn or die shortly after birth. Beta-thalassaemia sufferers fall into three categories: beta-thalassaemia minor (where patients have a heterozygous abnormality in the beta-globin gene); intermedia (with a homozygous or mixed heterozygous abnormality) and major (with a homozygous abnormality). Beta-thalassaemia minor sufferers are usually asymptomatic though they may have a mild microcytic anaemia. Beta-thalassaemia intermedia patients present with a variety of symptoms including hepatosplenomegaly, skeletal deformities, gallstones and leg ulcers, but patients will survive into adulthood even without treatment. Individuals with beta-thalassaemia major present in early infancy with failure to thrive and a transfusion dependent severe anaemia. Chronic disease usually causes a normochromic normocytic anaemia but may present with a microcytic hypochromic picture.

Question 83: Acromegaly

Regarding a person with acromegaly presenting for transsphenoidal hypophysectomy, which of the following statements is MOST LIKELY to be true?

a) The patient is more likely to be male than female
b) Males with acromegaly are as likely to suffer from obstructive sleep apnoea as females
c) Patients with acromegaly are more likely to have a distal rather than a proximal myopathy
d) They are likely to have raised adrenocorticotrophic hormone (ACTH) levels
e) They are likely to have raised levels of insulin-like growth factor-1 (IGF-1)

Answer: e

Explanation
Patients with acromegaly can present in a number of ways, but as an anaesthetist one is most likely to encounter them just prior to pituitary surgery as over 90% are secondary to a benign growth hormone (GH) secreting tumour. Of these tumours, 25% also secrete prolactin. The remaining 10% of cases are secondary to either ectopic GH production or due to excess growth hormone-releasing hormone (GHRH). This may be from either a hypothalamic tumour or ectopic GHRH production by tumours of the pancreas, kidneys or lungs. Growth hormone induces the synthesis of peripheral

IGF-1, which acts by inducing cell proliferation and reducing apoptosis hence, over time, leading to the characteristic features associated with the condition. Due to local destruction of the anterior pituitary gland by the tumour, production of other pituitary hormones (e.g. adrenocorticotropic hormone and thyroid stimulating hormone) may be reduced. Diagnosis is made by initial measurement of IGF-1 levels and if this is abnormal proceeding to measurement of GH levels during a standard glucose tolerance test and if this is abnormal, pituitary imaging by MRI scan. Anaesthetic implications of this condition are multiple but include raised intracranial pressure, cardiovascular disease (the most frequent cause of death in untreated acromegaly with up to 50% of patients dying before the age of 50), potential for difficult intubation, obstructive sleep apnoea (more common in males than females) and a proximal myopathy.

Reference

Melmed S. Medical progress: acromegaly. *New Engl J Med* 2006; **355**(24): 2558–73.

Question 84: Toxicology and blood gases

A patient is brought into the resuscitation room with a reduced conscious level. He was recognised as having been admitted a week earlier with deliberate self-poisoning. His blood gases were as follows: pH 7.01; PaO_2 9.8 kPa; $PaCO_2$ 6.1 kPa; HCO_3^- 12 mEq/L; base excess −18; anion gap 9 mEq/L.

Which one of the following is the patient MOST LIKELY to have been poisoned with?

a) Amitriptyline
b) Methadone
c) Paroxetine
d) Ethanol
e) Organophosphates

Answer: e

Explanation

Severe amitriptyline poisoning typically has a mixed respiratory and metabolic acidosis. Methadone poisoning will manifest itself as a respiratory acidosis. Poisoning in which paroxetine is the only agent taken generally produces mild symptoms such as vomiting and tremor. Paroxetine poisoning would not usually produce any derangement of arterial blood gases. Rarely, the patient may develop a 'serotonin syndrome' in which cognitive or behavioural changes (such as agitation or coma), autonomic changes (such as hyperthermia and tachycardia) and neuromuscular instability (such as hyperreflexia and trismus) are found. Ethanol would show a respiratory acidosis with a raised anion gap. Organophosphate overdose is a common method of suicide around the world. It is particularly prevalent in rural settings where organophosphate pesticides are easy to access. Organophosphates inhibit both cholinesterase and pseudocholinesterase, leading to an accumulation of acetylcholine at synapses. This manifests itself as overstimulation of nicotinic and muscarinic receptors. Typically, the patients get respiratory distress with tachypnoea following respiratory muscle weakness, pulmonary oedema and reduced respiratory drive. They present with a combined metabolic and respiratory acidosis. Treatment is with atropine and oximes.

Question 85: Systemic lupus erythematosus

Regarding systemic lupus erythematosus (SLE), the following statements are correct EXCEPT which one?

a) There is a 10:1 female preponderance, particularly affecting women of child-
bearing age

b) Patients with SLE and isolated lupus anticoagulant antibody are clinically coagulopathic contraindicating central neuraxial blockade
c) Peri-partum high dose steroid therapy may be necessary
d) Pregnant patients are at increased risk of pregnancy-induced hypertension, regardless of their pre-pregnancy renal status
e) More than 50% of patients with SLE have demonstrable psychiatric or neurological abnormalities including seizures and cerebrovascular events

Answer: b

Explanation

Systemic lupus erythematosus is an immune-mediated multisystem inflammatory disorder where autoantibodies are responsible for a diverse range of tissue damage and thus clinical manifestations. The condition's impact on coagulation is complex and not entirely intuitive. Patients may be coagulopathic or thrombophilic. Those patients with only the lupus anticoagulant IgG (or sometimes IgM) have prolonged activated partial thromboplastin time (APTT) in vitro, but do not have a bleeding tendency and the use of central neuraxial blockade is acceptable. However, caution must be exercised because prolonged APTT may also be caused by clinically relevant coagulopathies secondary to autoantibodies to clotting factors II, VII, VIII, IX and X. Pancytopenia is not uncommon with active disease. Hypercoagulable patients may present on anticoagulant therapy and liaison with a haematologist, well in advance of anaesthetic involvement, is prudent. Aside from the haematological manifestations, SLE is considered a connective tissue disorder although these abnormalities rarely impact on the anaesthetist here. Neurological, renal and cardiopulmonary complications do have implications for anaesthesia. Glomerulonephritis, hypertension and proteinuria are all common, but even without these pregnant patients with SLE are at elevated risk of pregnancy-induced hypertension. Patients may have accelerated coronary artery disease and pulmonary infiltrates or fibrosis. Therapy for SLE aims to ameliorate manifestations and dampen immune activity. It is common that SLE patients will be on glucocorticoid treatment, especially during pregnancy. Suppression of the hypothalamo–pituitary–adrenal axis should be considered and steroid supplementation at the time of delivery administered if necessary.

Reference

Davies SR. Systemic lupus erythematosus and the obstetrical patient – implications for the anaesthetist. *Can J Anaesth* 1991; **38**(6): 790–5.

Question 86: High-frequency oscillatory ventilation

A patient with severe acute respiratory distress syndrome (ARDS) develops a pneumothorax requiring insertion of a chest drain. You decide to institute high-frequency oscillatory ventilation (HFOV). Regarding this case which of the following options is CORRECT?

a) Positive end expiratory pressure (PEEP) levels during HFOV would be similar to those in an optimal conventional ventilator strategy
b) Tidal volumes employed in HFOV are generally only 1 to 2 mL/kg more than the physiological dead-space volume
c) Maximum ventilation frequency may be up to 300 per minute
d) On commencement of HFOV a drop in cardiac output and central venous pressure and a rise in pulmonary artery pressure would be expected
e) The tidal volume generated during HFOV is directly related to both the driving pressure and ventilator frequency, both of which are controlled by the operator

Answer: a

Explanation

High-frequency oscillatory ventilation (HFOV) delivers small tidal volumes at extremely high frequencies (anywhere from 3 to 15 Hz). Tidal volumes are usually 1 to 3 mL/kg less than the physiological dead space but gas exchange still occurs via a number of mechanisms including direct bulk flow, molecular diffusion, cardiogenic mixing and pendelluft, the latter due to regional differences in lung compliance and airway resistance. When initiating HFOV the frequency, I:E ratio, driving pressure and mean airway pressure are all set by the operator with the tidal volumes generated being directly related to the driving pressure and inversely related to the frequency. The potential advantages of HFOV over conventional ventilation include the delivery of smaller tidal volumes thus limiting alveolar overdistension, the application of a higher mean airway pressure (mPaw) than in conventional ventilation so promoting more alveolar recruitment and the maintenance of a constant mPaw during inspiration and expiration, thus preventing end-expiratory alveolar collapse. Patients treated with HFOV generally have an early and non-persistent increase in pulmonary artery occlusion pressure, a small persistent increase in central venous pressure and a small decrease in cardiac output compared with baseline. A small number of studies show that the use of HFOV in adult patients with ARDS is associated with improvements in oxygenation, without a significant reduction in mortality. Application of HFOV early in the course of ARDS may be associated with improved outcome but more trials are needed.

Reference

Krishnan JA, Brower RG. High-frequency ventilation for acute lung injury and ARDS. *Chest* 2000; **118**(3): 795–807.

Question 87: Estimated glomerular filtration rate

The following are used by a laboratory to calculate an estimated glomerular filtration rate EGFR EXCEPT for which one?

a) Age
b) Weight
c) Ethnic group
d) Local variations in serum creatinine measurement
e) Gender

Answer: b

Explanation

Estimated glomerular filtration rate (eGFR) has become the standard value used to quantify renal function. It is used to define a patient's degree of chronic kidney disease and in the calculation of nephrotoxic drug doses. eGFR can be calculated by the clinician by visiting online calculators, entering the patient's serum creatinine measurement and details of gender, age and ethnicity. A more accurate estimate is obtained by local laboratories who also take into consideration variations in measurement experienced within the local laboratory. It is still only an estimate and the standard formula for calculation is not accurate for children, pregnant women and people at the extremes of body habitus such as the malnourished or Class III obesity.

Reference

The Renal Association. eGFR calculator. Online at www.renal.org/eGFRcalc/GFR.pl (Accessed 30 October 2009)

Question 88: Pulmonary oedema

A 35-year-old male presents to the intensive care unit with respiratory failure requiring mechanical ventilation. His chest X-ray shows bilateral pulmonary infiltrates. Which of the following statements makes a diagnosis of non-cardiogenic pulmonary oedema MOST LIKELY?

a) The presence of peribronchial cuffing
b) Even or central radiographic distribution of the pulmonary oedema
c) The presence of septal lines
d) The presence of an air bronchogram
e) The presence of pleural effusions

Answer: d

Explanation

While pulmonary oedema may be relatively easy to diagnose, clinically elucidating the underlying cause is often far more taxing. These causes may be divided into cardiogenic and non-cardiogenic. The former is caused by a rapid increase in hydrostatic pressure in the pulmonary capillaries leading to increased transvascular fluid filtration. This in turn develops secondary to elevated pulmonary venous pressure from increased left ventricular end-diastolic pressure and left atrial pressure. The latter develops secondary to an increase in the vascular permeability of the lung leading to an increase in movement of fluid and protein into the lung interstitium and air spaces. Differentiation into non-cardiogenic and cardiogenic is based on a combination of history, physical examination, radiography, echocardiography and data from invasive cardiac output devices. Chest radiography is simple and used ubiquitously in this group of patients, but oedema may not even be visible until the amount of lung water increases by 30%. In addition other radiolucent material, such as pus and blood, may give a similar radiographic image and there are many technical problems associated with chest radiography in the critically ill that reduce both the sensitivity and specificity, e.g. incorrect penetration, rotation, degree of inspiration and PEEP. Radiographic features supporting a non-cardiogenic cause of pulmonary oedema are: normal heart size; normal or balanced vascular distribution; a patchy or peripheral distribution of the oedema; the absence of peribronchial cuffing; septal lines; pleural effusions and lastly the presence of air bronchograms. It is the presence of air bronchograms that is the MOST suggestive and thus the best answer here.

Reference

Ware LB, Matthay MA. Clinical practice: acute pulmonary edema. *New Engl J Med* 2005; **353**(26): 2788–96.

Question 89: Xenon

Regarding xenon, the following statements are true EXCEPT which one?

a) Xenon has analgesic as well as anaesthetic properties
b) Xenon may protect against hypoxic neuronal injury
c) A worldwide conversion to xenon use for anaesthesia would be beneficial with respect to climate change
d) Xenon's first reported use as an anaesthetic was in 1951
e) Xenon has a blood:gas partition coefficient of 0.115

Answer: c

Explanation

Xenon intermittently arises in MCQs. Xenon emerged as an anaesthetic agent in 1951 without gaining popularity or widespread use. It still interests examiners and researchers alike, as in many ways it resembles the perfect anaesthetic agent. It is an agent with rapid onset and offset due to its very low blood:gas partition coefficient, with a very low side-effect profile and can be extracted from the atmosphere. At 0.3 MAC it is equianalgesic to nitrous oxide. Current research has demonstrated a serendipitous tendency for xenon to halt excitotoxicity. This is the spiralling cell death that occurs in damaged neuronal tissue, especially when made hypoxic.

The main reason xenon has not caught on is cost. It is very expensive to purify (£100 000 per cylinder) and a large producer of carbon emissions as a one megawatt compressor has to run for one hour to produce one litre of xenon. It is therefore thought that the environmental impact of these emissions would not be offset by the cessation of release of current anaesthetic vapours.

Question 90: Wegener's granulomatosis

A previously fit and well 31-year-old male patient requiring ventilation for severe respiratory failure characterised by haemoptysis and hypoxia was found to have diffuse pulmonary haemorrhage. He also tested positive for haematuria and proteinuria. His tests for c-ANCAs (classical antineutrophil cytoplasmic antibodies) were positive, confirming the diagnosis of Wegener's granulomatosis. Once the diagnosis has been made, which one of the following would be the PREFERRED drug therapy?

a) Cyclophosphamide i.v. 1 g/day
b) Methylprednisolone i.v. 30 mg/day
c) Ciclosporin i.v. 200 mg/day
d) Azathioprine i.v. 250 mg/day
e) Methotrexate i.v. 7.5 mg/week

Answer: a

Explanation

Even though both high dose intravenous steroids and cyclophosphamide are used in the acute management of organ-threatening Wegener's granulomatosis, the answer to this question is cyclophosphamide as it is usually the specific definitive treatment for this condition and the dose of methylprednisolone is too low. Ciclosporin has been used in the management of patients with Wegener's granulomatosis who have not been successfully treated with cyclophosphamide and steroids. Azathioprine and methotrexate are both used in the longer term management of Wegener's granulomatosis, once the patient is in remission, as they are less toxic.

Question 91: Drugs in porphyria

You are working in the developing world and a patient with known acute intermittent porphyria presents for emergency surgery. Which one of the following pharmaceuticals would it be best to AVOID in this patient?

a) Suxamethonium
b) Halothane
c) Aspirin
d) Pancuronium
e) Ropivacaine

Answer: e

Explanation

The porphyrias are an example of pharmacogenetics in anaesthesia. Porphyrins (of which the most significant in humans is haem) are essential molecules concerned with oxygen transport and handling in the cell. They are manufactured via a sequence of enzyme-catalysed reactions from glycine and succinyl CoA. Congenital deficiencies in these enzymes lead to accumulation of porphyrin precursors, or porphyrinogens, which are responsible for clinical manifestations of the condition. The porphyrin biosynthesis pathway is very efficient and normally <2% of the precursors are produced in excess of that required for haem synthesis. The principal rate-limiting enzyme is δ-Aminolaevulinic acid (ALA) synthetase, which catalyses the initial combination of glycine and succinyl CoA. ALA synthetase is under tight negative feedback control via haem concentrations. If haem concentration falls, the enzyme is disinhibited and the biosynthesis pathway is encouraged. In the various types of porphyria, there are deficits in subsequent enzymes in the pathway. Acute attacks are precipitated by a drop in haem concentration prompting ALA synthetase to produce δ-ALA. Subsequent enzymes are then unable to continue the pathway. As haem is a pivotal component in cytochrome P450, enzyme-inducing drugs will increase demand for haem, drop its concentration and thereby induce an attack of porphyria. Unfortunately drugs to avoid are not limited to the usual quoted 'enzyme inducers' because there are a multitude of mechanisms by which administered drugs may reduce haem concentration or induce ALA synthetase. Drugs are classified by international consensus as *use, avoid, use with caution* and *use with extreme caution only*.

Reference

James MF, Hift RJ. Porphyrias. *Br J Anaesth* 2000; **85**(1): 143–53.

Question 92: Elective neurosurgery

Which one of the following statements is TRUE regarding anaesthesia for routine elective neurosurgery?

a) Desflurane is the agent of choice for many neuroanaesthetists
b) Dense neuromuscular blockade is required for a craniotomy
c) Permissive hypothermia is usually employed for cerebral protection
d) Resection of cortex is profoundly stimulating
e) A central venous catheter is mandatory for a craniotomy in a head-up position

Answer: a

Explanation

This question will be simple for those candidates who have clinical experience of neuroanaesthesia, but frustrating for those who have used standard textbooks to prepare for their exam. A consequence of modular training is that it is not uncommon that a candidate will be sitting their Final FRCA before completion of each of the anaesthetic sub-specialties. It is worthwhile trying to arrange some study leave accompanying a neuroanaesthetist for a routine neurosurgery list, as some of the historical mantras of neuroanaesthesia will be dispelled.

The concern over volatile anaesthetic agents is that they abolish cerebral autoregulation and cause a vasodilation that in turn increases intracranial pressure. This is counterbalanced by the fact that they reduce cerebral metabolism and reduce oxygen demand thus protecting neurones. Historically isoflurane was the agent of choice as its disruption in these respects was the least. In fact, all agents will diminish autoregulation in a dose-dependent fashion. Examination of data and graphs for percentage change in cerebral blood flow when compared to end-tidal agent concentration shows that at 0.5 minimum alveolar concentration (MAC) of isoflurane, sevoflurane, desflurane and even halothane there is minimal increase in cerebral blood flow over baseline. At 1 MAC of halothane, cerebral blood flow is increased to 250% of baseline and should therefore be avoided for neuroanaesthesia. However, for desflurane, isoflurane and sevoflurane at concentrations of around 1 MAC there is only a slight increase in cerebral blood flow (desflurane > isoflurane > sevoflurane). If a remifentanil infusion is used then analgesia may be titrated to cover particularly stimulating stages of a craniotomy, it is MAC sparing (so a full MAC of volatile agent is seldom required and the cerebral blood flow effects not seen) and dense neuromuscular blockade is not required as with adequate infusion rates spontaneous respiration, coughing and even response to laryngeal stimulation (by the endotracheal tube if the patient's head is moved) is abolished. Given the intricacy of the surgery it is of course mandatory that there is no movement (or potential movement) of the surgical field. The advantage of combining remifentanil and desflurane for a neuroanaesthetic is that rapid recovery allows early neurological assessment for potential deficit.

Application of Mayfield pins, dissection of the scalp (without local anaesthetic) and incision of the dura are very stimulating. The cortex is insensate and for the large part of the craniotomy stimulation is minimal.

Although an arterial line is required, a central venous catheter is rarely necessary (although this seems to be institution dependent). The use of central venous catheters for emergency aspiration of venous air embolism is attractive theoretically but may be practically prohibited. Hypothermia may be used in head injuries and some emergency work, but not for routine elective neurosurgery.

Question 93: Mechanism of action of inotropic drugs

The following drugs are correctly paired with their mechanism of action EXCEPT which one?

a) Dopexamine – dopamine and beta-adrenergic agonist
b) Prenalterol – beta-adrenergic agonist
c) Digoxin – inhibition of sodium–potassium ATPase pump
d) Bucladesine – phosphodiesterase inhibitor
e) Istaroxime – calcium channel stimulator

Answer: e

Explanation

There are a number of inotropic drugs currently under investigation. Very few of these will ever make it into mainstream clinical practice, and finding an agent that is both effective and safe when administered in the short or long term seems a long way off. The commonest inotropic agents currently in use work either by dopamine or adrenergic agonism or a combination of both. All of these agents have significant side effects. Several new classes of inotrope are under development including calcium channel stimulators, sodium channel stimulators, new sodium–potassium ATPase pump inhibitors, anti-endothelin agents, myosin activators, synthetic atrial natriuretic peptides, vasopressin antagonists and sodium–calcium exchange inhibitors. Within critical care a number of agents have been trialled with varying degrees of success. Most data exist about the phosphodiesterase inhibitors, e.g. amrinone, milrinone and bucladesine. They work by inhibiting type III phosphodiesterase thus preventing degradation of cAMP. As well as having an inotropic effect they cause vasodilation making their use somewhat challenging. Istaroxime, a sodium–potassium ATPase inhibitor has some promising animal data behind it. CK-1827452 is a cardiac myosin receptor entering human trials. Unlike the beta-adrenergic receptor agonists and phosphodiesterase inhibitors it does not increase intracellular calcium concentration or shorten ejection systolic time, so may have a much better safety profile. Ularitide (a synthetic atrial natriuretic peptide) has been used in the treatment of acute heart failure with mixed success. A number of other agents are entering phase I clinical trials.

Reference
Tavares M, Rezlan E, Vostroknoutova I, Khouadja H, Mebazza A. New pharmacologic therapies for acute heart failure. *Crit Care Med* 2008; **36**(1 Suppl): S112–20.

Question 94: Obstetric emergencies

Amniotic fluid embolism (AFE) is an obstetric emergency. Which one of the following statements is TRUE?

a) Polyhydramnios is a proven risk factor
b) AFE most commonly occurs during caesarean section
c) Regarding symptoms of AFE, headache is more common than chest pain
d) Presence of foetal squamous cells in the pulmonary vasculature is diagnostic
e) Delivery of the baby is not a priority in terms of improving maternal outcome

Answer: c

Explanation
Amniotic fluid embolism (AFE) is the peri-partum translocation of amniotic fluid, foetal cells and debris into the maternal circulation. There are no proven risk factors for AFE but polyhydramnios is an association. Of AFE cases, 70% occur during labour, 19% during caesarean section and 11% following vaginal delivery. Presenting symptoms (in order of frequency) are dyspnoea, cough, headache and chest pain. Presence of foetal squamous cells in the pulmonary vasculature is neither sensitive nor specific, but was once considered diagnostic. Management priorities are early recognition, immediate resuscitation and delivery of the baby. Life-threatening complications include cardiorespiratory collapse and haemorrhage secondary to disseminated intravascular coagulation.

Reference
Dedhia J, Mushambi M. Amniotic fluid embolism. *Contin Educ Anaesth Crit Care Pain* 2007; **7**(5): 152–6.

Question 95: Serum amylase

A 38-year-old woman who is hypotensive and has severe abdominal pain requires review. She has a raised serum amylase. Which of the following is the LEAST LIKELY to explain her symptoms and biochemical findings?

a) Perforated duodenal ulcer
b) Ruptured ectopic pregnancy
c) Diabetic ketoacidosis
d) Myocardial infarction
e) Acute pyelonephritis

Answer: e

Explanation
Amylase is a digestive enzyme that usually acts extracellularly to cleave starch into monosaccharides by hydrolysis of internal alpha-1,4-glycoside bonds resulting in the production of maltose and oligosaccharides. A variety of organs and secretions contain amylase activity, including the pancreas, salivary glands, fallopian tubes and cyst

fluid, testes, lungs, thyroid, tonsils, breast milk, sweat, tears and some malignant neoplasms (e.g. myeloma, phaeochromocytoma and carcinoma of the breast). The first two organs account for over 90% of the amylase produced. Electrophoresis shows that serum amylase is of two main types, P-type amylase from the pancreas, and S-type amylase from the salivary glands. Patients with acute pancreatitis usually have a raised amylase level but it may be normal even in the most severe cases of pancreatic necrosis and raised in many other conditions hence the use of serum lipase as a diagnostic test for acute pancreatitis. Other intra-abdominal pathologies causing raised amylase levels include inflammatory disease of the small intestine, mesenteric infarction, intestinal obstruction, appendicitis, abdominal aortic aneurysm and peritonitis, all of which usually result in increased P-type isoamylase. Serum amylase levels will also be raised in patients with liver and renal failure due to decreased clearance. Ruptured ectopic pregnancy, myocardial infarction and diabetic ketoacidosis are among other, non-GI tract causes of raised serum amylase level but not acute pyelonephritis.

Question 96: Adrenal cortex

Regarding hormone production in the adrenal cortex, the following statements are true EXCEPT which one? (CRH: corticotropin releasing hormone; ACTH: adrenocortico-trophin hormone)

a) Secretion of cortisol is under the exclusive control of the hypothalamopituitary CRH–ACTH axis
b) ACTH stimulates aldosterone secretion
c) Hyperkalaemia is a major stimulus to aldosterone secretion
d) Etomidate inhibits 17α-hydroxylase in the zona glomerulosa
e) Urinary cortisol metabolites give a reliable representation of cortisol secretion

Answer: d

Explanation
The adrenal cortex consists anatomically and functionally of three distinct zones, from superficial to deep, the zona glomerulosa, zona fasciculata and zona reticularis, which are responsible for the production of mineralocorticoids, glucocorticoids and androgens respectively. The precursor of all steroids produced here is cholesterol and subsequently pregnenolone, but then the synthetic pathways diverge and the steroid molecule ultimately produced depends on the enzymes to which it is exposed. The enzymes are of the cytochrome P450 superfamily and in each cortical zone are found those isoforms necessary for the production of the target steroid. The zona glomerulosa is deficient in 17α-hydroxylase hence it produces aldosterone whose biosynthesis does not require that enzyme. Etomidate inhibits 11β-hydroxylase and 17α-hydroxylase, both required for the production of cortisol in the zona fasciculata. Consequently, etomidate produces adrenal suppression, which after a single induction dose is of debated significance but if infused is associated with poor outcome. For this reason etomidate has been withdrawn for administration by intravenous infusion and in some countries it has been withdrawn altogether. Whereas cortisol secretion is responsive only to changes in ACTH level, aldosterone secretion can be influenced by angiotensin II, hyperkalaemia and ACTH. Cortisol secreted by the zona fasciculata and to a lesser extent the zona reticularis is 80% protein-bound in the plasma to a specific α_2-globulin. It undergoes hepatic reduction in phase I then conjugation with glucuronides during phase II. The glucuronides of cortisol are excreted renally. In the presence of normal hepatic and renal functions, measurement of urinary cortisol metabolites does give a true impression of glucocorticoid secretion.

Question 97: Distribution of cardiac output

At rest and during light, moderate or heavy exercise the distribution of cardiac output through specific vascular beds varies. For a typical 70 kg male, the following statements are true EXCEPT which one?

a) During heavy exercise, the cerebral blood flow is 750 mL/min
b) At rest, renal blood flow is 450 mL/min per 100 g of tissue
c) At rest, skeletal muscle receives 20% of total cardiac output
d) During heavy exercise, coronary blood flow increases eight-fold
e) During heavy exercise, splanchnic blood flow falls to around 1% of total cardiac output

Answer: d

Explanation

The distribution of cardiac output at rest and during exercise is to some extent intuitive, with blood flow being diverted to rapidly respiring tissues, sacrificed to those tissues less important during exercise and preserved unchanged to those tissues whose tolerance of relative ischaemia is poor (i.e. the central nervous system). Beware of confusing the factors by which cardiovascular and respiratory variables can be elevated. Minute ventilation can increase 30-fold; however, increase in cardiac output is a more modest five-fold, from around 5 L/min at rest to a maximum in the region of 25 L/min. The greatest proportional increase in blood flow during exercise is unsurprisingly through skeletal muscle. At rest, skeletal muscle receives around 1000 mL/ min, which although representing 20% of cardiac output when considered relative to total muscle mass supplied (34 kg) is only 2.9 mL/min per 100 g of tissue. During heavy exercise, skeletal muscle blood flow can increase 20-fold to 20 L/min (80% of cardiac output and 58 mL/min per 100 g). Compare this to the kidneys, which at rest also receive 1000 mL/min (20% of cardiac output), but given their much smaller mass, this represents 450 mL/min per 100 g. This is second only to the carotid bodies in terms of blood flow per mass of tissue. During exercise, renal blood flow can fall to 250 mL/min, at that stage just 1% of cardiac output. Splanchnic blood flow falls similarly. Coronary blood flow is 250 mL/min at rest and increases to a maximal 1000 mL/min during heavy exercise (a four-fold increase), thus as a proportion of total cardiac output it remains fairly consistent, which is also intuitive, given the determinants of coronary blood flow. As mentioned above, cerebral blood flow remains at 750 mL/min at rest or during exercise (54 mL/min per 100 g), but obviously as a proportion of total cardiac output, it falls from 15% at rest to 3% during heavy exercise.

Question 98: Statistical analysis

You have collected data on the blood pressure of 40 patients both pre- and post-admission to the critical care unit. You now wish to analyse this data. Which of the following statistical tests would be the MOST APPROPRIATE?

a) Mann-Whitney U test
b) Spearman's rank correlation coefficient
c) Kruskal–Wallace one-way analysis of variance
d) Paired Student's t-test
e) Wilcoxon signed-rank test

Answer: d

Explanation

There are many examples in medicine of continuous data (blood pressure, cholesterol, ejection fraction, etc.) There are a number of statistical methods for analysing this data, which can be divided into two main groups based on whether or not assumptions are made about the data that is being examined. Some distributions of data are described by quantities called parameters, for example the mean, standard deviation or variance, and methods that use distributional assumptions are called parametric methods. These methods (including various t-tests, and analysis of variance for comparing groups – also known as ANOVA) make the assumption that the data are normally distributed and also that the spread of the data is uniform either between the groups or across the range of values being examined. Non-parametric statistical tests (including those in Options (a), (b), (c) and (e)) do not require the data to follow a particular distribution and work by analysing the rank order of the data rather than the measurements themselves. Broadly speaking they are less powerful statistical tests unless the number of observations involved is large. It is possible to convert non-normally distributed data to make it suitable to be analysed by the more powerful parametric statistical tests.

Question 99: Intensive care unit-acquired weakness

The following statements regarding intensive care unit (ICU)-acquired weakness are true EXCEPT which one?

a) The incidence of critical illness polyneuropathy among septic shock patients on the ICU is 80%
b) Muscles of facial expression are spared by critical illness polymyopathy
c) Presence of normal deep tendon reflexes does not eliminate the diagnosis of critical illness polyneuropathy
d) Persistent hyperglycaemia is an independent risk factor for ICU-acquired weakness
e) Electrophysiological studies typically show a reduced nerve conduction velocity

Answer: e

Explanation

Acquired weakness is common among intensive care unit patients especially in those who have suffered systemic inflammatory conditions with multiorgan dysfunction. The exact aetiology remains to be elucidated but the demonstration of cytokine-initiated skeletal muscle breakdown does imply a chemical messenger-mediated process. The distinction between critical illness polyneuropathy and critical illness polymyopathy depends on detailed electroneurography, needle electromyography and a muscle biopsy. The exact clinical relevance of these invasive studies is debated given that therapeutic interventions are limited and are not specific to either variant. Focus should be on recognition of the at-risk population, preventative measures and, once symptomatic, exclusion of other (even pre-morbid) neurological conditions before arriving at the diagnosis. Risk factors are sepsis and other causes of systemic inflammation, multiorgan dysfunction, predicted prolonged immobility or ventilator dependence, hyperglycaemia and use of corticosteroids or non-depolarising muscle relaxants. Preventative measures involve avoiding those risks if possible and using minimal sedation techniques with frequent sedation holds to reduce complete immobility. Passive muscle exercises, ventilator-weaning regimens and optimising electrolytes and nutrition are also beneficial. In those patients who are able to co-operate with physical examination, serial neurological examination demonstrating symmetrical weakness with facial muscle sparing may obviate the need for invasive studies providing a slow improvement is demonstrable. In other circumstances, electrophysiological studies with or without muscle biopsy are required for diagnosis. In both critical illness polyneuropathy and myopathy, nerve conduction velocity is normal. However, in the neuropathy, compound muscle action potential and sensory nerve action potential are reduced. Differential diagnoses to be considered are diabetic neuropathy, porphyria, Guillian–Barré syndrome, myasthenic syndromes, subacute combined degeneration of the cord or muscular dystrophy. Also recall that low plasma phosphate, sodium, and potassium concentrations can be responsible for significant muscular weakness.

Reference
Schweickert W, Hall J. ICU-acquired weakness *Chest* 2007; **131**(5): 1541–9.

Question 100: Multiple sclerosis

Multiple sclerosis relapse is more commonly found to occur in all of the following situations EXCEPT which one?

a) Post-partum
b) Following influenza immunisation
c) In the spring and summer
d) Following periods of stress
e) Following hyperpyrexia

Answer: b

Explanation

Multiple sclerosis is an autoimmune disease characterised by demyelination of the central nervous system. Progression of the disease takes many forms but typically will involve either new symptoms occurring following acute attacks (relapsing) or slowly occurring over time (progressive). A number of factors have been shown to have associations with or to cause relapses. Pregnancy is protective against relapses in the third trimester, but once delivery has occurred is associated with relapse. There is no evidence showing an association between influenza immunisation and multiple sclerosis relapse. Relapse does have a seasonal variation and is associated with stress and raised temperature.

Reference
Confavreux C, Suissa S, Saddier P, Bourdès V, Vukusic S. Vaccinations and the risk of relapse in multiple sclerosis. Vaccines in Multiple Sclerosis Study Group. *New Engl J Med* 2001; **344**(5): 319–26.

Question 101: Non-obstetric surgery during pregnancy

A 23-year-old female presents on a Sunday evening with acute appendicitis and is booked for urgent appendicectomy. She is Caucasian and has been a UK resident all her life. She is 19 weeks pregnant. She was previously fit and well although has noticed some peripheral oedema and dyspnoea on exertion recently. On examination, she is found to be unwell, pyrexial (39.5 °C) and tachycardic. On praecordial auscultation, a mid- to late-systolic murmur at the left sternal edge is audible. Her electrocardiogram shows left axis deviation, some premature beats and some inconsistent T-wave changes. An echocardiogram cannot be performed until Monday morning. Her electrolytes are normal and she has been adequately volume resuscitated by the surgical team. Which one of the following statements regarding conduct of anaesthesia is TRUE?

a) Surgery should not be delayed until a cardiology opinion can be given
b) Coagulopathy of pregnancy necessitates availability of blood component therapy
c) Nitrous oxide should be avoided as there is evidence that, as a potent inhibitor of methionine synthetase, foetal detriment may be incurred
d) Awareness should be avoided by the use of slightly elevated concentrations of volatile anaesthetic agent, given the increased minimum alveolar concentration (MAC) associated with pregnancy
e) The prophylactic use of terbutaline, as a tocolytic, is recommended to avoid precipitating miscarriage

Answer: a

Explanation

The clinical features described are normal in pregnancy. The majority (97%) of murmurs detected in pregnancy are physiological and this murmur does not have sinister features. Of the other 3%, patients have often had exposure to infectious disease outside the UK. Furthermore, up to 93% of healthy pregnant women without structural heart disease have been shown to have an audible murmur of the type described at some stage during their pregnancy. The ECG changes are also normal in pregnancy. This patient is clearly toxic from her appendicitis and having been pre-optimised already, the greatest risk to mother and foetus is further delay. Pregnancy results in a thrombophilic state so careful attention must be paid to thromboprophylaxis. Theoretically nitrous oxide should be avoided for the reasons stated, but there is no evidence that the foetus is harmed if it is used. Minimum alveolar concentration decreases by up to 30% by 12 weeks gestation. There is no evidence for prophylactic tocolytics. Non-steroidal anti-inflammatory drugs must be avoided to avoid premature closure of the ductus arteriosus.

It should be noted that if a healthy pregnant woman presents to her midwife with these features (and without a pressing surgical emergency) the risk–benefit balance is altered: a high index of suspicion should be maintained and the murmur investigated.

Reference

Walton N, Melachuri V. Anaesthesia for non-obstetric surgery during pregnancy. *Contin Educ Anaesth Crit Care Pain* 2006; **6**(2): 83–5.

Question 102: Applied ultrasound

Regarding the physics of ultrasound, which one of the following statements is CORRECT?

a) Application of a direct current causes piezoelectric materials to vibrate
b) The speed of sound conduction through the human body is 940 m/s
c) Differences in acoustic impedance of different tissues causing refraction of the incident beam is the basis of ultrasound imaging in the body
d) For most applications in anaesthesia, e.g. vessel cannulation and regional anaesthesia, A-mode display format is employed
e) Anisotropy is an example of an ultrasound artefact where the echoic amplitude of a structure varies with the angle of insonation

Answer: e

Explanation

The basis of ultrasound imaging in the body is the reflection of sound pulses beyond the range of our hearing off the interface between tissues of different acoustic impedances. Return is best when the angle of incident sound (or insonation) is at 90° to the interface to be imaged. Refraction (the alteration of path direction on transition from one medium to another) only occurs when the angle of incidence is different to 90° and there is a significant change in the speed of sound between two media. The speed of sound through body tissues is fairly consistent at 1540 m/s (940 nm is the wavelength of the infrared LED in a pulse oximeter). Most ultrasound scanners used by anaesthetists use pulsed-wave emission and display in 2-D mode. A-, B- and M-mode display modalities give a highly detailed cross-section in one plane of the structure and, in M-mode, display its change over time. The application of an alternating current to a piezoelectric crystal causes it to vibrate (DC causes it to deform only). Pulsed-wave emission means that the probe will alternate between 'transmitting' and 'listening' tasks rapidly but will not do both at once. The frequency of the sound emitted in each pulse will be in the order of MHz (depending on the desired penetration), the pulse duration is typically 1 to 3 microseconds, and the pulse repetition frequency is how many pulses it will transmit per second while listening in between. This is between 1 and 10 kHz, which makes the gap for listening between pulses between 0.1 and 1.0 ms. This is mentioned to highlight that the probe spends much more time listening than transmitting. The sciatic nerve is highly anisotropic and will be bright at a 90° angle of insonation but virtually disappear at 80° or 100°.

Question 103: Femoral neck fractures

Regarding the clinical management of older patients with fractures of the femoral neck, the following are recognised targets EXCEPT which one?

a) Surgical fixation should be within 24 hours of admission unless there are clear reversible medical conditions
b) Patients should be admitted to an appropriate ward area within four hours of presentation
c) A preoperative electrocardiogram is mandatory
d) Addressing analgesic need is a clinical priority
e) Patients with a normal plain radiograph but a strong clinical suspicion of a fracture should undergo urgent supplementary imaging (MRI, CT or bone isotope scan)

Answer: a

Explanation
Although the topic of this question may seem suited to a surgical exam, the pivotal role of the anaesthetist in the pre-assessment and pre-optimisation of these often frail patients plus their involvement in theatre-list planning means familiarity with this subject is essential. The National Institute of Health and Clinical Excellence is in the process of producing a complete guideline of recommended practice for these patients. Until its publication the recognised standards are those of the British Orthopaedic Association Standards for Trauma (BOAST). As they stand, the target time for surgical fixation is 48 hours; however, local protocols may vary and indeed this may be revised to 24 hours in due course.

Reference
British Orthopaedic Association Standards for Trauma. BOAST 1: Hip fracture in the older person. British Orthopaedic Association, September 2007. Online at www.boa.ac.uk/default.aspx?ID=280 (Accessed 30 October 2009)

Question 104: Oxygen measurement

Regarding spectrophotometric oximetry, which one of the following statements is CORRECT?

a) 660 nm is the wavelength of light emitted by one of the LEDs in the apparatus because this is one of the isobestic points of the pertinent absorption spectra
b) While placed on the ear, approximately 30% of absorbed energy is due to the pulsatile component of the tissue
c) Venous blood in the tissues does not contribute to the absorption of the red and infrared light
d) Of all the potential colours of nail varnish, red-coloured nail varnish will disrupt the pulse oximeter to the greatest extent
e) Oximetry may determine relative proportions of carboxyhaemoglobin and methaemoglobin

Answer: e

Explanation

Oximetry is the technique by which the proportions of different varieties of haemoglobin in a sample are determined by examining the pattern with which red and infrared light successfully traverse the sample. It can be applied in vitro where a haemolysed sample may be exposed to a number of wavelengths of light and analysis of the absorption spectra allows determination of various haemoglobin combinations (deoxyhaemoglobin, oxyhaemoglobin, carboxyhaemoglobin, methaemoglobin) or in vivo as pulse oximetry where historically only deoxyhaemoglobin and oxyhaemoglobin are measured giving a quantification of oxygen saturation in arterial blood. In fact, there are now commercially available non-invasive monitors that may also determine other haemoglobins. The extent to which haemoglobin and oxyhaemoglobin absorb light varies according to the wavelength of the incident light. At around 700 nm, red light is absorbed well by deoxyhaemoglobin, but not by oxyhaemoglobin. This is intuitive as on visual inspection, deoxygenated blood appears dark and less red than oxygenated blood. This is because the red light is being absorbed. Oxygenated blood appears bright red because it does not absorb red light so well (thus we see it as red); however, at around 1000 nm it absorbs infrared light more than deoxygenated blood. By selecting light-emitting diodes (LEDs) with wavelengths in this region (and 660 nm and 940 nm), maximum discrepancy allows greatest sensitivity. The isobestic points are those wavelengths at which absorption by both types of haemoglobin are identical. The tissue composite through which the light travels is largely non-pulsatile: tissue, venous blood and that volume of arterial blood that is non-pulsatile. The component of the composite of interest is just the pulsatile component of the arterial blood. This forms a very small proportion of total absorption. Red nail varnish disrupts the signal least as it does not absorb the red light (hence it appears red to the eye).

Question 105: Drowning

Regarding drowning, the following statements are true EXCEPT which one?

a) Absence of water in the lungs at post mortem confirms a diagnosis of 'dry drowning', usually caused by laryngospasm
b) In the UK, 25% of cases of drowning occur in salt water
c) Atypical drowning may involve a sudden stopping of the heart on immersion in cold water
d) The incidence of cervical spine injury in drowning events is 1 in 200
e) Aspiration of as little as 200 mL of water by an 80 kg man may increase intrapulmonary shunt from 10% to 75%

Answer: a

Explanation

Drowning is a major cause of death worldwide and accounts for around 400 deaths per year in the UK. The majority of victims are under 25 years old. In 2003, the International Liaison Committee on Resuscitation (ILCOR) published the recommendations from a consensus conference on the uniform reporting of data from drowning. A drowning event was defined as a process resulting in respiratory impairment following immersion or submersion in a liquid. The report recommended abandoning the terms 'near drowning' and 'secondary drowning'. The mechanism of death in drowning is complex.

The majority of cases of drowning feature hypoxaemia following washout of pulmonary surfactant, alveolar collapse and intrapulmonary shunting. This may progress to ARDS in the following 72 hours. There used to be a lot of concern about whether the drowning had occurred in fresh water or salt water. This was thought to produce different profiles of electrolyte disturbance, but is now considered to only rarely be clinically relevant. Of drowning deaths, 15% are atypical and feature laryngospasm with minimal water entering the lungs or sudden cardiac standstill on immersion in cold water. However, the presence or absence of water in the lungs at post mortem does not indicate whether water was inhaled or not. The absence of water in the lungs may just indicate that the water has been absorbed and ILCOR also recommended that the term 'dry drowning' should be avoided. The most important factor determining the outcome following a drowning event remains the quality of immediate care the victim receives, with the target being rapid correction of hypoxaemia through rescue breathing or positive pressure ventilation.

References

Idris AH, Berg RA, Bierens J, *et al.* Recommended guidelines for uniform reporting of data from drowning: the 'Utstein style'. *Circulation.* 2003; **108**(20): 2565–74.

Soar J, Deakin CD, Nolan JP, *et al.* European Resuscitation Council. European Resuscitation Council guidelines for resuscitation 2005. Section 7. Cardiac arrest in special circumstances. *Resuscitation* 2005; **67**(Suppl 1): S135–70.

Question 106: Bodybuilder

A patient is admitted for incision and drainage of buttock abscesses. He is a 39-year-old professional bodybuilder who was competing in a national bodybuilding tournament four days ago. He is 185 cm tall and weighs 100 kg. He admits that his abscesses are due to long-term abuse of injected anabolic steroids administered into the buttock. Compared to a healthy male matched for age, height and weight who takes moderate exercise for 30 minutes three times a week, which of the following is LEAST LIKELY to be found in this patient?

a) A higher risk of developing atrial fibrillation
b) A higher anaerobic threshold
c) A higher risk of pressure sores
d) A faster emergence from volatile anaesthesia
e) A higher risk of venous thromboembolism

Answer: b

Explanation

From the history, there are two key points that need to be flagged up about the patient. First, he is a competition-prepared bodybuilder and, second, he is on parenteral anabolic steroids. Steroid abuse is common with a conservative estimate of 10 to 15% of regular gym attendees using anabolic steroids. Competitive bodybuilders train hard on high-calorie, protein-rich, low-fat diets in between competitions then go on to very low-calorie diets in the period leading up to competition. They reduce their body fat down to as low as 2 to 4% to improve muscle definition. At this level even the fat pads in their feet are reduced in size, so they are particularly at risk of pressure sores. In this condition, body builders are easily fatigued and so would perform less well than the comparison male who exercises regularly. The low body fat would also produce a faster emergence from volatile anaesthesia. Because of the illegal nature of steroid use, there are not and are never likely to be any randomised controlled trials looking at their side effects in the bodybuilding community. Information from case reports and series would suggest that bodybuilding and steroid abuse puts the patient at risk of a wide range of side effects. These may include palpitations, arrhythmias, left ventricular hypertrophy, hypertension, clotting abnormalities, hypercholesterolaemia, and both functional and structural abnormalities of the liver.

Reference

Kam PC, Yarrow M. Anabolic steroid abuse: physiological and anaesthetic considerations. *Anaesthesia* 2005; **60**(7): 685–92.

Question 107: Blood transfusion

From the *Serious Hazards of Transfusion Reports (SHOT) 1996–2008*, which one of the following conditions has resulted in the HIGHEST number of deaths in which a transfusion reaction was felt to be either causal or contributory?

a) Transfusion-related acute lung injury
b) Incorrect blood component transfused
c) Acute transfusion reaction
d) Transfusion-transmitted infections
e) Transfusion-associated graft versus host disease

Answer: a

Explanation

The first SHOT report looked at transfusion complications from data collected in 1996/1997. Since then, reports have been produced initially biannually and since 2003 on an annual basis. SHOT has a number of aims including the building of an evidence base of transfusion hazards, to make evidence-based and targeted recommendations for improvements in transfusion practice and to work with the national and international bodies responsible for transfusion safety. Reporting is voluntary but strongly encouraged by a number of organisations including the Department of Health as is advocated in their document 'Better Blood Transfusion'. To aid reporting SHOT, in conjunction with the Medicines and Healthcare products Regulatory Agency (MHRA), have set up an internet-based reporting system called SABRE (Serious Adverse Blood Reactions and Events). In time it is expected that reporting will become compulsory. Indications from the reports are that both the number of serious adverse events and the mortality directly related to transfusion have fallen since reporting first began. In total SHOT has recorded 125 deaths of which the most (40) have been attributed to transfusion-related acute lung injury (TRALI). This is likely to change as the number of reported TRALIs has fallen dramatically since the inception of TRALI reduction strategies in 2003–4. Incorrect blood and component transfusion, acute transfusion reaction, graft versus host disease and transfusion-transmitted infection (in that order) make up the rest of the 'top five' transfusion-related deaths.

Reference

Serious Hazards of Transfusion (SHOT) website. Online at www.shotuk.org (Accessed 30 October 2009)

Question 108: Prognosis following cardiac arrest

A patient is admitted to the intensive care unit following an out-of-hospital ventricular fibrillation cardiac arrest. He was sedated and cooled for 24 hours and is now 72 hours post event. Which of the following is NOT invariably associated with a poor outcome (i.e. a Glasgow Outcome Scale score of three or less)?

a) Absent bilateral N20 response from the primary somatosensory cortex at 72 hours post event
b) Extensor posturing to noxious stimulus at 72 hours post event
c) Absence of a corneal response at 72 hours post event
d) Myoclonic status epilepticus at 24 hours post event
e) Significantly elevated levels of S100 (glial protein) post cardiac arrest

Answer: e

Explanation

A patient's outcome following cardiac arrest is improved by cooling post event. However, a proportion of these patients still die or are left with a significant neurological disability. A comatose state (otherwise known as anoxic-ischaemic encephalopathy) post resuscitation is associated with poor prognosis, but within this group a small proportion will make a good neurological recovery. Most studies that have assessed predictors of outcome in this patient group have as an objective the reliable prediction of an outcome better than a Glasgow Outcome Scale score of three or less. This scale gives scores of one to five (one = dead; two = vegetative state; three = severe disability; four = moderate disability; and five = a good recovery) and a score of three or less is considered a poor prognosis. A number of clinical signs are associated with poor prognosis and a subgroup of these are invariably associated with poor prognosis. The latter group includes an absent pupillary response 72 hours post event (but not on admission to hospital), a motor response to noxious stimuli that is no better than extensor posturing (i.e. a decerebrate response or no response) at 72 hours and an absent corneal response also at 72 hours. Myoclonic status epilepticus usually presents as bilaterally synchronous twitches of limb, trunk, or facial muscles and is most commonly detected at 24 hours. Its presence is, likewise, invariably a marker of a poor outcome. The measurement of somatosensory evoked potentials (SSEPs), especially the N20 response from the primary somatosensory cortex, has emerged as an extremely accurate predictor of a poor outcome in patients with anoxic-ischaemic encephalopathy. Bilateral absence of the N20 response 72 hours post event is again invariably associated with poor outcome. Several chemicals are released from the brain into the blood and cerebrospinal fluid after cardiac arrest, including neuron-specific enolase and S100 (glial protein). The former shows a strong correlation with outcome, the latter far less so. The measurement of other clinical variables has insufficient predictive value to be as useful in clinical practice, i.e. they may be associated with poor outcome but the correlation is less strong than those above. These include age, sex, cause of cardiac arrest, type of arrhythmia, total arrest time, body temperature on admission and duration of CPR.

Reference

Young G. Clinical practice. Neurologic prognosis after cardiac arrest. *N Engl J Med* 2009; **361**(6): 605–11.

Question 109: Diabetes mellitus

Regarding the anaesthetic considerations of patients with diabetes mellitus, the following are correct EXCEPT which one?

a) The National Institute of Health and Clinical Excellence recommends preoperative urinalysis for ASA 2 patients with cardiovascular comorbidity
b) The Alberti regime initially involves 500 mL of 10% dextrose with 10 mmol of potassium chloride and 10 units of rapid acting soluble insulin infused at 100 mL/h
c) Patients with diabetes are prone to gastroparesis and thus pulmonary aspiration of gastric contents
d) Glycosylation of collagen in cervical and temporomandibular joints may render laryngoscopy difficult
e) Autonomic dysfunction is detectable in 40% of patients with diabetes mellitus Type 1

Answer: a

Explanation

Options (c) and (d) are well known facts and should be considered in clinical practice and quoted in viva responses regarding the challenges that face the anaesthetist in the peri-operative management of the patient with diabetes. Similarly the Alberti regime is something to be learned and should not trip up the informed candidate in this case.

This leaves (a) and (e), which might be the correct answers. A candidate may scour endocrinology texts to confirm or refute the value of 40% in (e); however, examiners are well aware that different sources will quote a variety of values but that these will likely be in a range about a mean. In cases such as these, if the branch is false, it is likely to be so by an order of magnitude (e.g. 4%) or at least double or half (80% or 20%) in order to acknowledge that sources vary. If the value appears to be close to the one the candidate has learned (or even sounds sensible) it is more than likely to be true because if it were false it would be *very* false.

By exclusion, therefore, this leaves (a) as the correct answer. It seems intuitive good practice to perform urinalysis for glucose, protein and ketones in a preoperative patient with diabetes. In the extensive document published by NICE in June 2003 there is no specific mention of this. Authorities involved in compiling the recommendations did not reach consensus on the value of preoperative urinalysis. This answer can be reached by exclusion without memorising the content of the NICE guidelines; however, it would be worth the candidate having an overview of the recommendations and in particular those that seem counterintuitive.

Reference
National Collaborating Centre for Acute Care. Preoperative tests. The use of routine preoperative tests for elective surgery. Evidence, methods and guidance. NHS/NICE, June 2003. Online at www.nice.org.uk/nicemedia/pdf/Preop_Fullguid eline.pdf (Accessed 30 October 2009)

Question 110: Withdrawn drugs

All of the following drugs were withdrawn or had their licence removed because of cardiovascular adverse effects at therapeutic doses EXCEPT which one?

a) Cisapride
b) Aprotinin
c) Droperidol
d) Co-proxamol
e) Rofecoxib

Answer: d

Explanation
Cisapride was withdrawn in 2000. This prokinetic agent was found to prolong the QT interval and had been associated with 125 reported fatalities worldwide. The risks were thought to outweigh the benefits. Aprotinin was withdrawn from the formulary in 2008. A 2006 study by Mangano *et al.* demonstrated a doubling in the incidence of serious renal damage. Congestive heart failure increased by 50% and strokes by 180%. This was followed up by the BART study, which was halted following demonstration of significantly increased mortality in the aprotonin-treated group. Droperidol is a dopamine receptor antagonist that also prolongs the QT interval. It was withdrawn in the UK in 2001 and has remained so up to the time of going to press. It is, however, currently being relaunched throughout Europe. Co-proxamol is a combination of paracetamol and dextropropoxyphene. It causes respiratory depression and cardiac arrhythmias in overdose. It has some undesirable non-cardiovascular adverse effects at therapeutic doses, such as dizziness and dependence, and some undesirable drug interactions, such as with carbamazepine. Rofecoxib was removed from the formulary in one of the most expensive drug withdrawals ever. Worldwide turnover of rofecoxib in the year prior to withdrawal had exceeded $2 billion. The VIGOR study and the

APPROVE study demonstrated an increase in stroke and myocardial infarction in patients on rofecoxib.

References
Mangano DT, Tudor IC, Dietzel C. The risk associated with aprotinin in cardiac surgery. *N Engl J Med* 2006; **354**(4): 353–65.
BART Investigators. A comparison of aprotinin and lysine analogues in high-risk cardiac surgery. *N Engl J Med* 2008; **358**(22): 2319–31. Online at http://content.nejm.org/cgi/content/full/358/22/2319 (Accessed 30 October 2009)

Question 111: Rivaroxaban

Regarding rivaroxaban, which one of the following statements is TRUE?

a) It is a new oral direct thrombin inhibitor
b) It is a pro-drug
c) At therapeutic doses, it has a superior effect on venous thromboembolism rate compared to enoxaparin
d) At therapeutic doses, it produces lower rates of bleeding complications compared to enoxaparin
e) It has a half-life of two to four hours

Answer: c

Explanation
Rivaroxaban and dabigatran are new anticoagulants that may have an important role in patient care. They are administered orally, avoiding painful injections and have a relatively fast onset of action (one to four hours post ingestion). Rivaroxaban is a direct factor Xa inhibitor and therefore stops the production of thrombin while allowing existing thrombin to produce haemostasis. Dabigatran is a pro-drug that becomes a direct thrombin inhibitor and so may stop existing thrombin from contributing towards clot formation. In therapeutic trials (RECORD trials 1 to 4), rivaroxaban had a better effect on venous thromboembolism rate than enoxaparin, and had a mildly raised but not statistically significant rate of bleeding complications. Rivaroxaban's half-life is 7 to 9 hours with factor Xa activity not returning to normal for 24 hours, allowing once-daily dosing. This is important knowledge to have when timing such activities as surgery or removal of an epidural catheter, as rivaroxaban has no reversal agent and its effects are difficult to assess through standard laboratory tests.

Reference
RECORD4 Investigators. Rivaroxaban versus enoxaparin for thromboprophylaxis after total knee arthroplasty (RECORD4): a randomised trial. *Lancet* 2009; **373**(9676): 1673–80.

Question 112: Conn's syndrome

In primary hyperaldosteronism (Conn's syndrome) which one of the following is MOST LIKELY to be found on routine blood investigations?

a) High potassium, low sodium and high hydrogen ions
b) High potassium, low sodium and low hydrogen ions
c) Low potassium, low sodium and high hydrogen ions
d) Low potassium, high sodium and high hydrogen ions
e) Low potassium, high sodium and low hydrogen ions

Answer: e

Explanation

Conditions such as Conn's syndrome are loved by examiners, as they are a pathology that makes the candidate think clearly about normal physiology. In clinical practice they are rarely seen by anaesthetists, but this piece of information is of little solace sitting in the exam room. It is also a condition much loved by physicians, as it is one of the few causes of hypertension that you can do something about.

Aldosterone maintains circulating volume by retaining sodium. An excess of aldosterone will lead to an excess of renal re-absorption of sodium in exchange for potassium. There then may be increased secretion of hydrogen ions in the collecting duct in response to the hypokalaemia. In the real world of clinical medicine, patients with Conn's syndrome do present with hypokalaemia and alkalosis, but rarely have hypernatraemia.

Question 113: Failed intubation

A 21-year-old woman has acute appendicitis and requires general anaesthesia for an appendicectomy. Thorough pre-oxygenation is undertaken and a rapid sequence induction of anaesthesia is performed using 5 mg/kg of thiopentone and 1.5 mg/kg of suxamethonium while a trained assistant applies 30 N of cricoid pressure. After three attempts at tracheal intubation it has not been possible to intubate the trachea.

According to the Difficult Airway Society guidelines, which one of the following options is the most appropriate action to be taken NEXT?

a) Have one last (fourth) attempt at intubation
b) Check and optimise the patient's head and neck position
c) Request that the assistant perform backwards–upwards–rightwards pressure
d) Recognise that this is a failed intubation and move to 'Plan B'
e) Ventilate via a facemask

Answer: e

Explanation

It is essential to be familiar with the Difficult Airway Society guidelines on management of failed intubation. There are separate, slightly dissimilar, guidelines for intubation of the trachea in the presence of high or low risk of aspiration of stomach contents. Clearly there are certain sensible behaviours and their precise order can be debated so this question is based on the suggested order of the Difficult Airway Society. As the guidelines stand it is suggested that during a rapid sequence induction, no more than three attempts at tracheal intubation should be made in order to prevent delay in acknowledging failure and moving on toward a solution. Where there is low risk of aspiration, it is suggested that no more than four attempts should be made. The patient's head and neck position should be optimised before pre-oxygenation is commenced and re-checked after the first failed attempt. However, after three failed attempts, options such as re-positioning, using a different laryngoscope blade, external laryngeal manipulation or use of an introducer should be abandoned in favour of moving on through the algorithm. The objective (Plan C) should be to maintain oxygenation while awakening the patient – this may be with a facemask although a supraglottic device may become necessary. There is no 'Plan B' (secondary tracheal intubation plan) here, as attempts to intubate the trachea have been abandoned. Plan B applies where there is a low risk of aspiration of stomach contents.

Reference

Difficult Airway Society. Rapid sequence induction – Guidelines. Online at www.das. uk.com/guidelines/rsi.html (Accessed 30 October 2009)

Question 114: Gas analysis

The following methods can be used, clinically or experimentally, to detect carbon dioxide, EXCEPT for which one?

a) Infrared light spectroscopy
b) Infrared photoacoustic spectroscopy
c) Raman spectroscopy
d) Polarography
e) Chromatography

Answer: d

Explanation

Three techniques may detect all gases pertinent to anaesthesia (oxygen, carbon dioxide, nitrous oxide, nitrogen and volatile anaesthetic agents). They are mass spectrometry, Raman spectroscopy and gas chromatography. Oxygen may also be detected by polarography (Clarke electrode), fuel cell and paramagnetism. Molecules with two dissimilar atoms (carbon dioxide, nitrous oxide and volatile anaesthetic agents) may be detected by infrared light spectroscopy and infrared photoacoustic methods. Finally, volatile anaesthetic agents may also be measured by piezoelectric resonance.

Question 115: Heparin-induced thrombocytopenia (HIT)

Regarding heparin-induced thrombocytopenia (HIT) the following statements are true EXCEPT which one?

a) The patient receiving low molecular weight heparin is less likely to develop HIT than the patient receiving unfractionated heparin
b) A diagnosis of HIT is more likely if the platelet count falls to $50 \times 10^9/L$ than falls to $10 \times 10^9/L$
c) The assays used to make a diagnosis of HIT have a higher specificity than they do sensitivity
d) A patient with HIT is more likely to develop thrombosis than a similar patient without HIT
e) Prophylactic platelet transfusions should be avoided in a patient with HIT

Answer: c

Explanation

Heparin-induced thrombocytopenia is defined as a decrease in platelet count during or shortly after exposure to heparin. There are two types of HIT. HIT type 1 affects up to 10% of patients receiving treatment with heparin, is non-immune, is characterised by a mild and transient asymptomatic thrombocytopenia and disappears when the heparin is withdrawn. HIT type 2 is immune mediated and associated with thrombosis. The latter occurs in 1 to 5% of patients receiving unfractionated heparin. The risk is much lower with low molecular weight heparin. The increased thrombosis risk is due to the development of an antigen complex of heparin and platelet factor 4 (PF4). This leads to increased platelet activation thus predisposing to thrombosis. As the assays used to diagnose HIT are extremely sensitive but not specific it is important to limit testing to those patients deemed at highest risk of HIT type 2. Various HIT scoring systems exist to determine those patients who should be tested. These are based around the '4Ts' – Thrombocytopenia, Timing, Thrombosis and the absence of oTher explanations. Mortality in HIT type 2 is high and treatment other than general supportive care starts with immediate cessation of heparin administration. Danaparoid, epoprostenol, lepirudin or argatroban may be used as alternative anticoagulants. There may be possible treatment benefit with plasmapheresis, aspirin, clopidogrel and glycoprotein IIb/IIIa inhibitors. Platelet transfusion and warfarin should both be avoided.

Reference
Arepally G, Ortel TL. Clinical practice. Heparin-induced thrombocytopenia. *New Engl J Med* 2006; **355**(8): 809–17.

Question 116: Carbohydrate-rich beverages

The preoperative administration of carbohydrate-rich beverages has been shown to reduce all the following EXCEPT which one?

a) Risk of significant aspiration
b) Postoperative nausea and vomiting
c) Insulin resistance
d) Length of hospital stay
e) Anxiety

Answer: a

Explanation
Following questioning of old received wisdom that all patients should be kept nil by mouth for six hours for solids and four hours for clear fluids pre-operatively, a number of research projects have examined the impact of allowing the consumption of carbohydrate-rich (CHO) beverages two to three hours before induction. Post-operative nausea and vomiting (PONV), insulin resistance, thirst and anxiety have all been shown to be improved by CHO drinks. In a small randomised controlled study by Noblett *et al.* (2006), a significant decrease in hospital stay was demonstrated. No study has yet proven an increased aspiration risk.

Reference
Noblett SE, Watson DS, Huong H, *et al.* Preoperative oral carbohydrate loading in colorectal surgery: a randomised controlled trial. *Colorectal Dis* 2006; **8**(7): 563–9.

Question 117: U waves

The following are recognised causes of a U wave on an electrocardiogram EXCEPT which one?

a) Congenital long QT syndrome
b) Hypercalcaemia
c) Flecainide
d) Thyrotoxicosis
e) Hypokalaemia

Answer: c

Explanation
A U wave is a small wave on the ECG, which begins after the T wave terminates. The U wave usually has the same polarity as the T wave. A number of hypotheses explain their presence on an ECG. These include U waves representing repolarisation of the Purkinje fibres or that they may represent delayed after-potentials. They occur with the disturbances outlined above, on exposure to adrenaline or as part of digitalis toxicity. They are sometimes seen following an intracranial haemorrhage or mitral valve pro-lapse. They can be found with Class Ia and III antiarrhythmic agents. Flecainide is a Ic

agent and does not cause U waves. Inverted U waves are sometimes seen following myocardial infarction or fluid overload of the left ventricle and have a high specificity for demonstrating significant underlying disease.

Question 118: Throat pack insertion

The National Patient Safety Agency (NPSA) recommends a number of methods to reduce the risk of a throat pack (TP) being inadvertently left *in situ*. As part of these recommendations they suggest that one of two methods be used in all cases. Which of the following options contains BOTH of these suggested methods?

a) Placing a visible label on the patient stating a TP is *in situ* and removing it when the TP is removed, or placing a label on the airway device (LMA or endotracheal tube) stating a TP is *in situ*.
b) Tying one end of the TP to the airway device, or recording insertion and removal of the TP as part of the formal swab count
c) Recording insertion and removal of the TP as part of the formal swab count, or performing a formalised two-person check of the insertion and removal of the TP
d) Leaving part of the TP protruding externally, or putting a visible label or mark on the patient stating a throat pack is *in situ*
e) Recording insertion and removal of the TP as part of the formal swab count, or attaching the TP securely to the artificial airway device

Answer: c

Explanation
A joint working party including the National Patient Safety Agency (NPSA), the Royal College of Anaesthetists, and the Association of Anaesthetists of Great Britain and Ireland has examined the evidence for and methods to prevent the inadvertent retention of throat packs (TPs). Of 63 270 recorded incidents in 2006 and 2007 the NPSA identified 38 that were related to TPs of which one resulted in moderate harm to the patient. Twenty-four of the incidents were related to inadvertent retention, the rest related to the act of insertion itself. The report questioned the need for a TP in the vast majority of cases. The working party recommended six methods to reduce TP retention, and that two methods should be employed for each TP insertion. Of these, one of either recording the TP insertion as part of the formal swab count, or performing a formalised two-person check of TP insertion and removal should be used in each case. The other four methods are putting a label or mark on the patient, putting a label or mark on the airway device, securely attaching the TP to the airway device, or leaving part of the TP protruding externally.

Reference
National Patient Safety Agency website. Online at www.npsa.nhs.uk (Accessed 30 October 2009)

Question 119: Non-invasive ventilators

According to the British Thoracic Society guidelines on non-invasive ventilation (2002), essential features of a non-invasive ventilator include the following EXCEPT which one?

a) A disconnection alarm
b) Internal battery with power for at least one hour
c) Sensitive flow triggers
d) Rate capability of at least 40 breaths/min
e) Pressure control

Answer: b

Explanation

According to British Thoracic Society guidelines, the seven essential features of a non-invasive ventilator are a disconnection alarm, sensitive flow triggers, rate capability of at least 40 breaths/min, pressure control, a pressure capability of at least 30 cmH$_2$O, a capability of supporting flows of at least 60 L/min, and assist-control and bi-level pressure support modes. An internal battery was one of a further ten desirable features.

Reference

British Thoracic Society Standards of Care Committee. Non-invasive ventilation in acute respiratory failure. *Thorax* 2002; **57**(3): 192–211. Online at www.brit-thoracic.org.uk/Portals/0/Clinical%20Information/NIV/Guidelines/NIV.pdf (Accessed 30 October 2009)

Question 120: Myasthenic syndromes

Which one of the following clinical features is MOST LIKELY to distinguish myasthenia gravis from Lambert–Eaton myasthenic syndrome?

a) Aged 55 at onset of symptoms
b) An improvement of strength with the administration of intravenous edrophonium
c) Involvement of facial muscles
d) Finding of immunoglobulin G antibodies to the nicotinic acetylcholine receptor
e) Presence of deep tendon reflexes

Answer: d

Explanation

Myasthenia gravis (MG) is an autoimmune disorder of the neuromuscular junction involving autoantibodies to the post-synaptic acetylcholine receptor. Given the amount of receptor redundancy at this site, receptors need to be reduced to less than 30% of their quantity in health before the typical weakness is manifest. Most commonly bulbar and eye muscles are affected but a fluctuating degree of generalised muscle weakness is seen, which at its greatest extreme (Grade IV) requires mechanical ventilation. Lambert–Eaton myasthenic syndrome (LEMS) is also an autoimmune disorder of the neuromuscular junction involving immunoglobulin G autoantibodies but these are to the pre-synaptic voltage-gated calcium channels, which ultimately cause defective release of acetylcholine from the terminal button of the motor neurone. It is associated with small cell lung cancer and the distribution of the weakness tends to favour proximal muscles of the lower limb. However, facial muscle weakness, diplopia and ptosis are seen with LEMS and this feature is not a reliable distinguisher. Classically, tendon reflexes are present in MG and absent in LEMS; however, LEMS weakness improves with exercise of the muscle at which point tendon reflexes may return. Myasthenia gravis weakness worsens with sustained or repeated use of the muscle – the so-called fatiguability. Edrophonium is a cholinesterase inhibitor, which via increasing the quantity of acetylcholine at the neuromuscular junction will cause a transient improvement of symptoms in MG. However, it is not uncommon for edrophonium to have a similar effect in LEMS. In LEMS, autonomic dysfunction is sometimes noted, in particular a dry mouth and, of course, if there is an underlying malignancy the patient may be cachectic and complain of B-symptoms. The presence of anti-acetylcholine receptor autoantibodies would allow the confident diagnosis of MG rather than LEMS (however, it is only identified in 90% of cases).

Question 121: Soda lime

Regarding the soda lime in a circle system, the following statements are true EXCEPT which one?

a) The granule diameter is 3 to 4 mm
b) If it contains Titan Yellow, the colour change will be from deep pink when fresh to off-white when exhausted
c) It will contain water even in an unopened packet prior to use
d) It will always contain calcium hydroxide
e) As it is used there will be a steady decline in the amount of sodium hydroxide present

Answer: e

Explanation

Soda lime is made up of calcium hydroxide (approximately 95% and always present), sodium hydroxide and sometimes some potassium hydroxide (e.g. in Baralyme). In addition there will be some silicates for binding, water (even prior to first use) and a colour indicator. Titan Yellow causes the soda lime to turn from deep pink to off-white (fresh to exhausted), and Ethyl Violet causes a change from white to purple (fresh to exhausted). Soda lime is capable of absorbing approximately 25 L of CO_2 per 100 g. Carbon dioxide reacts with sodium (and potassium) hydroxide to form sodium carbonate. This then reacts with calcium hydroxide to reform the sodium hydroxide and produce calcium carbonate. Thus it is only at the very end of soda lime's active life that the sodium hydroxide concentration falls. This reaction is exothermic and produces water, both of which may be beneficial especially at low flows as it will humidify and warm the inspired gases.

Question 122: Paediatric advanced life support

A 15 kg two-year-old boy is being anaesthetised, spontaneously breathing on a laryngeal mask airway, for exploration and repair of a small umbilical hernia. The child is otherwise fit and well. Thirty minutes into the procedure, for no apparent reason, the child develops a bradycardia of 30 bpm and end-tidal CO_2 falls to zero. With regard to the choice of uncuffed endotracheal tube (internal diameter in mm) for initial intubation attempt, the bolus dose of intravenous adrenaline, and setting for the manual monophasic defibrillator, which of the following options describes the BEST practice?

a) 4.0 endotracheal tube, 300 mcg adrenaline, defibrillator set to 30 joules
b) 4.5 endotracheal tube, 150 mcg adrenaline, defibrillator set to 60 joules
c) 4.0 endotracheal tube, 150 mcg adrenaline, defibrillator set to 60 joules
d) 4.5 endotracheal tube, 150 mcg adrenaline, defibrillator set to 30 joules
e) 4.0 endotracheal tube, 300 mcg adrenaline, defibrillator set to 60 joules

Answer: b

Explanation

The age-based formula for endotracheal tube size of (age in years/4) + 4 is well known and well validated for children aged over one year. This formula gives a figure of 4.5. It is recommended that at least a tube size larger and smaller should be available. The problem with age-based formulae is that children come in such a range of sizes for any given age. This child, at 15 kg by two years old, is on the 95th centile on the UK growth charts, so having an even larger tube available would be wise. The intravenous bolus dose of adrenaline is 10 mcg/kg. The 2005 Paediatric Advanced Life Support guidelines recommend an initial shock with 4 joules/kg. The previous guidelines had recommended 2 to 4 joules/kg but this has now been adjusted up to the higher figure as higher energies effectively defibrillated children with negligible adverse effects.

Reference
Paediatric Advanced Life Support. Resuscitation guidelines. Resuscitation Council (UK), 2005. Online at www.resus.org.uk/pages/pals.pdf (Accessed 30 October 2009)

Question 123: Methylene blue
Regarding methylene blue, the following statements are true EXCEPT which one?

a) It has been used in cases of anaphylaxis previously unresponsive to standard treatment
b) It has been used in combination with light to treat psoriasis
c) It has been used to treat arsenic poisoning
d) It has been used to treat methaemoglobinaemia
e) It has been used to treat malaria

Answer: c

Explanation
Methylene blue has had many uses in medicine. It has been used successfully in the treatment of anaphylaxis resistant to all other therapies, with light in the treatment of psoriasis, in managing methaemoglobinaemia and treating malaria. Its main historical indication in the management of poisons was to treat potassium cyanide toxicity. Cyanide inhibits mitochondrial cytochrome oxidase, causing cytotoxic hypoxia. Methylene blue is not now recommended as it may reverse treatment with nitrites, releasing free cyanide. It is not used in the treatment of arsenic poisoning. Methylene blue sometimes contains small quantities of arsenic as an impurity. This has been put forward as an explanation for the gastrointestinal symptoms some patients experience when treated with methylene blue.

Question 124: Arterial supply of the spinal cord
Regarding the arterial supply of the spinal cord, the following statements are true EXCEPT which one?

a) There are two posterior spinal arteries and one anterior spinal artery, all derived from the vertebral arteries
b) The great anterior radicular artery (spinal artery of Adamkiewicz) most often arises at T10 on the left
c) Some radicular arteries derive their supply from intercostal arteries
d) The pia mater does not cover the spinal vasculature
e) The anterior inferior spinal cord is more vulnerable to ischaemia than the posterior cord

Answer: d

Explanation
The anterior spinal artery is unpaired, being formed by a branch from each vertebral artery anastomosing at the level of the foramen magnum. The two posterior spinal arteries are variably described as originating from the vertebral arteries or sometimes via the posterior inferior cerebellar arteries. These are branches of the vertebral arteries so Option (a) remains correct. These three arteries run the length of the spinal cord, augmented in a segmental fashion by radicular arteries at most (usually 21) spinal

levels. The origin of the radicular arteries depends on the vertebral level at which they contribute to the anterior and posterior spinal arteries, thus they are derived from the vertebral, deep cervical, intercostal and lumbar arteries. Those radicular arteries that do not contribute to the longitudinal arteries directly supply the cord at that level. Posteriorly, a dense plexus of arterial anastomoses confer more reliable supply of oxygenated blood. Anteriorly, the single spinal artery means occlusion or hypoperfusion risks ischaemia. One radicular artery dominates supply to the inferior two thirds of the cord. This is known as the radicularis magna, great anterior radicular artery or spinal artery of Adamkiewicz. Aortic or spinal surgery or traumatic spinal cord injury may disrupt this supply with the consequence of flaccid paraplegia and symmetrical loss of pain and temperature perception below the level of the ischaemia, as these pathways run in the anterior part of the cord. The great anterior radicular artery arises in the lower thoracic or upper lumbar levels, but with greatest frequency arises on the left at T10. The pia mater is closely adherent to the substance of the cord, but does cover the spinal vessels and ensheathes the anterior spinal artery.

Question 125: Prostaglandins in pregnancy

A 23-year-old severely asthmatic primigravida suffers a major post-partum haemorrhage due to uterine atony following a vaginal delivery. As well as appropriate therapy of major haemorrhage she receives syntometrine intramuscularly, syntocinon intravenously as a bolus and then by infusion. Which one of the following would be the MOST SUITABLE agent for further pharmacological management of her condition?

a) Carboprost
b) Mifepristone
c) Misoprostol
d) Alprostadil
e) Dinoprostone

Answer: c

Explanation

All of the options are synthetic prostaglandin analogues except mifepristone, which is a competitive antagonist at the progesterone receptor (it is used in the induction of medical abortion and should be avoided in asthmatics). Carboprost (Hemabate®) is prostaglandin $F_{2\alpha}$ and although is a suitable treatment for post-partum haemorrhage as an intramuscular injection, it should be avoided in severe asthmatics because of its side effect of bronchospasm. Dinoprostone (prostaglandin E_2 – Prostin E2®) is used as a vaginal gel or pessary in the process of induction of labour. It should also be used with caution in asthmatics. Misoprostol (Cytotec®) and alprostadil (Prostin VR®) are both analogues of prostaglandin E_1 and do not carry the same cautions for treatment of asthmatics. Alprostadil is used on the paediatric intensive care unit for maintaining patency of the ductus arteriosus in neonates with a duct-dependent circulation. Misoprostol is encountered in gastroenterology for prevention of peptic ulcers, but is also used in obstetrics orally, sublingually or often rectally as a second- or third-line agent in post-partum haemorrhage.

Question 126: Herbal remedies

Which of the following DECREASES the anticoagulant effect of warfarin?

a) Garlic
b) Glucosamine
c) Echinacea

d) Evening primrose oil
e) St John's wort

Answer: e

Explanation

St John's wort is a herbal remedy used for earaches and depression. It contains around ten active ingredients. It is an enzyme inducer of cytochrome P450 and can therefore increase the metabolism and decrease the effect of warfarin. All of the other four herbal remedies have some level of evidence to support an increase in anticoagulant activity or contribute towards anticoagulation.

Question 127: Beta-adrenoreceptor antagonists

Which one of the following statements regarding β-blockers is TRUE?

a) When using esmolol, a loading dose of 0.1 mg/kg intravenously over one minute is reasonable
b) Propranolol has high oral bioavailability
c) Atenolol has high β_1 receptor selectivity
d) Metoprolol has low lipid solubility thus its absorption and bioavailability are limited
e) Labetalol antagonises α_1:β adrenoreceptors with a ratio of 1:7 when administered orally

Answer: c

Explanation

β-blockers are all competitive antagonists and demonstrate varying degrees of selectivity for the β_1 adrenoreceptor. This 'cardioselectivity' is advantageous as β_2 antagonism could potentially result in bronchoconstriction. Cardioselectivity can be expected from atenolol, esmolol and metoprolol at moderate therapeutic doses but is lost at higher doses. Propranolol and metoprolol are both highly lipophilic and are well absorbed from the gut; however, for both drugs, significant first-pass metabolism limits their bioavailability. Labetalol antagonises α_1:β adrenoreceptors with a ratio of 1:7 when administered intravenously; when given orally the ratio is 1:3. With esmolol, a loading dose of 0.1 mg/kg would be unlikely to exert a clinically detectable effect. A bolus of 0.5 mg/kg is the recommended starting point and often needs repeating five minutes later before an infusion is started at 50 to 200 mcg/kg per min. Beware of the widely different presentation concentrations of esmolol where 10 mL may contain 100 mg (10 mg/mL) or 2.5 g (250 mg/mL).

Reference

Peck T, Hill S, Williams M. *Pharmacology for Anaesthesia and Intensive Care*, 2nd edn. London: Greenwich Medical Media, 2004; pp.213–20.

Question 128: Approaches to regional anaesthetic blockade of the brachial plexus

Which one of the following statements regarding approaches to the blocking of the brachial plexus is TRUE?

a) The axillary approach alone is sufficient for all aspects of awake hand surgery
b) The interscalene approach blocks the plexus at the level of the trunks
c) The vertical infraclavicular approach has the highest rate of pneumothorax
d) An advantage of the supraclavicular approach is, being more distal, phrenic nerve block is not a complication

e) The subclavian perivascular approach relies on the plexus being immediately posterior to the subclavian artery as it crosses the first rib in between the scalenus anterior and medius

Answer: e

Explanation

The axillary approach to the brachial plexus is attractive because of the relative ease of the technique and low complication rate, but has some significant disadvantages. It will often spare the intercostobrachial and musculocutaneous nerves thus tourniquet pain in awake patients can be a problem if not addressed separately. The single-shot technique can also spare the radial nerve, again rendering it unsuitable for complete anaesthesia for hand surgery. These problems can be overcome with ultrasound-guided targeted nerve blocks at the same level. The interscalene approach blocks the plexus at the level of the roots and is likely to miss C8 and T1 giving rise to ulnar sparing. It is therefore excellent for shoulder surgery but should not be used as sole anaesthesia for hand surgery. The supraclavicular approach has the highest rate of pneumothorax (5% in one series) but when ultrasound guided it reliably blocks the whole of the brachial plexus as the hour-glass nature of the plexus means that the trunks and proximal divisions are closely related here. It is sometimes referred to as the 'spinal of the arm'. Back-tracking of the local anaesthetic means that phrenic nerve block is still encountered. The subclavian perivascular approach is a landmark variant of the supraclavicular block.

Question 129: Gas analysis

Which one of the following gases is paramagnetic?

a) Nitrogen
b) Nitrous oxide
c) Nitric oxide
d) Nitrogen dioxide
e) Dinitrogen tetroxide

Answer: c

Explanation

The only paramagnetic gases used in anaesthesia and intensive care are oxygen and nitric oxide. The application of this principle is used in the paramagnetic oxygen analyser – the concentration of oxygen in a mixture of gases may be measured regardless of the other constituents of the mixture (providing one of them is not nitric oxide). The same cannot be said of other methods of gas analysis where reliability is impaired with particular constituents of a gas mixture. Some of the other gases in the question are higher oxides of nitrogen produced as byproducts in the manufacture of nitrous oxide. They must be removed before supply of nitrous oxide as they have serious toxicity if inhaled.

Question 130: Altitude anaesthesia

While working abroad, at an altitude of 5000 m, it becomes necessary to administer a general anaesthetic with an FiO_2 of 0.9, to a healthy patient who lives locally. The operating theatre is heated and equipped with an anaesthetic machine that uses variable orifice flowmeters and a Tec5 isoflurane vaporiser, out of circuit. Regarding your anaes-thetic management, the following statements are true EXCEPT for which one?

a) The delivered concentration of isoflurane will be more than that shown on the dial of the vaporiser
b) The oxygen rotameter will accurately read the delivered flow of oxygen

c) The alveolar concentration of isoflurane will need to be higher than at sea level to achieve the same degree of anaesthesia

d) The partial pressure of isoflurane in the vaporiser is the same as it would be if you returned with the same vaporiser to sea level

e) The patient's oxygen saturation is more likely to be 90% than 96%

Answer: b

Explanation

In individuals living at altitude a number of compensatory changes occur including hyperventilation, increased erythropoietin secretion, increased 2,3-diphosphoglycerate, adaptation of the respiratory centre to a lower $PaCO_2$ and an increase in peripheral capillaries. At altitude there are a number of issues pertinent to giving an anaesthetic. The first is that although the FiO_2 remains constant at any altitude the PO_2 decreases the higher you go. The sigmoid-shaped oxyhaemoglobin dissociation curve compensates for this, maintaining haemoglobin saturation in the high nineties up to about 3000 m when the PO_2 hits the steep part of the curve and haemoglobin saturation starts to fall. The position of the oxyhaemoglobin dissociation curve does not shift much as the respiratory alkalosis shifts it to the left and the hypoxia shifts it to the right. In terms of delivering an inhalational anaesthetic agent at altitude it is important to remember a few basic principles. The first is that the saturated vapour pressure of a volatile agent, while affected by temperature, is unaffected by atmospheric pressure hence at altitude the partial pressure of the isoflurane in the vaporiser is the same as at sea level. This means that the delivered concentration (or minimum alveolar concentration (MAC)) of isoflurane the patient receives will be more than is dialled up due to the drop in atmospheric pressure (as explained by Dalton's law). However, the action of an anaesthetic agent depends on the effect site concentration, which is determined by the alveolar partial pressure not the concentration. Although the MAC is up, the effect will be the same so dialling up the same amount as at sea level will have the same effect. At altitude due to the reduced atmospheric pressure there are fewer gas or vapour molecules per unit volume. This means that at a given flow rate dialled up on a rotameter fewer molecules pass the bobbin per unit time, therefore the bobbin will under-read at altitude due to fewer molecules hitting the underside of the bobbin per unit time.

Question 131: Ventilators in the operating theatre

You are ventilating a patient in theatre using a simple bag-in-bottle ventilator connected to the common gas outlet. You are using a fresh gas flow of 1 L/min, a circle breathing system and volume control ventilation mode. Using spirometry connected to your anaesthetic machine you note a tidal volume of 500 mL, a respiratory rate of 12 breaths per minute and an I:E ratio of 1:2. You need to rapidly affect a change in circuit concentration of volatile anaesthetic agent. You increase your fresh gas flow to 4 L/min. You leave all the ventilator settings unchanged. One minute later, what delivered minute volume would you expect the spirometry to be registering?

a) 5 L/min
b) 6 L/min
c) 7 L/min
d) 8 L/min
e) 9 L/min

Answer: c

Explanation

This question regards gas flow coupling in bag-in-bottle ventilators. As these are still among the commonest ventilators used on anaesthetic machines it is a phenomenon that can be witnessed in our daily work. Fresh gas flow is delivered into the bellows of the ventilator, which are themselves contained within a glass chamber (so the bellows can be visualised to be filling and moving appropriately). A separate gas source provides an intermittent pneumatic pressure into the chamber, which when applied to the bellows causes them to collapse (to a controllable extent), ejecting a proportion of their contents into the breathing system. A spill valve in the chamber then opens during expiration allowing the pressure to drop and the bellows to refill from the fresh gas flow. During inspiration the volume delivered to the breathing circuit will be that volume set on the ventilator (and consequently delivered to the chamber) PLUS whatever volume of fresh gas flow is delivered to the bellows and circuit during this inspiratory phase. This is because during inspiration the spill valve in the chamber is closed to allow the necessary pressurisation of the chamber such that the fresh gas flow, which is being delivered continuously, must enter the bellows and breathing system thus augmenting the volume delivered on that breath. In the example here, the fresh gas flow has been increased by 3 L/min. With an I:E ratio of 1:2, one third of every minute is spent in inspiration, during which time the fresh gas flow is added to the set volume. One third of 3 L is 1 L, so our measured minute volume will be seen to increase by 1 L/min. Prior to the increase it was 500 mL × 12 = 6 L/min, so now it is 7 L/min.

Incidentally, during the expiratory phase once the volume to the bellows is restored any excess fresh gas flow will be vented to the scavenging (to avoid pressurising the system), which is neither economical nor environmentally sound.

Question 132: Surgical risk-assessment tools

A 55-year-old man is awaiting a transjugular intrahepatic portosystemic shunt procedure. Considering the Child–Pugh classification of liver disease, of the following clinical features, which one does NOT score two points?

a) Ascites controlled with diuretics
b) Encephalopathy grade II
c) Bilirubin 42 micromol/L
d) Albumin 27 g/L
e) INR 2.4

Answer: e

Explanation
The Child–Pugh (or Child–Turcotte–Pugh) score is a risk-stratification tool used to predict mortality associated with surgical procedures on patients with liver disease, although originally was described for use with patients awaiting portocaval shunt surgery. Five criteria each score one to three points giving a summed score with a minimum of five and a maximum of fifteen. A score of five to six is labelled Child's A, seven to nine is Child's B and ten to fifteen is Child's C with a progressively worse prognosis and mortality as the score rises. Other factors determining outcome are the patient's comorbidity and the nature of the proposed surgery. An INR of 2.4 would score three points. The patient in the question would, with those features described, score eleven translating to Child's C liver disease and a peri-operative mortality of >75% (for intra-abdominal surgery). Child's C one-year mortality, without intervention, is 50%. In many spheres the Child–Pugh score is being replaced by the MELD score (Model for End-stage Liver Disease). This excludes subjective assessment of the degree of ascites and encephalopathy, requiring only the patient's bilirubin, INR and creatinine (adjusted for use of renal replacement therapy). These data are inserted into a formula as their natural logarithms and a score is generated. Originally introduced for prognostication following transjugular intrahepatic portosystemic shunt (TIPS), MELD has been applied and validated to most surgeries

contemplated for patients with active liver disease. Transjugular intrahepatic porto-systemic shunt is associated with poor outcome if the MELD score is >24, thus historically would be avoided in these circumstances. Regarding the patient in the question, their serum creatinine would have to be less than 140 micromol/L to achieve a MELD score of <24.

Question 133: Lumbar plexus

Regarding the anatomy and regional anaesthesia of the lumbar plexus, the following statements are true EXCEPT which one?

a) The lumbar plexus is described as being derived from spinal nerve roots T12–L4
b) The genitofemoral nerve is of L1–2 spinal root origin
c) The lumbar plexus is embedded in the psoas major muscle
d) A lumbar plexus block combined with a proximal sciatic nerve block can provide complete anaesthesia for all leg and foot surgery
e) As the skin on the back is less sensitive, a lumbar plexus block is one which is better tolerated by patients without the need for sedation/analgesia

Answer: e

Explanation

Sources vary on the spinal nerve roots that contribute to the lumbar plexus but plenty, including *Gray's Anatomy*, include a branch from T12 contributing to the subcostal nerve. Other sources identify L1–L4 only. The spinal roots exit the intervertebral foraminae and penetrate the psoas major muscle in which they make some of their divisions and coalitions. When performed well by an experienced practitioner, combined with a sciatic nerve block and allowing at least 20 minutes onset time, the block is adequate for sole anaesthesia for the leg and foot. A lumbar plexus block provides excellent analgesia for hip surgery but due to the many components of innervation of the hip, complete anaesthesia for hip surgery cannot be guaranteed. The lumbar plexus block is emerging as a block amenable to ultrasound-guided regional anaesthesia but currently is mostly performed with a peripheral nerve stimulator. As the needle passes through the paravertebral muscles and into psoas major, the stimulation of these large muscles is distinctly uncomfortable and a small dose of alfentanil is recommended as well as some sedation as necessary.

Question 134: Anaphylaxis triggers

The MOST COMMON cause for an anaphylactic reaction under anaesthesia is which one of the following?

a) Antibiotics
b) Latex
c) Neuromuscular blocking drugs
d) Colloid solutions
e) Radiocontrast media

Answer: c

Explanation

Neuromuscular blocking drugs account for around 60 to 75% of anaphylactic reactions under anaesthesia. After that comes latex and then antibiotics, although the incidence of latex anaphylaxis is reducing.

Question 135: Jehovah's Witness

A 30-year-old Jehovah's Witness presents for emergency surgery. Which of the following options is likely to be LEAST ACCEPTABLE to this patient during the peri-operative period?

a) Transfusion of pre-operatively donated autologous blood
b) Transfusion of human albumin solution
c) Epidural blood patch
d) Intraoperative cell salvage
e) Cardiac bypass

Answer: a

Explanation

An adult patient with capacity is entitled to refuse to consent to medical treatment for good reason, bad reason or no reason at all, and no opinion should be attributed to a patient simply because they are a member of a religious group. Patients are entitled to change their minds at any time and the only thing that matters is what treatment the patient wishes to have at the time when the decision has to be taken. Due to an interpretation of several biblical texts the established Jehovah's Witnesses' view is that an individual's life is represented by their blood and that the prohibition of blood transfusion is a deeply held core value and a sign of respect for the sanctity of life. As a result of this a number of treatments are either regarded as unacceptable or a matter for personal belief. The former group includes transfusion of whole blood, packed red cells, white cells, plasma, platelets and preoperative autologous blood collection and storage for later reinfusion (also known as pre-deposit). The latter group includes blood salvage (intra- and postoperative, e.g. intraoperative cell salvage or blood collected in drains), haemodilution, haemodialysis, and cardiac bypass, blood 'fractions' of plasma or cellular components (e.g. albumin, immunoglobulins, clotting factors), transplantation, including solid organ, bone, tissue, etc, and epidural blood patch. Jehovah's Witnesses often have advanced directives detailing their specific beliefs and requests and these should be identified wherever possible.

Reference

Management of Anaesthesia for Jehovah's Witnesses, 2nd edn. Association of Anaesthetists of Great Britain and Ireland, 2005. Online at www.aagbi.org/publications/guidelines.htm (Accessed 30 November 2009)

Question 136: Anaesthesia in a patient with porphyria

A patient with known variegate porphyria presents with suspected acute appendicitis and requires a laparoscopy. The patient is fasted, in pain and extremely anxious. Which one of the following options describes the BEST peri-operative management?

a) Fluid: Hartmanns + 10% glucose; Premedication: Midazolam; Induction agent: Propofol; Maintenance anaesthetic agent: Isoflurane
b) Fluid: Hartmanns; Premedication: none; Induction agent: Thiopentone; Maintenance anaesthetic agent: Propofol
c) Fluid: Hartmanns + 10% glucose; Premedication: none; Induction agent: Propofol; Maintenance anaesthetic agent: Sevoflurane
d) Fluid: 5% dextrose; Premedication: none; Induction agent: Propofol; Maintenance anaesthetic agent: Isoflurane
e) Fluid: Hartmanns + 10% glucose; Premedication: none; Induction agent: Thiopentone; Maintenance anaesthetic agent: Isoflurane

Answer: a

Explanation

The porphyrias are due to deficiencies in activity of one or more of the enzymes required for normal haem synthesis, which results in an overproduction of porphyrins and porphyrin precursors. Most types of porphyria are inherited, although the most common type, porphyria cutanea tarda, is usually an acquired disorder associated with liver disease and iron overload. Porphyrias can be classified in a number of ways but from an anaesthetic point of view classification by whether or not they cause acute symptoms is of most use as those that do are the only ones of major anaesthetic relevance. The porphyrias causing acute symptoms are acute intermittent porphyria, variegate porphyria, hereditary coproporphyria and plumboporphyria. Symptoms of an acute attack vary but include abdominal pain, autonomic disturbance, electrolyte abnormalities, neuropsychiatric manifestations and neuromuscular weakness. A number of factors precipitate or exacerbate attacks, including starvation, poor intake of carbohydrates, drugs, alcohol, smoking, infections and other forms of stress. Although the pathogenesis is not completely understood, it appears likely that many aspects of such an attack are due to adverse effects of excess 5-aminolevulinic acid (ALA), which is structurally similar to γ-aminobutyric acid, the major inhibitory neurotransmitter. Diagnosis is made by the measurement of ALA and porphobilinogen in urine or serum. A variety of drugs are known to precipitate attacks and an up-to-date list may be found via the website listed below. For the purposes of answering this question the patient should have a source of carbohydrate perioperatively, hence Option (b) is false. Thiopentone is on the list of drugs that carry a risk of precipitating a porphyric crisis, so ruling out Option (e). Hyponatraemia is known to precipitate a crisis, so fluid therapy consisting of solely 5% dextrose would be unwise, thus ruling out Option (d). Option (c) is incorrect as Sevoflurane may carry some risk (see website) and the lack of a premedication will increase the risk of anxiety precipitating a crisis.

References

James MF, Hift RJ. Porphyrias. *Brit J Anaes* 2000; **85**(1): 143–53.
University of Queensland Department of Medicine website. Online at www.uq.edu.au/porphyria (Accessed 30 November 2009)

Question 137: Temperature measurement

Regarding temperature measurement, the following statements are true EXCEPT which one?

a) Rectal temperature tends to be higher than oesophageal temperature
b) Oesophageal probes most commonly incorporate a thermistor to transduce temperature to electrical changes
c) A thermopile is a collection of thermocouples connected in parallel
d) Tympanic membrane thermometers often employ the Seebeck effect
e) Miniaturised temperature measurement probes typically have response times of around one second

Answer: e

Explanation

Given the importance of intraoperative temperature management and temperature measurement incorporated into other devices, familiarity with thermometers will not be limited to the Primary exam. Local bacterial fermentation in the rectum renders its temperature slightly higher than core temperature. Oesophageal temperature may also be falsely lowered if the probe (which does indeed incorporate a thermistor) is too superficially inserted, as the proximal oesophagus is subject to the cooling effect of respiratory gas exchanges in the trachea. The lower third (sometimes quoted as 35 to 45 cm insertion depth) is in closer proximity to the great vessels and thus the core temperature of interest. Nasopharyngeal temperature measurement is accurate if an airway management device has eliminated cooling gas flow in the nasopharynx that might otherwise lower measured temperature. Tympanic membrane thermometers transduce infrared radiation (produced by most objects at around body temperature) to measurable electrical change either via a thermopile or a pyroelectric sensor. A thermocouple employs the Seebeck effect (the induction of a potential difference at the junction of two dissimilar metals that varies with temperature). When connected in parallel the sensitivity and response time are improved and this is called a thermopile. A pyroelectric sensor involves a crystal of variable measurable polarisation where the degree of polarisation varies with the level of infrared radiation to which it is exposed. Temperature probes miniaturised for use in, for example, intravascular catheters must have a much faster response time (e.g. 100 ms) in order to be useful for thermodilution techniques.

Question 138: Ankle block

The following nerves must be anaesthetised when performing regional anaesthesia of the foot. Which nerve is readily amenable to location using the peripheral nerve stimulator?

a) Superficial peroneal (fibular) nerve
b) Deep peroneal (fibular) nerve
c) Tibial nerve
d) Sural nerve
e) Saphenous nerve

Answer: c

Explanation

The ankle block can be performed by a surface landmark technique or be ultrasound guided. The approach to the component nerves is different according to the technique selected. This is because the level at which the nerves are blocked using the surface landmark technique precludes easy ultrasonographical visualisation. The nerves are either too indistinct there or the footprint of the probe prevents consistent skin contact. For this reason, ultrasound-guided ankle blocks involve anaesthetising the saphenous nerve at the medial knee, the superficial peroneal at the lateral calf, the deep peroneal on the lower third of the shin (lateral to the anterior tibial artery) and the sural and tibial nerves in similar locations to the landmark technique. The tibial nerve is located just posterior to the palpable pulse of the posterior tibial artery and peripheral nerve stimulation here will cause plantar-flexion of the toes. The saphenous and sural nerves are purely sensory. As well as its cutaneous sensation role, the superficial peroneal nerve gives motor supply to peroneus longus and brevis. The lateral branch of the deep peroneal nerve innervates the extensor digitorum brevis muscle, although the deep peroneal nerve is largely sensory, supplying skin of the first webspace and innervation to many of the small joints of the foot. Despite their motor components, peripheral nerve stimulation of the peroneal nerves is not described.

Question 139: Measurement of biopotentials

Regarding the measurement of biopotentials, which one of the following statements is TRUE?

a) Signal-to-noise ratio must be minimised to optimise fidelity of displayed biopotential

b) Electrocardiogram electrodes generate potential as well as conduct current
c) Input impedance at the amplifier must be minimised in order to maximise the potential measured
d) The bandwidth of frequencies over which an electromyogram must consistently amplify is 0.5 to 100 Hz
e) Gain and common-mode rejection ratio are measured in Sone units

Answer: b

Explanation

Capacitance and inductance coupling as well as extrinsic electromagnetic interference are responsible for unwanted frequencies that disrupt the transmission and reception of biopotentials, which are small in magnitude. The use of physical shields and electronic filters serves to maximise signal-to-noise ratio to reduce disruption of the displayed potential. With electrocardiogram electrodes, the combination of a metal and its chloride (usually silver) making electrical contact with tissues containing electrolytes (which may conduct current) means that chemical changes at the interface may render the electrodes the equivalent of an electrochemical cell. They may generate their own potential and where conduction is available, current will flow. Electrodes may become polarised as a result of this process. Input impedance to an amplifier must be large to avoid a step-down effect on the measured potential. It is the electrode impedance that must be small; 0.5 to 100 Hz is the necessary bandwidth for accurate reception and display of an electrocardiogram. Electromyograms have extremely sharp spikes that require a very high frequency capability in their processing because Fourier analysis of the waveform reveals very high frequency harmonics. The Sone is a unit of perceived loudness. Sound intensity is often expressed in decibels, which is also the unit used to express gain and common-mode rejection ratio.

Question 140: Hepatitis B

A British anaesthetist working in the United Kingdom suffering a needle stick injury with a bloody, hollow sharp from a patient known to have hepatitis B, has serum tests at ten weeks post-inoculation. Which of the following is LEAST LIKELY to be found?

a) Positive for antibody to hepatitis B surface antigen
b) Positive for IgM for anti-hepatitis D virus
c) Positive for anti-hepatitis B surface antigen
d) Positive for hepatitis B virus DNA
e) Positive for hepatitis B e antigen

Answer: b

Explanation

Anti-hepatitis B surface antigen is found early in the disease and may test positive before symptoms start. It often disappears from the blood during the recovery phase from the disease, around five months after exposure. Hepatitis B e antigen (HBeAg) is only detected when the virus is present. Once recovery starts and the viral load falls, HBeAg levels drop off until it becomes undetectable at around the three-month stage. It is often used to indicate whether a patient is infective. Hepatitis B virus DNA is generally on the wane by the three-month stage but remains detectable longer than HBeAg. It is a more sensitive test of the presence of hepatitis virus in the serum than HBeAg. Both of these markers of the presence of virus may persist if the person goes on to develop chronic contagious hepatitis B. Antibody to hepatitis B surface antigen typically is found from 24 weeks after exposure. However, it is also found following immunisation with hepatitis B vaccine, which is widespread throughout British health-care workers at high risk of needle stick injury. Hepatitis D infection may be detected by testing for IgM that is anti-hepatitis D virus. Hepatitis D is found in patients with hepatitis B, so infection with hepatitis B puts a person at risk of concomitant infection with hepatitis D. In a recent study, however, only 13% of hepatitis B positive patients tested positive for hepatitis D.

Question 141: Sodium nitroprusside

Regarding the drug sodium nitroprusside (SNP), the following statements are correct EXCEPT which one?

a) SNP ultimately causes vasodilation via increased concentration of intracellular cyclic guanylate monophosphate (cGMP)
b) Dicobalt edetate has a place in the management of toxicity induced by SNP
c) Vitamin B12 deficiency may predispose to SNP toxicity
d) SNP causes increased right-to-left intrapulmonary shunt
e) Thiocyanate, produced during one pathway of SNP metabolism, is non-toxic

Answer: e

Explanation

Sodium nitroprusside is metabolised in the erythrocytes. Sodium nitroprusside and oxyhaemoglobin react to produce methaemoglobin plus nitric oxide and five molecules of cyanide ions. It is the nitric oxide that is responsible for the clinical effect of the drug, and the cyanide ions and their metabolites that potentially cause toxicity. Nitric oxide is usually produced in the vascular endothelial cells via the action of nitric oxide synthetase (inducible or constitutive) on L-arginine, an amino acid. In vascular smooth muscle cells, nitric oxide avidly binds and activates guanylyl cyclase, which dephosphorylates guanylate triphosphate (GTP) to cyclic guanylate monophosphate (cGMP). It is the cGMP that precipitates a number of intracellular events that result in smooth-muscle relaxation and thus vasodilation. Some of the cyanide ions produced combine with the evolved methaemoglobin to produce cyanomethaemoglobin, which is non-toxic. Residual cyanide ions combine with vitamin B12 to form the non-toxic cyanocobalamin; others are converted in the liver mitochondria by rhodanase to thiocyanate via the addition of a sulphydryl moiety. Thiocyanate itself is toxic and when these pathways of elimination are exhausted, cyanide ions accumulate further contributing to the toxicity. If toxicity develops, SNP therapy should be discontinued and the cyanide chelator dicobalt edetate administered. Depleted sulphydryl stores may be supplemented via the infusion of sodium thiosulphate. Intrapulmonary shunt may be worsened by SNP by causing pulmonary vasodilation thus disrupting hypoxic pulmonary vasoconstriction.

Question 142: Invasive arterial blood-pressure monitoring

Regarding invasive arterial blood pressure monitoring, which one of the following statements is TRUE?

a) An overdamped waveform underestimates diastolic pressure
b) An anacrotic notch is a sign of severe aortic stenosis
c) A rapid systolic upstroke is associated with a high systemic vascular resistance
d) The dicrotic notch appears later in the waveform complex if measured at the radial artery compared to the dorsalis pedis
e) Critical damping refers to the perfect level of damping and is the desired set-up for the system

Answer: b

Explanation

An overdamped waveform underestimates systolic pressure and overestimates diastolic pressure. The opposite is the case for an underdamped waveform. An anacrotic notch is a sudden fall on the upstroke of the arterial waveform and is seen in severe aortic stenosis limiting the upstroke. A slow systolic upstroke is associated with a high systemic vascular resistance or poor myocardial contractility. The waveform changes morphology the further it travels away from the heart with the dicrotic notch appearing later in the complex. Optimal damping in the context of arterial lines refers to the perfect level of damping and is the desired set-up for the system. Critical damping (a damping coefficient of 1.0) is when deflection returns as quickly as possible to the null point without any overshoot. However, a critically damped system would have a slow response time and may not show maximal amplitude. Optimal damping (damping coefficient 0.69 or thereabouts) is a compromise between underdamping and overdamping. Underdamping allows some degree of overshoot in order to maximise response time and allows accurate display of magnitude. Overdamping keeps resonance to a minimum.

Question 143: Mental capacity

Which of the following scenarios would give you MOST CONCERN that the patient lacked capacity to consent for the given procedure?

a) A 51-year-old understands the risks of delaying the surgery for her aggressive bowel cancer but still maintains that she does not want an operation that may cure her

b) For the fourth successive time a 63-year-old agrees to have surgery for a large incarcerated inguinal hernia, but on arriving in the anaesthetic room panics at the thought of the anaesthetic and refuses to have the operation

c) A 38-year-old woman who is 16 weeks pregnant with worsening signs and symptoms of acute appendicitis has the risks and benefits of surgery including the risks to the foetus explained. She refuses to have surgery as she believes any medicines, including anaesthetics, may damage her baby

d) An 87-year-old with mild dementia who is conversational and orientated but prone to being forgetful asks you twice to repeat the risks you have explained to him about the anaesthetic for his dynamic hip screw surgery

e) A 24-year-old with depression thought to be at high risk of suicide who has benefited from electroconvulsive therapy (ECT) in the past, refuses ECT against the recommendations of two senior psychiatrists. Six months earlier, the patient, during a period when considered by her mental health team to be of sound mind, had legally signed an advanced directive stating that she did not wish to ever have ECT again

Answer: e

Explanation

The Mental Health Act (1983 and amended in 2007) and the Mental Capacity Act (2005) are important pieces of legislation that underpin the legal position regarding consent. An anaesthetist at Final FRCA level should have some grasp of the main points of these acts. A patient should be assessed as to whether they have capacity, and, if they do, they are the only ones who can consent for a planned procedure with only a very few exceptions. Capacity is based on determining whether the patient understands what a treatment involves including the risks and benefits, can understand the impact of not receiving the treatment, can then retain and consider the information and communicate their decision back to the medical team. If the patient has capacity, they are allowed to make what doctors might consider to be bad decisions, such as in the patient with bowel cancer refusing surgery. A pregnant woman has substantial rights to refuse any treatment even if it may be to the detriment of the foetus. The gentleman returning to theatre is complicated. He has capacity at the initial consent discussion and then suffers a panic attack. The question is whether a panic attack, which is a psychiatric diagnosis in which insight is usually preserved, removes capacity. This is controversial and right at the border of a possible answer. As this is a 'single best answer' question, and we are looking for the patient that would *most* concern us, let's keep looking. The elderly gentleman for hip surgery may lack capacity, but it would be too early to say from the information given. He may be hearing impaired, he may just need information imparted in a slow methodical manner or he may need formal assessment of capacity. Finally we arrive at the last scenario. This is a complex ethical and legal problem. However, the question asks you whether the patient has capacity, not whether her advanced directive allows her to decline electroconvulsive therapy (ECT). With severe depression she almost certainly lacks capacity. Regarding ECT, the amended 2007 Mental Health Act brought in two new safeguards. These were that if a patient has capacity, they may refuse treatment with ECT unless in an emergency, and that if a detained patient had signed a valid advanced directive opposed to ECT, then they cannot be treated with it, except in an emergency. It is clear that the decision about capacity in this question is fairly straightforward, but the decision about whether ECT should proceed is not.

Reference
The Mental Health Acts are a fairly stodgy read. A good summary may be found online at www.patient.co.uk/doctor/Consent-To-Treatment-(Mental-Capacity-and-Mental-Health-Legislation).htm (Accessed 30 November 2009)

Question 144: Teeth

At preoperative assessment it is noticed that a patient's top teeth appear to be abnormally anterior to their bottom teeth. When asked to close their mouth, the tip of their top central incisors is 12 mm anterior to the tip of their bottom central incisors. Which one of the following terms BEST describes the patient's condition?

a) Overbite
b) Malocclusion
c) Micrognathia
d) Overjet
e) Overclosure

Answer: d

Explanation
It is important to be able to recognise and accurately describe abnormal dentition. This scenario describes a substantial overjet. Overclosure is when the mandible rises an excessive vertical distance on occlusion, such as through the wearing down of teeth through grinding. Overbite is when the top incisors overlap the bottom incisors in a vertical plane and is commonly used incorrectly to describe an overjet. This patient may well have micrognathia and this is a cause of overjet, but there is not enough evidence to make that assumption here. Malocclusion is a broader term that describes all the dental conditions in which the teeth misalign on mouth closure. This patient does have a malocclusion, but describing it as such adds little.

Question 145: Severe sepsis

A 69-year-old, 80 kg male is admitted to the intensive care unit with respiratory failure secondary to a lower respiratory tract infection. He has his trachea intubated and mechanical ventilation of the lungs is commenced. He has a PiCCO cardiac output monitor sited; an internal jugular central venous catheter and urinary catheter are also inserted. He receives antibiotics, intravenous fluid resuscitation and an infusion of noradrenaline. Three hours following admission to hospital, some of his clinical measurands are as follows: heart rate 110 bpm; mean arterial blood pressure 66 mmHg; central venous pressure 10 mmHg; arterial oxygen saturation 93%; central venous oxygen saturation 68%; cardiac index 2.5 L/min per m^2; urine output 30 mL/h; pH 7.23; PaCO$_2$ 6.0 kPa; PaO$_2$ 9.1 kPa; HCO$_3^-$ 19 mmol/L; base excess −6.2 mmol/L; lactate 3.2 mmol/L; haematocrit 0.31; FiO$_2$ 0.7; MV 7.2 L/min; plateau pressure 29 cmH$_2$O. Which one of the following should be prioritised for the patient to receive NEXT?

a) Increased rate of noradrenaline infusion
b) Dobutamine infusion
c) Further intravenous fluid
d) Infusion of packed red cells
e) Increased minute ventilation

Answer: c

Explanation

During the management of septic shock, mechanically ventilated patients should have a higher target central venous pressure: 12 to 15 mmHg whereas the target would be 8 to 12 mmHg in spontaneously ventilating patients. Low central venous pressure should prompt a fluid challenge of crystalloid or colloid. This may increase this patient's cardiac output sufficiently to increase his central venous pressure, urine output (to >0.5 mL/kg/h) and central venous oxygen saturation (to >70%). A mean arterial pressure of >65 mmHg is adequate and the noradrenaline need not be increased, as to do so may jeopardise microvascular flow. Dobutamine may be introduced if the cardiac output is low (as manifest via a number of indicators) and filling pressures are elevated but supranormal levels should not be targeted. Red cells may be transfused to maintain a haemoglobin concentration of >7 g/dL or a haematocrit of >0.3 but not before, unless there are mitigating circumstances. Increasing minute ventilation may risk increasing plateau pressure above 30 cmH$_2$O, further increasing the likelihood of acute respiratory distress syndrome. Permissive hypercapnia is acceptable where the pH is not grossly deranged. The candidate should be familiar with the 2008 surviving sepsis guidelines (see below).

Reference

Dellinger RP, Levy MM, Carlet JM et al. Surviving Sepsis Campaign: International guidelines for management of severe sepsis and septic shock: 2008. Crit Care Med 2008; 36(1): 296–327.

Question 146: Features of local anaesthetic toxicity

The following statements regarding the features of local anaesthetic toxicity are true EXCEPT which one?

a) Prilocaine toxicity may cause the pulse oximeter to read 85%
b) At a plasma lidocaine concentration of 5 mg/mL, tinnitus may be present
c) As toxicity develops, inhibitory pathway inhibition at first causes excitation
d) Unconsciousness may precede convulsions
e) Cardiac resting membrane potential is made more negative

Answer: b

Explanation

At a plasma concentration of 5 mcg/mL, tinnitus may well be present, but at a thousand times this level (as in Option (b)) the patient would not survive to report this symptom. Published data relates the increasing severity of manifestations of local anaesthetic toxicity to plasma concentrations of lidocaine. At 5 mcg/mL circumoral paresthesia, light-headedness and numbness of the tongue would also be expected. At 5 to 10 mcg/mL, unconsciousness, muscle twitches or visual disturbance might be seen; at 10 to 20 mcg/mL we might see convulsions, myocardial depression and coma; and at >20 mcg/mL we would expect arrhythmias, respiratory arrest and cardiac arrest.

Prilocaine, when metabolised to O-toluidine, can produce methaemoglobinaemia, which distorts pulse oximetry (but not the co-oximeter in a standard arterial blood gas analyser). Cardiac toxicity is via a number of mechanisms, not least of which is as a membrane stabiliser, local anaesthetics will hyperpolarise myocardial and conduction cells. This causes a prolonged PR interval, widened QRS complex and a prolonged ST segment before tachyarrhythmias supervene.

Reference

Smith T. Systemic toxic effects of local anaesthetics. *Anaesth Intens Care* 2007; **8**(4):155–8.

Question 147: Basic SI units

Which of the following is NOT a basic SI unit?

a) Candela
b) Kelvin
c) Mole
d) Newton
e) Ampere

Answer: d

Explanation

The basic SI units (Système Internationale d'Unités) are the metre, kilogram, second, kelvin, candela, mole and ampere. The candidate must know these and their definitions. All other units are derived and may be expressed in terms of these seven basic units. It is an interesting paper exercise to consolidate understanding of the subject by choosing any derived unit then by application of the laws of physics and conversion factors, prove that the unit may be expressed in terms of these basic seven units. For example, prove that $1\,\text{mmHg} = 133.3\,\text{kg/m/s}^2$ or that $1\,\text{ohm} = 1\,\text{kg.m}^2/\text{s}^3/\text{amp}^2$.

Question 148: Discharge following day surgery

Following a day case procedure under general anaesthesia, which one of the following is NOT a criterion for approval of discharge from the day surgery unit?

a) Able to ambulate unassisted
b) No pain or mild pain controllable with oral analgesia
c) Agreed carer for 24 hours
d) No bleeding or minimal bleeding or wound drainage
e) Stable vital signs for one hour

Answer: a

Explanation

The British Association of Day Surgery publishes guidelines for discharge procedures from day surgery units on which, it is suggested, local guidelines should be based. The guidelines have the objective of ensuring safe, best practice but are pragmatic in their application of common sense. If a patient is unable to walk pre-operatively, insisting on postoperative ambulation may lead to prolonged admission. Also, if the patient has had lower limb orthopaedic surgery, many of which procedures may be performed as day cases, they will need assistance to ambulate but are perfectly fit for discharge. The main factors to consider when assessing suitability for discharge are vital signs, cognitive orientation, pain control (and analgesia to take home), wound status, nausea and vomiting, activity level (self-care/ambulation), micturition, oral intake, escort home and carer for 24 hours, written and verbal instructions and a 'safety-net' (i.e. 'what to do if . . . '). These have been structured into scoring systems where a patient must achieve a threshold score before being labelled suitable for discharge. However, the British Association of Day Surgery does not recommend these scoring systems over a simple tick list.

Reference

Cahill H, Jackson I, McWhinnie D. Guidelines about the discharge process and the assessment of fitness for discharge. British Association of Day Surgery Handbook Series. Online at: www.daysurgeryuk.org/bads/ (Accessed 30 November 2009)

Question 149: Calcium channel blocking drugs

Which one of the following statements regarding calcium channel blocking drugs is TRUE?

a) Most of these drugs act on the T-type calcium channel
b) Nifedipine acts mainly by negative inotropy
c) Nimodipine is a class III calcium channel blocking drug
d) Verapamil is a suitable treatment for supraventricular tachycardia
e) Heart block caused by calcium channel blocking drug overdose is treated with atropine

Answer: d

Explanation

Calcium ion flux is fundamental to excitable tissues. In the cardiovascular system, myocardial contractility, autorhythmicity and vessel tone may all be reduced by blocking calcium channels. They are classified according to their predominant effects. Class I: negative inotropy and chronotropy – useful for hypertension, angina and supraventricular tachycardia (e.g. verapamil). Class II: reduction in vessel tone with minimal direct cardiac effect except reflex tachycardia (e.g. nifedipine, nimodipine, nicardipine). Class III: negative inotropic effects (e.g. diltiazem). They mostly act on L-type channels and in overdose heart block is usually resistant to atropine. Overdose would be treated with intravenous calcium chloride, glucagon and catecholamines.

Reference

Yentis S, Hirsch N, Smith G. *Anaesthesia and Intensive Care A to Z: An Encyclopaedia of Principles and Practice*, 3rd edn. London: Elsevier, 2004; p.84.

Question 150: Haemophilia

A 31-year-old male with known haemophilia A presents with a fracture of his left tibia sustained while playing football. The orthopaedic surgeons propose operative application of an external fixation frame. The patient is unable to grade the severity of his haemophilia but has had two knee haemarthroses in the previous seven years. As part of the preoperative preparation of this patient, which one of the following should be administered intravenously?

a) Fresh frozen plasma
b) Cryoprecipitate
c) Recombinant factor VIII concentrate
d) Recombinant factor IX concentrate
e) Desmopressin

Answer: c

Explanation

Haemophilia A is an X-linked recessive inherited coagulation disorder resulting in a congenital deficiency or absence of clotting factor VIII. One in 5000 males are affected, but the extent to which factor VIII plasma concentration is reduced dictates the severity of clinical manifestation. One in 100 000 females are symptomatic carriers with a demonstrable mild-to-moderate bleeding tendency; however, the functional gene on the unaffected X chromosome in females makes severe bleeding diathesis very rare. Factor VIII is involved in the intrinsic coagulation pathway, so activated partial thromboplastin time is prolonged. Diagnosis is made by demonstrating reduced plasma factor VIII concentrations. Unaffected individuals will have a plasma factor VIII concentration of 0.5 to 1.5 units/mL (termed 50 to 150% activity). Mild haemophiliacs have 4 to 50% activity, moderate have 1 to 4%, and severe haemophiliacs have <1% of normal factor VIII activity. Patients with greater than 10 to 15% activity tend to be asymptomatic. Spontaneous bleeding is unlikely at levels greater than 5%. Haemorrhagic manifestations include haemarthroses, soft tissue haematomas and intracranial haemorrhages. Platelets, vasculature, extrinsic pathway and final common pathway are not affected, thus bleeding time, platelet count and prothrombin time will be normal. Significant haemarthroses indicate at least moderate disease and the planned surgery may well involve reasonable blood loss. The preoperative objective would be to raise plasma factor VIII concentration to 1 unit/mL (100%) with factor VIII concentrate, before proceeding. This is a recombinant engineered product that avoids the infective risks of blood component therapy that were previously associated with haemophilia. Cryoprecipitate would be a second-line alternative; it is sometimes used prior to dental procedures in moderate haemophiliacs. Desmopressin can be used to prevent bleeding complications in mild haemophiliacs.

Paper C

Question 151: Eponymous laws of physics

The following statements regarding the laws of physics applied to anaesthesia are true EXCEPT which one?

a) Darcy's law is analogous to Ohm's law
b) Henry's law relates quantity of dissolved gases to their partial pressure
c) Laplace's law relates pressure, tension and radius of curvature of a tube, sphere or bubble
d) Hooke's law can be applied to the resonance witnessed in underdamped arterial blood pressure recording
e) Charles' law is often quoted in association with Boyle's law

Answer: d

Explanation

Many of the laws of physics arise in anaesthetic textbooks to explain some of the physical phenomena witnessed. Unsurprisingly, the laws and formulae associated are often simplified in anaesthetic texts from how they appear in their true form in physics textbooks, where they sometimes seem inaccessibly complicated to the occasional physicist.

In fluid dynamics, when we observe that flow is directly proportional to driving pressure and is inversely proportional to the resistance to that flow, we are quoting a simplification of Darcy's law. Laplace's law should include a term for wall thickness but the statement in Option (c) is still correct. Hooke's law simply states that within its elastic limit, the length of a spring is directly proportional to the load applied to it. Hooke also experimented with oscillating springs with loads attached and introduced concepts of natural frequency and resonance – relevant to invasive pressure monitoring but his law cannot be applied to this. Charles' law and Boyle's law are both ideal gas laws.

Question 152: Polycystic kidney disease

Regarding polycystic kidney disease the following statements are true EXCEPT which one?

a) Autosomal dominant polycystic kidney disease is one of the most common inherited disorders in humans
b) Clinical manifestations usually present in the third or fourth decade of life

c) Hepatic cysts, diverticular disease and cardiac valvular abnormalities are associated with polycystic kidney disease
d) Flank pain is a recognised, although uncommon, complaint
e) Pregnancy in autosomal dominant polycystic kidney disease is not associated with higher rates of complications from extrarenal manifestations

Answer: d

Explanation
The genetic mutation for autosomal dominant polycystic kidney disease (ADPKD) is very common. Prevalence of the mutation is variably quoted as between 1 in 200 to 1 in 1000 depending on source. Other common genetic disorders are familial combined hyperlipidaemia, familial hypercholesterolaemia, Huntington's disease and cystic fibrosis. There are two genotypes responsible for the condition: PKD1 (90% of cases, chromosome 16) and PKD2 (10% of cases, chromosome 4). Progressive expansion of bilateral renal tubular cysts disrupts kidney function. Patients present with pain, hypertension, haematuria and subsequently renal failure. Given its prevalence and progressive nature, it is a common cause of end-stage kidney failure necessitating dialysis. Pain in the back, flank or abdomen is virtually universal in patients with the condition. The extrarenal manifestations are either cystic, with similar pathophysiology, or result from altered connective tissue architecture. Hepatic cysts are the most common and although hepatic function tends to be preserved, complications arising from the physical presence of hepatic cysts are a significant cause of morbidity and mortality. Other extrarenal manifestations are as in Option (c) plus, of course, an association with intracranial aneurysms, which occur in around 10% (80% of which are unilateral and in the anterior circulation) of adult patients with ADPKD. Although the condition can reduce fertility, even before chronic kidney disease has developed, female patients with ADPKD may present for obstetric care. It has been demonstrated that they are not at higher risk of complications related to extrarenal manifestations, but parturients with known intracranial aneurysms should be managed as special cases.

References
Perrone RD. Extrarenal manifestations of ADPKD. *Kidney Int* 1997; **51**(6): 2022–36.
Torra R. Polycystic kidney disease. *eMedicine* 17 September 2009. Online at http://emedicine.medscape.com/article/244907-overview (Accessed 30 November 2009)

Question 153: Smoking

A 51-year-old man currently smokes 20 cigarettes a day, has a 40-pack-year history, asthma and is scheduled for elective inguinal hernia repair. Which of the following statements regarding the effects of his cigarette smoking is INCORRECT?

a) On average, compared to an identical non-smoker his morphine dose requirement will be increased
b) On average, compared to an identical non-smoker his vecuronium dose requirement will be increased
c) On average, compared to an identical non-smoker he is less likely to suffer post-operative nausea and vomiting
d) On average, compared to an identical non-smoker his paracetamol dose requirement will be increased
e) If he were to stop smoking, his therapeutic theophylline dose is likely to be reduced

Answer: d

Explanation

Over 4800 separate substances have been found in cigarette smoke, and the health risks of cigarette smoking are well documented. Cigarette smoke may interfere with both the action and metabolism of a wide range of medications, some of which are relevant to anaesthetic practice. Central to this is the cytochrome P450 (CYP) multi-enzyme system of which there are around 30 CYP enzymes responsible for drug metabolism. Polycyclic aromatic hydrocarbons (PACs) in cigarette smoke react with these enzymes, in general inducing them, thus affecting the metabolism of a number of drugs including paracetamol, codeine and theophylline. It is only the last whose dose is significantly affected. In addition, PACs also have an effect on a membrane-bound glycoprotein called uridine diphosphate-glucuronosyltransferase (UGT). UGT partially metabolises codeine and morphine as well as being involved in the glucuronidation of a number of drugs including non-steroidal anti-inflammatory drugs, amitriptyline and temazepam. It has consistently been shown that smokers have an increased requirement for opiates in the postoperative period. Smoking decreases the potency of aminosteroid muscle relaxants (vecuronium > rocuronium) and of interest, greater than ten hours' abstinence from cigarette smoking decreases atracurium requirements, probably secondary to removal of a nicotinic effect at the neuromuscular junction. The incidence of postoperative nausea and vomiting is reduced in smokers as is, interestingly, the prevalence of ulcerative colitis.

Reference

Sweeney BP, Grayling M. Smoking and anaesthesia: the pharmacological implications. *Anaesthesia* 2009; **64(2)**: 179–86.

Question 154: Lactic acidosis

Regarding lactate metabolism, the following statements are true EXCEPT which one?

a) A proportion of plasma lactate is produced by both erythrocytes and the heart
b) Ethanol excess produces a Type B lactic acidosis
c) Sepsis produces a Type B_1 lactic acidosis
d) Hyperlactaemia is variably associated with acidaemia
e) Lactate is metabolised by the liver, kidneys and skeletal muscle

Answer: a

Explanation

The end product of glycolysis is pyruvate. If pyruvate is unable to enter an aerobic energy production pathway (e.g. as AcetylCoA into the Kreb's cycle) then it is converted into lactate. Hyperlactaemia is defined as plasma lactate concentration >2 mmol/L. It may arise in a number of circumstances, both physiological and pathophysiological, and it may or may not be associated with an acidaemia depending on concurrent metabolic challenges and an intact buffering system. Lactic acidosis is a metabolic acidosis caused by accumulation of lactic acid in the plasma either caused by tissue hypoxia (Type A) or by failure to clear lactate, without overt tissue hypoxia (Type B). Type A, as caused by tissue hypoxia, may be considered in terms of hypoxaemic, stagnant, anaemic and cytotoxic causes. Type B occurs when there is no evidence of tissue hypoperfusion or oxygenation deficit. It may be subcategorised into B_1 (common metabolic derangements): sepsis, renal failure, liver failure, diabetes, malignancy; B_2 (toxic causes): metformin, paracetamol, aspirin, ethanol, methanol, ethylene glycol, catecholamines, cyanide, cocaine, etc.; B_3 (other causes): tonic-clonic seizures, disorders of carbohydrate metabolism. Producers of lactate are the erythrocytes (as they only generate energy via anaerobic glycolysis and do not possess mitochondria), gut, brain and skeletal muscle, although when lactate concentration exceeds 4 mmol/L skeletal muscle becomes an overall metaboliser of lactate. Lactate is metabolised back to pyruvate (which can potentially enter gluconeogenesis) by the liver (50%), heart, kidneys and skeletal muscle if necessary. Cardiac substrate utilisation is split between carbohydrate and fat energy sources. Considering it in terms of myocardial oxygen consumption: 60% is used in fatty acid consumption, 20% in glucose and 20% in lactate consumption. The heart uses entirely aerobic energy production pathways but when challenged with ischaemia, lactic acid is not cleared from the myocardial cell into the plasma – it accumulates, the myocardial cell becomes acidotic, cellular processes cease and the cell dies. So the heart does not contribute to plasma lactate levels but reduces them.

Question 155: Obstructive sleep apnoea

Regarding obstructive sleep apnoea (OSA), the following statements are true EXCEPT which one?

a) Diagnosis is not dependent on polysomnography analysis
b) Hypopnoea is defined as >50% reduction in air flow for more than ten seconds
c) OSA syndrome is diagnosed by the presence of more than five episodes of apnoea or hypopnoea in every hour of sleep
d) Polysomnography may reveal arterial blood pressure of 240/120 mmHg during the arousal phase after an apnoeic episode
e) A neck circumference of greater than 17 inches (42 cm) is the most significant predictor for the presence of OSA

Answer: c

Explanation
Apnoea is complete cessation of air flow, and hypopnoea is defined as >50% reduction in air flow for more than ten seconds. Obstructive sleep apnoea (OSA) is defined as more than five episodes of apnoea or hypopnoea in every hour of sleep. The obstructive sleep apnoea syndrome is diagnosed when OSA is accompanied by the presence of daytime symptoms such as somnolence, morning headaches, poor concentration or loss of libido. Of the many risk factors for OSA, obesity is the most common where simple mechanics dictate that during sleep, with associated reduction in muscle tone, the weight of peripharyngeal fat can no longer be supported. Various components of pharyngeal anatomy partially obstruct the airway. Polysomnography is the gold standard for diagnosis but is expensive and not universally available. Often diagnosis can be made on the basis of history alone: an obese, somnolent patient with loud snoring and witnessed apnoeas is very likely to have obstructive sleep apnoea syndrome. Overnight pulse oximetry or a simple device to measure cardiorespiratory variables can be used at home or on the ward and are a suitable alternative to full polysomnography. Polysomnography involves overnight monitoring of heart rate, blood pressure, pulse oximetry, air flow at the nose, respiratory rate, electroencephalogram, electromyogram and electrooculogram. The anaesthetist should be familiar with the physiological consequences of OSA and the challenges a patient with OSA may pose in the peri-operative period.

Reference
Williams J, Hanning C. Obstructive sleep apnoea. *Contin Educ Anaesth Crit Care Pain* 2003; **3**(3): 75–8.

Question 156: Awake intubation techniques

Regarding awake tracheal intubation, the following statements are true EXCEPT which one?

a) Xylometazoline is a useful agent for nasal vasoconstriction
b) During a translaryngeal block, remifentanil sedation, to minimise coughing, is desirable
c) For a 70 kg patient the maximum safe dose of cocaine is 1 mL of a 10% solution
d) Lidocaine applied topically has its potential plasma concentration reduced by first-pass metabolism
e) Superior laryngeal nerve block may be performed via a needle insertion point 1 cm inferior and 2 cm anterior to the prominent cornu of the hyoid

Answer: b

Explanation

Sedation techniques have the objective of rendering the procedure more tolerable for the patient, not acting as an antitussive. They should be conscious throughout if it is to be described as a true awake technique. Coughing is necessary during a translaryngeal block via cricothyroid puncture in order to disperse local anaesthetic to both supra-glottic and subglottic mucosa. The maximum safe dose of cocaine is 1.5 mg/kg and given there are 100 mg/mL in a 10% solution this equates to 0.015 mL/kg or for a 70 kg patient, 1.05 mL. A significant proportion of lidocaine applied topically to the pharynx and larynx is swallowed, thus first-pass metabolism does limit plasma concentrations to lower than would be expected if it was subjected to complete transmucosal absorption. There are many transcutaneous laryngeal nerve blocks described, including the approach in Option (e); however, they are losing popularity due to the effective anaesthesia achieved with 'spray-as-you-go' techniques that eliminate the requirement for injections.

Reference

Sudheer P, Stacey M. Anaesthesia for awake intubation. *Contin Educ Anaesth Crit Care Pain* 2003; **3**(4): 120–3.

Question 157: Necrotising fasciitis

A 61-year-old diabetic patient in the emergency department has developed signs of a systemic inflammatory response in the 90 minutes since she arrived with a painful, red, swollen ankle. She scratched her ankle yesterday. In the hour since triage, she has become rapidly unwell and the rash has spread up her leg to the knee, with the skin looking indurated, purple and blistering.

Along with resuscitating the patient, initial management should involve which of the following options?

a) Administer intravenous imipenem and arrange a computerised tomography (CT) scan
b) Administer intravenous imipenem and urgently call the general surgeons
c) Administer intravenous benzylpenicillin and arrange a magnetic resonance imaging (MRI) scan
d) Administer intravenous gentamicin and metronidazole and arrange a CT scan
e) Administer intravenous benzylpenicillin and urgently call the general surgeons

Answer: b

Explanation

The history and examination in this patient are highly suggestive of the diagnosis of necrotising fasciitis (NF). Typically NF starts with a trivial injury, leads to the initial development of trivial signs such as pain, swelling, cellulitis and pyrexia, then may rapidly progress on to skin discolouration (purple or blue), blistering, crepitus, the discharge of 'dishwater' fluid and a systemic inflammatory response with multiorgan dysfunction. At-risk groups include the elderly, diabetic or chronic renal failure patients, intravenous drug abusers and the immunosuppressed. Although streptococci are the most common organism found in NF, the infection is usually polymicrobial, with a single organism responsible in only 15% of cases. The antimicrobial plan in the initial treatment of NF is to provide broad-spectrum antibiotic cover, which may be changed once sensitivities are known. The mainstay of treatment is surgical. The patient should be taken to theatre without delay for exploration and debridement of all non-viable tissue. This should occur synchronously with resuscitation. Imaging is only of use when the clinical findings are subtle or equivocal. Delaying surgery for MRI or CT scan in advanced progressing NF is generally inadvisable.

Reference

Hasham S, Matteucci P, Stanley PR, Hart NB. Necrotising fasciitis. *BMJ* 2005; **330**(7495): 830–3.

Question 158: Renal replacement therapy

Following emergency surgery a patient remains ventilated on the critical care unit. He needs a low dose noradrenaline intravenous infusion and now requires renal replacement therapy. He is to be commenced on continuous venovenous haemodiafiltration (CVVHDF). Which of the following flow rates of the total effluent (the sum of the dialysate and ultrafiltrate) of CVVHDF is the LOWEST that can still be considered effective for optimum renal replacement therapy?

a) 10 mL/kg of body weight per hour
b) 20 mL/kg of body weight per hour
c) 30 mL/kg of body weight per hour
d) 40 mL/kg of body weight per hour
e) 50 mL/kg of body weight per hour

Answer: b

Explanation

The main questions that must be answered when considering a patient with acute renal failure for renal replacement therapy (RRT) are when to start, what is the most appropriate method, the best dialysis membrane and the amount of fluid removal and dialysate. There has been considerable recent work on the latter and initially it was thought that higher doses were associated with a reduction in mortality. This, intuitively, would seem to make sense given the lack of efficiency of RRTs when compared to the native kidneys and the high catabolic state of most critically ill patients. Balanced against this is the increased risk of hypotension associated with higher rates of RRT. In 2008, a well constructed, multicentre trial concluded that a dose of 20 mL/kg/h was as effective as a higher dose. The trial results showed no difference between the 20 mL/kg/h dose and a more intensive dose of RRT on mortality; time to, or improved recovery of renal function; or the rate of non-renal organ failure. In the intensive treatment group there were more episodes of hypotension, hypophosphataemia and hypokalaemia. It is important to note that the patients receiving continuous RRT in this group received CVVHDF and not continuous venovenous haemofiltration (CVVH). However, there is no research suggesting that the addition of dialysis to CVVH is in any way detrimental.

References

Bonventre JV. Dialysis in acute kidney injury – more is not better. *N Engl J Med* 2008; **359**(1): 82–4

VA/NIH Acute Renal Failure Trial Network. Intensity of renal support in critically ill patients with acute kidney injury. *N Engl J Med* 2008; **359**(1): 7–20.

Question 159: Subarachnoid haemorrhage

Regarding the management of a patient who has had a subarachnoid haemorrhage, which one of the following statements is MOST CORRECT?

a) Systolic blood pressure should be carefully controlled within narrow limits
b) Hypervolaemia, haemodilution and hypertension ('triple H' therapy) should be introduced if cerebral oedema is suspected
c) Following procedural aneurysm management, prophylactic anticonvulsants should be administered
d) After an aneurysm has been coiled, aspirin and heparin are administered
e) Nimodipine 60 mg i.v. four-hourly for 21 days is used as prophylaxis against cerebral vasospasm

Answer: d

Explanation

Following subarachnoid haemorrhage (SAH), the range of mean arterial blood pressure over which cerebral blood flow is autoregulated is narrowed or lost altogether. Cerebral perfusion is thus pressure dependent so reducing blood pressure risks watershed infarction, especially in jeopardised regions where autoregulation is completely absent. There is no evidence that treatment with antihypertensives positively impacts on the outcome, but in the clinical setting, blood pressure is rarely allowed to remain above 200/110 mmHg for long. Although not evidence based, triple H therapy is widely used for the prevention of secondary cerebral ischaemia caused by vasospasm, should it occur. It is unusual for an SAH to present with seizures and this is the only circumstance in which anticonvulsants will be administered. Calcium channel antagonists may have a neuroprotective effect and do reduce incidence of vasospasm. The regimen is as described in Option (e), except the drug is given enterally, not intravenously. If the patient is unable to swallow, the nimodipine is crushed, suspended in 0.9% saline and delivered down the nasogastric tube. Counterintuitive as it seems in a patient who has presented with haemorrhage, anticoagulation is crucial following coiling because although the objective is to induce clotting in the aneurysmal sac, if the clot extends into the parent artery, disastrous thrombotic infarct results.

Reference

van Gijn J, Rinkel GJ. Subarachnoid haemorrhage: diagnosis, causes and management. *Brain* 2001; **124**(2): 249–78.

Question 160: Tracheostomy

One complication at the time of insertion of surgical or percutaneous dilational tracheostomy is bleeding. The following are true of peritracheal anatomy EXCEPT which one?

a) The left brachiocephalic vein crosses from left to right, anterior to the trachea
b) The inferior thyroid veins run in the tracheoesophageal groove but form an anterior plexus
c) About 50% of people will have a thyroid ima artery
d) The thyroid isthmus lies anterior to the trachea at the level of the second and third tracheal rings
e) The jugular venous arch lies anterior to the trachea superior to the manubrium

Answer: c

Explanation

Frustratingly for performing the procedure and learning for examinations, there is considerable variation of normal anatomy around the trachea. The low rate of moderate or severe peri-procedure haemorrhage associated with percutaneous tracheostomy should not permit complacency with respect to this potential complication. Figures quoted for the frequency of the presence of a thyroid ima artery are around 10%. It may originate from the aorta, right common carotid, subclavian or internal thoracic artery; it ascends in the midline and supplies the lower regions of the thyroid – usually compensating for the absence of one of the other thyroid arteries. The left brachiocephalic (or innominate) vein and the brachiocephalic artery do pass anterior to the trachea and although they are usually intrathoracic, absolute separating distance between the surgical field and these vessels may be small, especially in children. The thyroid isthmus can be formally identified and divided at surgical tracheostomy, but omitting this at percutaneous tracheostomy does not seem to cause problems, perhaps due to the direct pressure (tamponade) effect of the dilated, as opposed to incised, tissues. The anterior jugular vein may be singular and midline, paired and non-communicating, or paired and united anteriorly forming the jugular venous arch, which is suprasternal and anterior to the trachea.

Question 161: Muscle relaxants

Urgent attendance in the recovery room is required. A patient is hypoxic and has overt features of residual neuromuscular blockade. A dose of neostigmine metilsulfate and glycopyrronium bromide is administered and the patient recovers quickly. On reviewing the patient's anaesthetic and drug charts, which of the following is LEAST LIKELY to have prolonged the action of the vecuronium that had been given?

a) The presence of an intraoperative metabolic acidosis
b) The isoflurane used as the maintenance anaesthetic
c) The gentamicin given prior to induction
d) The lithium the patient has been on to treat his long-standing bipolar disorder
e) Serum potassium 6.1 mmol/L

Answer: e

Explanation

A number of drugs either prolong or enhance the effects of both non-depolarising muscle relaxants (NDMR) and suxamethonium. These include volatile anaesthetic agents, procainamide, aminoglycosides, clindamycin, the polymixin antibiotic colistin, propranolol, nifedipine, verapamil, lithium and parenteral magnesium. The mechanism for aminoglycoside prolongation of NDMRs is thought to be inhibition of calcium influx to the motor nerve terminals, which decreases the amount of acetylcholine released into the neuromuscular synapse. Both carbamazepine and phenytoin antagonise the muscle relaxant effects of NDMRs leading to accelerated recovery. In addition to drug interactions a number of physiological conditions have an effect on muscle relaxants. Hypothermia prolongs the action of both NDMRs and suxamethonium due to reduced drug metabolism and a metabolic acidosis prolongs the action of all except gallamine. Acute hypokalaemia increases the resting membrane potential thus potentiating the action of NDMRs and antagonizing the effect of suxamethonium. The reverse is true in hyperkalaemia. Hypermagnesaemia prolongs NDMR blockade via decreased acetylcholine release and stabilisation of the post-junctional membrane.

References

British National Formulary website. Online at www.bnf.org (Accessed 30 November 2009)

Dotan ZA, Hana R, Simon D, *et al*. The effect of vecuronium is enhanced by a large rather than by a modest dose of gentamicin as compared with no preoperative gentamicin. *Anesth Analg* 2003; **96**(3): 750–4.

Question 162: Chronic kidney disease

Regarding a patient with Stage 3 chronic kidney disease, which one of the following statements is TRUE?

a) They should have their haemoglobin maintained at 11 to 12 g/dL using iron supplements with or without erythropoietin
b) They should have their kidney function assessed every three months
c) They could be diagnosed during a period of acute kidney disease
d) If newly diagnosed, they should have a renal biopsy
e) They may have an average glomerular filtration rate of 25 mL/min per 1.73 m^2

Answer: a

Explanation
A patient with Stage 3 chronic kidney disease is functioning at about half of normal renal function. They should have their renal function assessed annually if stable or every six months if new or progressive. They would normally have a glomerular filtration rate (GFR) in the 30 to 59 mL/min/1.73 m^2 range. They cannot be diagnosed during acute kidney disease as they require a stable creatinine to make the diagnosis. If newly diagnosed, they should be investigated, but renal biopsy is only required if they have significant proteinuria or haematuria. A target haemoglobin of 11 to 12 g/dL is a starting point. This may need adjusting depending on level of exercise and the ease with which the target is reached.

Reference
Chronic kidney disease in adults: UK guidelines for identification, management and referral. Online at www.renal.org/CKDguide/full/UKCKDfull.pdf (Accessed 30 November 2009)

Question 163: The Valsalva manoeuvre

Regarding the Valsalva manoeuvre, which one of the following statements is TRUE?

a) Phase I involves raised intrathoracic pressure being transmitted to the aorta causing a transient decrease in blood pressure
b) Using a Valsalva manoeuvre therapeutically to terminate a supraventricular tachycardia takes advantage of Phase III physiology
c) Diabetic autonomic neuropathy disrupts the usual phases seen, most commonly by an exaggerated late hypertension
d) The Valsalva ratio is normally greater than 3
e) Congestive cardiac failure results in a square wave response

Answer: e

Explanation
The Valsalva manoeuvre is sustained intrathoracic pressure of 40 mmHg (54 cmH$_2$O) for 15 seconds. The candidate should be able to draw a graph of arterial blood pressure (or heart rate) against time, indicating the four phases of the Valsalva manoeuvre. The phases are quite intuitive if one considers how the intrathoracic pressure is transmitted to the great vessels, its effect on venous return and the normal function of baroreceptors. A bradycardia is expected during Phase IV. Autonomic neuropathy manifests as a

profound hypotension in Phase II and the absence of overshoot and bradycardia on release of airway pressure. In congestive cardiac failure, venous return is maintained throughout the manoeuvre secondary to an increased blood volume and increased peripheral venous pressure. As intrathoracic pressure rises, its transmission to the aorta causes a sustained rise in blood pressure, which terminates without overshoot on airway pressure release – the 'square wave response'. The Valsalva ratio (usually >1.5) is the longest R–R interval (bradycardia in Phase IV) divided by the shortest R–R interval during the manoeuvre.

Reference
Power I, Kam P. *Principles of Physiology for the Anaesthetist*, 1st edn. Bath: Arnold, 2000; pp. 157–8.

Question 164: Reporting a death to the coroner

Following the death of a patient, referral to the coroner or their deputy is mandatory in a number of situations. In which of the following situations is referral NOT mandatory?

a) A 52-year-old patient who has died six days after a proven myocardial infarction who was awaiting trial while on remand in prison
b) A 75-year-old man who has died of a subarachnoid haemorrhage with a past medical history including a diagnosis of pneumoconiosis
c) A 75-year-old woman admitted from a residential home with a bronchopneumonia and a core temperature of 34 °C
d) A 60-year-old patient with known COPD who had been discharged well following surgery three weeks previously and is then readmitted with bronchopneumonia from which they die two days later
e) A 40-year-old man who has died following admission for treatment of a urinary tract infection contributed to by a paraplegia sustained following an assault 20 years previously

Answer: d

Explanation
All deaths should be reported to the coroner if the death cannot be certified as being due to natural causes. Death should also be referred under a number of other circumstances. (1) If injury, whether it is self-inflicted, inflicted by another person or as a result of an accident, played a part in the death of the patient. (2) If there might have been something unnatural causing or accelerating the death, for example any disease contracted during employment, any death that is wholly unexpected or a death where there are allegations of poor or delayed treatment. (3) If there is any evidence of neglect on the part of the individual or carer(s), e.g. unexplained hypothermia or multiple bed sores. (4) If the deceased was 'in custody' at the time of death. (5) If there is no clinical history or evidence to satisfactorily establish the cause of death. (6) If there was any toxic substance involved. This includes all deaths from anaphylaxis secondary to therapeutic drugs and all alcohol-related deaths. (7) If death occurred within 24 hours of hospital admission whatever the cause. (8) If death occurred abroad and the body is repatriated to the United Kingdom.

The coroner does not need to be informed of every death within a specific timeframe. They should be informed if the patient failed to recover from the effects of the anaesthesia or if death may have been related to the surgery itself, e.g. bronchopneumonia three days following general anaesthetic for a laparoscopic colectomy.

Reference
The Intensive Care Society Working Group on Organ and Tissue Donation. Guidelines for adult organ and tissue donation. Online at www.ics.ac.uk (Accessed 30 November 2009)

Question 165: Removing epidurals

In the following options, $T_{1/2}$ is the half-life of the anticoagulant they are currently taking and T_{max} is the time taken from administration to reaching full activity. If a patient is anticoagulated and needs to have an epidural catheter removed, the ideal time between stopping the last dose of anticoagulant and starting the next dose of anticoagulant is:

a) $(3 \times T_{1/2}) + (8 \text{ hours} + T_{max})$
b) $(3 \times T_{1/2}) + (4 \text{ hours} - T_{max})$
c) $(2 \times T_{1/2}) + (8 \text{ hours} - T_{max})$
d) $(3 \times T_{1/2}) + (4 \text{ hours} + T_{max})$
e) $(2 \times T_{1/2}) + (8 \text{ hours} + T_{max})$

Answer: c

Explanation
Epidural catheter removal is a dangerous time for the anticoagulated patient. The challenge is to balance the risk of unwanted thrombus formation against the risk of epidural haematoma. With the new oral anticoagulants soon to be introduced into clinical practice, anaesthetists will need to be able to advise on when it is safe to remove catheters for individual cases. In the 2007 review article by Rosencher *et al.*, guidance was given for catheter removal for a patient on any anticoagulant with known pharmacology. Adherence to this formula should allow activity to fall to 25% after the two $T_{1/2}$ periods and the catheter can then be safely removed. After this period of time, elimination slows considerably so it takes a relatively long time off the anticoagulant to gain small returns in the ability to clot. The catheter is then removed and a period of time is required for a platelet plug to adequately solidify. This was thought to have happened by eight hours. However, eight hours' wait is not required before restarting the anticoagulant as it takes the T_{max} time to gain full activity. For some drugs this may be a considerable amount of time (three to four hours for low molecular weight heparin).

Reference
Rosencher N, Bonnet M-P, Sessler D. Selected new antithrombotic agents and neuraxial anaesthesia for major orthopaedic surgery: management strategies. *Anaesthesia* 2007; **62**(11): 1154–60.

Question 166: Phantom limb pain

A 20-year-old soldier is complaining of phantom limb pain (PLP) six months following lower-limb amputation. Which one of the following is INCORRECT regarding his condition and possible treatment options?

a) If he had had an epidural inserted prior to amputation his chances of developing PLP would have been reduced
b) The use of mirror therapy has been shown to reduce PLP in both upper- and lower-limb amputations
c) The incidence of PLP has been shown to be as high as 80%
d) The pain in PLP tends to be constant rather than intermittent
e) The incidence of PLP in adults is independent of age, gender and level of amputation

Answer: d

Explanation

Following limb amputation, virtually all amputees experience phantom sensations. These may or may not be painful. Pain is experienced by up to 80% of adults dependent on the group examined and is independent of gender, age and side or level of the amputation. Phantom limb pain is less common in children. Patients with a history of gangrene and/or infection and/or pre-amputation pain are at increased risk of PLP. Phantom limb pain tends to be intermittent and often seems to mimic the pre-amputation pain both in quality and location. The mechanism of PLP is not fully understood and is likely to be multifactorial including contributions from peripheral (e.g. neuroma formation), spinal cord (e.g. sensitisation of pain neurons via N-methyl-D-aspartic acid receptors) and brain elements (cerebral reorganisation). Treatment can often be difficult and may be divided into medical, non-medical and surgical. Medical options include tricyclic antidepressants, anticonvulsants, N-methyl-D-aspartic acid receptor antagonists, benzodiazepines, calcitonin and opioids. Non-medical treatments include mirror therapy (effective for both upper and lower limbs), transcutaneous electrical nerve stimulation, acupuncture, electroconvulsive therapy and hypnosis. Surgical options include neurectomy, stump revision, cordotomy, dorsal column stimulation and pallidotomy. Epidural insertion prior to amputation reduces the risk of developing PLP.

Reference

Nikolajsen L, Jensen T. Phantom limb pain. *Brit J Anaesth* 2001; **87**(1): 107–16.

Question 167: Tetanus

Regarding tetanus, the following statements are true EXCEPT which one?

a) May be diagnosed with the aid of the spatula test with high sensitivity and specificity
b) A patient who has survived the disease does not require further tetanus vaccination
c) Cardiovascular instability is best treated in intensive care with deep sedation
d) Musculoskeletal symptoms are caused by disruption of inhibitory neurotransmitter release by central nerves
e) Autonomic dysfunction may be successfully treated with magnesium

Answer: b

Explanation

Tetanus is a clinical condition caused by the tetanus toxin. This toxin is produced by *Clostridium tetani* and usually enters the body as a wound contaminant. It produces a characteristic clinical pattern of muscle spasm and autonomic instability, with life-threatening swings in cardiovascular status. The intensive care management of choice is pinned around deep sedation, as when light, the patient's instability is triggered by stimulation. The spatula test involves stimulation of the posterior pharyngeal wall with a soft-tipped stick. Positive test is biting down on the stick and negative is the gag reflex. Anyone suffering tetanus should be offered immunisation or a booster once they have recovered.

References

Thwaites CL, Farrar JJ. Magnesium as first line therapy in the management of tetanus *Anaesthesia* 2003; **58**(3): 286.

Taylor A. Tetanus. *Contin Educ Anaesth Crit Care Pain* 2006; **6**(3): 101.

Question 168: Acute abdominal emergencies

A 58-year-old Afro-Caribbean female presents with clinical and radiological features of ischaemic colitis. She does not speak English. She is clinically dehydrated, tachypnoeic and distressed. Her laboratory results are as follows: Hb 10.8 g/dL; WCC 18×10^{10}/L; Platelets 146×10^9/L; Urea 10.1 mmol/L; Creatinine 89 micromol/L; pH 7.32; $PaCO_2$ 3.4 kPa; PaO_2 8.8 kPa; Base excess –4.0 mmol/L; Lactate 2.4 mmol/L. Erect chest X-ray does not show gas under the diaphragm. The surgical team proposes an urgent laparotomy. Oxygen is applied and aggressive fluid resuscitation commenced. Which one of the following statements is the most appropriate action to take next?

a) Once fluid resuscitated, proceed to surgery
b) Provide analgesia and order more blood tests
c) Give urgent antibiotics, then proceed to surgery
d) Transfuse packed red blood cells to a target haematocrit of 0.4
e) Intubate and ventilate on the intensive care unit and observe initially

Answer: b

Explanation

Surgery is not indicated currently, and ventilation is not required at this stage. Sickle crises can present as an acute abdomen. The patient should be kept warm and given oxygen, intravenous fluid and analgesia while results of a Sickledex test and electrophoresis are awaited. These simple interventions and careful observation, perhaps in a high-dependency environment, are the appropriate conservative management of ischaemic colitis or a sickle crisis. Surgery is a last resort in severe cases. Ischaemic colitis often presents with bright red blood in the stools. This would account for her mild anaemia. Her haemoglobin level of 10.8 g/dL virtually eliminates sickle cell disease, but sickle cell trait (HBAS) is a possibility. HbSS homozygotes typically have a haemoglobin concentration of 6 to 8 g/dL. In sickle cell anaemia the proportion of adult haemoglobin is the important factor peri-operatively. The extent of sickling in conditions of hypoxaemia is proportional to the percentage of haemoglobin that is HbSS. A target HbA of 70% should be attained if the patient's haemoglobin is less than 7 g/dL or if heavy blood loss is anticipated. Antibiotics are sometimes used in severe ischaemic colitis but otherwise are not indicated.

Question 169: Peri-operative loss of vision

Occurring with an incidence of 1 per 7000 operations, which one of the following is the COMMONEST cause of peri-operative loss of vision in patients undergoing non-ocular surgery?

a) Cortical infarction
b) Retinal ischaemia
c) Corneal abrasion
d) Ischaemic optic neuropathy
e) Electromagnetic retinal injury

Answer: d

Explanation

In a recent publication, cases of blindness were reviewed among 126 666 anaesthetics. Seventeen cases of peri-operative blindness due to ischaemic optic neuropathy (ION) were found. ION accounts for about 80% of cases of peri-operative loss of vision. The most commonly associated operations were coronary artery bypass grafting and prone spinal surgery. Suggested reasons for these operations being high risk included anaemia, hypotension, facial and orbital oedema, and direct pressure on the globe

Reference

Sarah H, Tsai J, McAllister R, Smith, K. Perioperative ischemic optic neuropathy: a case control analysis of 126,666 surgical procedures at a single institution. *Anesthesiology* 2009; **110**(2): 246–53.

Question 170: Pre-eclampsia

Regarding risk factors for the development of pre-eclampsia, the following statements are true EXCEPT which one?

a) Pre-eclampsia is more likely to develop in women whose mothers had pre-eclampsia than in women whose mothers did not
b) Pre-eclampsia is more likely to develop in the daughters-in-law of women with a history of pre-eclampsia than in other women
c) Women with pre-existing chronic hypertension are more likely to develop pre-eclampsia
d) Among nulliparous women, black women have twice the risk of developing pre-eclampsia compared to white women
e) Nulliparous women who smoke have a similar risk of developing pre-eclampsia to non-smokers

Answer: e

Explanation

Pre-eclampsia and subsequent eclampsia cause an estimated 50 000 deaths worldwide per year. Causation is probably multifactorial but there does seem to be both a maternally transmitted and paternally transmitted genetic predisposition to pre-eclampsia. This is borne out by a number of observations. These include the facts that the daughters-in-law of women who suffered from pre-eclampsia are more likely to develop the condition themselves, and that a woman who becomes pregnant by a man who has already had a child with a different woman who during that pregnancy developed pre-eclampsia, has a risk of pre-eclampsia that is nearly twice as high as that of a woman whose partner does not have such a history. Other risk factors include race, pre-existing chronic hypertension, nulliparity, obesity, previous pre-eclamptic pregnancy, pre-existing diabetes mellitus and multiple pregnancy. Surprisingly, women who smoke cigarettes have a lower risk of pre-eclampsia even after confounding variables have been removed.

Reference

Broughton Pipkin F. Risk factors for preeclampsia. *New Engl J Med* 2001; **344**(12): 925–6.

Question 171: Anxious patient in recovery

You are asked to review a patient in the recovery room one hour after the end of an anaesthetic for manipulation of a forearm fracture. He is 43 years old, unkempt and is of no fixed abode. He has a past history of schizophrenia for which he is on 75 mg of chlorpromazine per day. He is a 20 cigarette a day smoker, drinks up to 100 units of alcohol a week and has previously taken intravenous heroin. He has been in hospital for 24 hours. He is anxious, sweating, hypertensive, tremulous and hyperreflexic. As you arrive at the bedside, he has a self-limiting tonic-clonic seizure for 30 seconds. None of these symptoms or signs were present before induction and he has no history of epilepsy.

Which one of the following is the MOST LIKELY explanation?

a) Alcohol withdrawal
b) Nicotine withdrawal
c) Heroin withdrawal
d) Emergence from anaesthesia
e) Side effects of excess chlorpromazine

Answer: a

Explanation

Tremor, agitation, anxiety, hypertension, hyperreflexia, sweating and gastric upset leading on to seizures, hallucinations and delirium are classic symptoms of alcohol withdrawal. This typically occurs within 6 to 24 hours after stopping drinking, and is most commonly seen by the anaesthetist presenting in the postoperative period. It is important to recognise, as it may be fatal if not treated appropriately. Nicotine withdrawal is typically characterised more by psychological than physical symptoms, so even though anxiety may be present, tremor and hyperreflexia usually are not. Heroin withdrawal may present with any of the initial symptoms, but rarely produces seizures. Anxiety and hypertension may be seen after emergence from anaesthesia, especially if the patient is in pain, but one hour post emergence, tremor and hyperreflexia are unlikely to be present. Excess chlorpromazine tends to produce sedation and hypotension with moderate antimuscarinic and extrapyramidal side effects. These signs would tend to be present before induction.

Question 172: Handwashing

When washing hands, which one of the following hand parts is MOST COMMONLY missed?

a) The thenar eminence
b) The lateral aspect of the index finger
c) The dorsum of the thumb
d) The hypothenar eminence
e) The knuckle at the base of the little finger

Answer: c

Explanation

Handwashing is of paramount importance and proven efficacy in reducing healthcare-associated infection. The College will always be looking for ways to ask handwashing questions. It is worth knowing about. Typically, the areas most frequently missed when handwashing are the thumb, especially the dorsal aspect; the fingerpads where the fingerprints are; and the lateral and medial surfaces of all the digits apart from the lateral aspect of the index finger and the medial aspect of the little finger.

Question 173: Postoperative nausea and vomiting risk

A 39-year-old patient presents for day case surgery. Which of the following is LEAST LIKELY to indicate that this patient is at risk of postoperative nausea and vomiting (PONV)?

a) The operation is laparoscopic sterilisation
b) The patient is female
c) The patient is a non-smoker
d) The patient had nausea following a rhinoplasty three years ago
e) The patient suffers from 'car-sickness'

Answer: a

Explanation

Risk factors for PONV were analysed and simplified in the seminal 1999 paper by Apfel *et al.*, which proposed a simple score containing just four factors. This scoring system has been further validated in a number of papers since publication. The factors predicting risk of PONV were female gender, non-smoking, the use of postoperative opioids, and previous history of PONV or motion sickness. Depending on the presence of none, one, two, three or all four risk factors, the predicted probability of PONV would be 10%, 21%, 39%, 61% or 78%, respectively. There was an association between type of operation and PONV, but this was thought to be due to the incidence of high-risk patients in the operative group rather than any causal relationship. For example, gynaecological surgery patients are female. Gynaecological laparoscopy produced an odds ratio of 1.63 with 95% confidence intervals of 0.86 to 3.09. Duration of surgery over one hour was shown to confer an increased risk, but is a less useful predictor as it can often only be assessed retrospectively.

Reference

Apfel CC, Läärä E, Koivuranta M, Greim CA, Roewer N. A simplified risk score for predicting postoperative nausea and vomiting. *Anesthesiology* 1999; **91**(3): 693–700.

Question 174: Ventilator-associated pneumonia

Which of the following is NOT considered a risk factor for the development of ventilator-associated pneumonia?

a) The presence of an orogastric tube
b) Acute respiratory distress syndrome (ARDS)
c) An *in situ* percutaneous tracheostomy
d) Treatment with muscle relaxants
e) Age >60 years

Answer: a

Explanation

Ventilator-associated pneumonia (VAP) is a leading cause of mortality among patients ventilated on a critical care unit and, dependent on the population studied, develops in up to 30% of mechanically ventilated patients. Its pathogenesis relies on both bacterial colonisation of the aerodigestive tract and the aspiration of contaminated secretions into the lower airways. Ventilator-associated pneumonia may be divided into early (usually within 48 to 72 hours) and late onset, with the former usually due to antibiotic-sensitive bacteria, e.g. *Haemophilus*, oxacillin-sensitive *Staphylococcus* and *Streptococcus pneumoniae* and the latter more frequently with antibiotic-resistant organisms, e.g. methicillin-resistant *Staphylococcus aureus* (MRSA), *Acinetobacter* and *Pseudomonas*. Risk factors for VAP may be divided into patient factors and intervention factors. Patient risk factors include advanced age; low serum albumin; chronic obstructive pulmonary disease; acute respiratory distress syndrome; reduced conscious level; ventilation following trauma, burns or a surgical procedure; sinusitis and large-volume gastric aspiration. Intervention risk factors include use of muscle relaxants, the presence of a nasogastric (not orogastric) tube, re-intubation, inappropriate use of antibiotic therapy, supine head position, prolonged nasal intubation, the use of positive end expiratory pressure and most importantly being mechanically ventilated in the first place (the longer the duration, the greater the risk, either via an endotracheal tube or tracheostomy). Prevention of VAP has been the subject of a National Institute of Health and Clinical Excellence document and as part of the Department of Health's Saving Lives campaign, a high-impact intervention has been produced that suggests a care bundle for the care of mechanically ventilated patients designed to prevent the development of VAP. This includes nursing the patient in a semi-recumbent position, routine use of selective oral decontamination (SOD), humidification of inhaled gases, strict infection control policies, venous thromboembolism and gastric ulcer prophylaxis, and the care of breathing tubing.

References

Chastre J, Fagon JY. Ventilator-associated pneumonia. *Am J Respir Crit Care Med* 2002; **165**(7): 867–903.

High Impact Intervention No. 5. Saving Lives: reducing infection, delivering clean and safe care. Care bundle for ventilated patients (or tracheostomy where appropriate). Online at www.clean-safe-care.nhs.uk/toolfiles/25_SL_HII_5_v2.pdf (Accessed 30 November 2009)

Question 175: Ear, nose and throat surgery

Regarding the provision of anaesthesia for ENT surgery, which one of the following statements is MOST CORRECT?

a) For microlaryngoscopy, a microlaryngoscopy tube (cuffed oral endotracheal tube, ID 5 mm) must be used
b) For functional endoscopic sinus surgery, given the operation's proximity to the patient's eyes, the eyes must be taped and padded
c) Of the various lasers available, carbon dioxide lasers do have the capacity to ignite endotracheal tubes
d) In myringoplasty using an overlay graft, use of nitrous oxide as part of the inhaled gas mixture is actually likely to be beneficial
e) In parotidectomy, neuromuscular blockade is recommended because coughing can cause surgical field disruption and significant haemorrhage

Answer: c

Explanation

Providing anaesthesia for ENT surgery has a number of procedure-specific nuances that are important to recall. Anaesthesia for microlaryngoscopy can involve a micro-laryngoscopy tube, but total intravenous anaesthesia and jet ventilation with a Sander's jet ventilator attached to the surgeon's laryngoscope is an equally valid option. Tracheal catheters and cricothyroidotomy techniques have also been described. For surgery where access is via the nose, the proximity of the optic nerves necessitates leaving the eyes uncovered so the surgeon is aware of movements of the globe and pupillary changes. Carbon dioxide lasers are ideal for laryngeal work because of their tissue penetration and destruction characteristics, but they can certainly ignite an endotracheal tube and special precautions are taken. As nitrous oxide diffuses into the middle ear potentially increasing pressure inside, an overlay myringoplasty graft can be disrupted. Theoretically, if an underlay graft is used, it would be held in place by the increased middle ear pressure but this can hardly be considered an indication for use of nitrous oxide (especially given the emetogenic nature of the surgery). In paro-tidectomy, the surgeon will employ facial nerve monitoring because of the immediate proximity of the facial nerve to operative site. Neuromuscular blockade will interfere with this monitoring. For this reason, remifentanil infusions are a commonly used alternative to neuromuscular blockade in this, and similar, circumstances.

Question 176: Haemodynamic monitoring

A pulmonary artery flotation catheter is being used to monitor a patient on the cardiac intensive care unit following cardiac surgery. Which one of the following variables BEST reflects left ventricular preload?

a) Pulmonary capillary wedge pressure
b) Left ventricular end-diastolic pressure
c) Left ventricular wall tension

d) Left ventricular end-diastolic volume
e) Mean pulmonary venous pressure

Answer: c

Explanation

In this question the presence of a pulmonary artery flotation catheter is a distraction, which if recognised and disregarded renders the question a simple one. The question does not ask for the variable measurable with the catheter that best reflects preload. There are many definitions of preload, but all of them aim to usefully express a myocardial fibre's pre-contraction stretch because it is this that is proportional to its subsequent power of contraction (according to Starling's Law). One way to express a fibre's pre-contraction stretch is to consider the left ventricular wall tension and indeed this would most accurately reflect left ventricular preload. A surrogate of that (and next best marker) is the left ventricular end-diastolic volume as it will vary as a function of the wall tension. However, the two may not vary linearly if wall compliance is dynamic such as in evolving ischaemia, diastolic dysfunction or manipulation of inotropic therapy. Left ventricular end-diastolic pressure can be a surrogate marker of the volume (and is next best) *if* compliance is fairly static (see above). If the tip of the pulmonary artery flotation catheter is in West zone 3 (where pulmonary artery pressure exceeds pulmonary venous pressure, which exceeds alveolar pressure) then there is an uninterrupted column of blood between the tip of the catheter and the left atrium, so from the pulmonary artery occlusion pressure we can infer the left atrial pressure. From this, in the absence of mitral valve disease the left ventricular end-diastolic pressure may be inferred. Remember that as a guide to volume resuscitation status the presence of high intrathoracic pressure (secondary to mechanical ventilation) and ventricular interdependence must also be considered.

Question 177: Cost of volatile anaesthetic

A hypothetical new anaesthetic vapour, jabetone, is presented as 600 g in a bottle costing £74.67. It has an atomic weight of 120 and a minimum alveolar concentration (MAC) of 2%. At a fresh gas flow of 1 L/min with an agent concentration of 2%, which one of the following options is the cost per hour?

a) 15 p/hour
b) 20 p/hour
c) 40 p/hour
d) 80 p/hour
e) 220 p/hour

Answer: d

Explanation

Jabetone comes in 600 g bottles. It has an atomic weight of 120, so a bottle contains 5 moles.

5 moles would make 5×22.4 L of vapour, i.e. 112 L.

If this were made up to a fresh gas containing 2% anaesthetic agent, it could make 50×112 L (i.e. 5600 L).

Therefore 5600 L of fresh gas would cost £74.67 or 7467 p.

1 L costs 7467/5600 pence.

A fresh gas flow of 1 L/min is 60 L/h and would therefore cost $60 \times 7467/5600$ p/hour, or 80p/hour. At current prices, this would make jabetone more expensive than isoflurane and cheaper than desflurane at 1 MAC and 1 L/minute fresh gas flow.

Question 178: Breathing systems

Regarding the eponymous descriptions of anaesthetic breathing systems the following statements are true EXCEPT which one?

a) A Lack is a co-axial Mapleson A
b) A Water's circuit is a Mapleson C
c) A Magill is a parallel Mapleson A
d) An Ayre's T-piece is a Mapleson E
e) A Bain is a co-axial Mapleson D

Answer: c

Explanation

Mapleson analysed and categorised anaesthetic breathing systems in 1954. He considered bidirectional systems without carbon dioxide absorption. Non-re-breathing systems and circle systems with carbon dioxide absorption were not included in the classification. The Magill system, described in the 1930s by Sir Ivan Magill, involves a reservoir bag on the inspiratory limb (i.e. afferent reservoir system – ARS), just downstream of the fresh gas flow. The adjustable pressure-limiting (APL) valve is at the patient end of the single limb rendering the point of application to the patient bulky and cumbersome. Lack described a modification that involves transferring the APL valve to adjacent to the reservoir bag via an expiratory limb that has identical length to the inspiratory limb. The expiratory limb may either run adjacent to the inspiratory limb to the APL valve (parallel Lack) or inside the inspiratory limb (coaxial Lack). The Magill and Lack systems are Mapleson A systems. Avoid confusing the coaxial Lack, which is a Mapleson A, with the Bain system, which is Mapleson D and where the inner tube is inspiratory, not expiratory. The Ayre's T-piece used in paediatric anaesthesia today is the Jackson–Rees modification of the original device, which did not have an open-ended reservoir bag. The original is classified Mapleson E. The modified version has subsequently been added as Mapleson F but was not included in the original classification. Mapleson D, E and F systems are termed efferent reservoir systems (ERS) because their reservoir facility is on the expiratory limb. The Water's circuit is a to-and-fro system that historically has been used with a soda lime carbon dioxide absorber but problems arose from inhalation of soda lime dust. It lacks a one-way valve so relies on high fresh gas flows to avoid re-breathing. It is portable and can be connected to wall oxygen, without need for a common gas outlet. It is therefore useful for manual ventilation outside the theatre environment.

Question 179: Signs of anaphylaxis

The following signs of anaphylaxis detected under anaesthesia are matched with the correct frequency EXCEPT which one?

a) Cardiovascular collapse 88%
b) Bronchospasm 36%
c) Cutaneous erythema 45%
d) Angioedema of the face 24%
e) Bradycardia 3%

Answer: e

Explanation

It is important to understand the likelihood of anaphylaxis presenting with or without certain signs. Erythema, which is widely looked for, is absent in 55% of cases of anaphylaxis. Bradycardia is an important feature found in 10% of cases of anaphylaxis under general anaesthesia. A suggested mechanism for bradycardia is the Bezold–Jarisch reflex, although there are other possible mechanisms such as transient sino-atrial node ischaemia. The usual physiological response to vasodilatation and reduced venous return is tachycardia. The Bezold–Jarisch reflex is a paradoxical effect in which following pooling of the intravascular volume into a dilated vascular tree and a reduction in venous return, tension receptors in the left ventricle send cardioinhibitory messages. These are the afferents in the reflex arc in which the final efferent pathway is the vagus nerve, which is stimulated by various nuclei in the brain stem. These inhibitory cardiac-sensory receptors are different from the baroreceptors we are used to considering, and part of the reflex may also include a reflex hypopnea. The brady-cardia should not be treated with atropine, but with intravenous fluid and adrenaline.

Reference
Working Party of the Association of Anaesthetists of Great Britain and Ireland. Suspected anaphylactic reactions associated with anaesthesia. *Anaesthesia* 2009; **64**(2): 199–211. Available online at www.aagbi.org/publications/guidelines/docs/anaphylaxis_2009.pdf (Accessed 30 November 2009)

Question 180: Opioid pharmacokinetics
Regarding the applied pharmacokinetics of opioids, which one of the following state-ments is TRUE?

a) When administered intrathecally or extradurally, diamorphine is less likely than morphine to produce a delayed respiratory depressant effect due to its high lipid solubility
b) Alfentanil has a quicker onset time than fentanyl because it is more lipid soluble
c) The duration of action of morphine is longer than fentanyl because it has a longer terminal elimination half-life
d) Morphine may demonstrate a secondary peak effect due to gastro-enteric recirculation
e) When compared to morphine at equipotent doses, alfentanil has a shorter duration because it is subject to a more rapid clearance than morphine

Answer: a

Explanation
The pharmacokinetic profile of opioids is frequently relevant in clinical practice and explains the selection of each drug in particular circumstances. The speed of onset is governed by the total dose that may reach the central nervous system in a particular time, and is governed not just by lipid solubility but by the un-ionised fraction of the drug dictated by its pKa (and ambient pH). Fentanyl is the most lipid soluble of the opioids (600 times that of morphine), which explains its rapid onset, but alfentanil is quicker (despite being only 90 times more lipid soluble than morphine) because alfentanil's pKa of 6.5 means it is 89% un-ionised at physiological pH (as opposed to 9% of fentanyl) thus it crosses the blood–brain barrier quicker than fentanyl. The relative lipid solubilities of the opioids, as a multiple of that of morphine, are, in order, as follows: fentanyl (600), diamorphine (200), alfentanil (90), remifentanil (50), pethidine (30) and morphine (1). When administered intrathecally or extradurally, morphine has a propensity to exhibit delayed respiratory depression as it slowly diffuses into the brain. Regarding the duration of action of the opioids, distribution plays as much of a part as metabolism in governing the rate at which plasma concen-tration falls and therefore the duration of clinical effect. Therefore protein-binding, volume of distribution, lipid solubility and clearance all influence decrement time. The

terminal elimination half-life of morphine is three hours, compared to three-and-a-half hours for fentanyl and the clearance of morphine is up to 30 times quicker. Morphine's longer duration of action is explained by its low lipid solubility and slow diffusion out of the central nervous system. Even though clearance of alfentanil is slow compared to morphine, its duration of action is short because being 90% protein bound its volume of distribution is small so it is subject to very little redistribution. Only highly lipid-soluble drugs show gastro-enteric recirculation but morphine may demonstrate entero-hepatic recirculation.

Question 181: Clinical application of the Monro–Kellie doctrine

Regarding neurophysiology in the healthy, supine, adult subject, the following statements are true EXCEPT for which one?

a) Brain parenchyma occupies 85% of the available intracranial volume
b) Cerebral blood volume accounts for 5 to 8% of the available intracranial volume
c) Cerebrospinal fluid occupies 7 to 10% of the available intracranial volume
d) Cerebrospinal fluid is produced at a rate of 0.1 to 0.2 mL/min
e) Intracranial pressure is 10 to 23 cmH$_2$O

Answer: d

Explanation

Cerebrospinal fluid (CSF) is produced at a rate of 0.35 to 0.4 mL/min (double the value in the question) or 500 to 600 mL/day. The total volume in the adult is 150 mL so it can be seen that it turns over three to four times every day. One third of this volume is in the spinal canal; two thirds is intracranial (but this proportion is quoted, depending on source, anywhere from 25%/75% to 50%/50%). This is worth recalling when performing lumbar puncture on the intensive care unit. Being too conservative with the volumes of CSF withdrawn potentially reduces sensitivity of analysis and is not warranted. In adults it is usually acceptable to remove 20 mL or even 30 mL of CSF at one time (with some exceptions). Intracranial pressure is 7 to 17 mmHg, which is 9.5 to 23.1 cmH$_2$O. This is relevant when comparing opening pressure measured with a manometer at time of lumbar puncture (measured in cmCSF) with, for example, the pressure readings from a Codman intracranial pressure monitor (measured in mmHg).

Reference

Fogarty-Mack P, Young W. Chapter 21: Neurophysiology. In: Hemmings J, Hopkins P, eds. *Foundations of Anesthesia: Basic Sciences for Clinical Practice*, 2nd edn. London: Mosby-Elsevier, 2006; pp. 245–56.

Question 182: Surgical emergencies

A 55-year-old overweight male presents during the evening. He was brought in by ambulance from a restaurant at which he had been at a celebration and had consumed a larger than average quantity of food and a large amount of alcohol. On leaving the restaurant he had vomited a small amount, but continued to retch and complained of severe left-sided chest pain. He soon developed haematemesis and subcutaneous emphysema in his neck. Which one of the following statements is TRUE?

a) Admiral Boerhaave was famously a victim of this syndrome when it was originally described
b) The mechanism described is the commonest aetiology of the resulting surgical pathology

c) Mackler's triad, suggestive of the diagnosis, is the combination of dysphagia, epigastric pain and melaena

d) Management here should be with two large-bore thoracostomy tubes and observation on ITU, although thoracotomy is a possibility

e) Time from onset of symptoms until treatment is a major determinant of mortality with the two variables being directly related

Answer: e

Explanation

This is a classical presentation of post-emetic oesophageal rupture or Boerhaave syndrome. Boerhaave was the Dutch physician, who in 1724 attended Grand Admiral Wassenaer of the Netherlands who had just suffered a similar presentation to the patient in the question. Admiral Wassenaer died within 24 hours and Dr Boerhaave described the syndrome. Mackler's triad is chest pain and subcutaneous emphysema following vomiting or retching. The triad suggested in Option (c) is too vague to be suggestive of one diagnosis. The commonest aetiology by far is iatrogenic. Instrumentation of the oesophagus ranges from diagnostic oesophagogastroduodeno-scopy (which is low risk) to oesophageal dilatation or stenting, which carries a high risk of the complication. Over half oesophageal perforations are iatrogenic; less than 20% are post-emetic; 90% of intrathoracic perforations are directed towards the left chest. Perhaps surprisingly, a case is made for conservative management in some cases, especially if delayed presentation. However, in this case, with such a short and clear-cut history, immediate thoracotomy, wash-out and repair is indicated to optimise the possible outcome. Mortality is high; higher still if the cause is post-emetic, and varies directly with time elapsed between insult and treatment. Mortality is around 25% if the perforation is addressed within 24 hours of onset, but over 60% if delay is greater than this.

Question 183: ASA score

A 93-year-old man presents for reduction and repair of a large inguinal hernia that has made buttoning up his trousers uncomfortable. He is a lifelong non-smoker and still works two mornings a week in his son's bookshop. He wears a hearing aid and has had a previous haemorrhoidectomy, which was followed by postoperative vomiting. He has a thin, weak left arm, which he rarely uses following a brachial plexus injury in a tram accident at the age of 22. According to the American Society of Anesthesiologists (ASA) criteria, which of the following would be his correct ASA score?

a) I
b) I E
c) II
d) II E
e) III

Answer: a

Explanation

The original ASA score was proposed in 1941 and appeared in its current form in 1963. The score is used to assess a patient's preoperative disease severity status. The possible scores are as follows: ASA I – a normal healthy patient; ASA II – a patient with mild systemic disease; ASA III – a patient with severe systemic disease; ASA IV – a patient with severe systemic disease that is a constant threat to life; ASA V – a moribund patient who is not expected to survive without the operation. An additional score of ASA VI has been added to account for a declared brain-dead patient whose organs are being removed for donor purposes. The ASA states that 'There is no additional information that will help you further define these categories.' Despite the fact that some consider age >75 years to be associated with sufficient normal age-related degenerative change that physiology is impaired to the extent of a mild systemic disease, thus age >75 is ASA II, there are no conditions attached for age in the ASA's criteria. The described patient has no systemic disease. His procedure is elective. The additional 'E' for emergency used to be defined as 'a surgical procedure, which, in the surgeon's opinion, should be performed without delay'. This has been modified to identify an operation, which, if delayed, would produce significant increased threat to the patient's life or body part.

Reference
ASA Physical Status Classification System. Definition available online at www.asahq. org/clinical/physicalstatus.htm (Accessed 30 November 2009)

Question 184: Tracheal intubation in morbidly obese patients

In morbidly obese patients which one of the following is the MOST RELIABLE predictor of difficult intubation?

a) Height
b) Body mass index
c) Mallampati score
d) Neck circumference
e) Thyromental distance

Answer: d

Explanation
Historically morbid obesity has been one of a number of factors associated with challenging tracheal intubation, prompting employment of awake fibreoptic techniques. This received wisdom has been challenged by those anaesthetists involved in providing anaesthesia for bariatric surgery. It is important to differentiate between a difficult airway, difficult mask ventilation, difficult laryngoscopy and difficulty in the physical act of passing an endotracheal tube into the trachea. Clearly the challenges are not synonymous and fortunately they are very rarely concurrently present in a particular patient. In circumstances where one challenge is present, adequate performance of the other tasks mean the potential crisis of 'can't intubate, can't ventilate' is rarely encountered. Notwithstanding this fact, the anaesthetist should be well versed in drills for this scenario and preferably rehearse their actions in simulations. Studies among bariatric surgical patients emphasise the importance of patient positioning, suggesting that adopting a semi-recumbent 'ramped' position improves ease of each of the tasks mentioned and perhaps historical associations with difficulty had not incorporated this practice. In the study cited, multiple factors associated with 'problematic intubation' were subjected to logistic regression analysis and only neck circumference showed a statistically significant association, with each 1 cm increase in neck circumference being associated with a 1.13-fold increase in odds of 'problematic intubation'. Five per cent of morbidly obese patients with a neck circumference of 40 cm (16in) posed a challenge, whereas this figure rose to 35% in morbidly obese patients with a neck circumference of 60 cm (24in). Of note, 99% of their subjects were intubated in three attempts or less, with conventional equipment.

Reference
Brodsky JB, Lemmens HJ, Brock-Utne JG, Vierra M, Saidman LJ. Morbid obesity and tracheal intubation. *Anesth Analg* 2002; **94**(3): 732–6.

Question 185: Syndrome of inappropriate antidiuretic hormone (SIADH) secretion

The following are recognised causes of the syndrome of inappropriate antidiuretic hormone secretion, EXCEPT for which one?

a) Prone positioning
b) Positive-pressure ventilation
c) Subarachnoid haemorrhage
d) Pain
e) MDMA or 'Ecstasy' ingestion

Answer: a

Explanation
Hyponatraemia is the most common electrolyte disturbance in hospitalised patients. Syndrome of inappropriate antidiuretic hormone (SIADH) secretion is the most frequent cause of hyponatraemia in a euvolaemic patient, although hyponatraemia associated with volume depletion of the extracellular fluid also commonly occurs. In humans the AD (antidiuretic) of SIADH refers to vasopressin. Rarely, in patients with SIADH, vasopressin levels may be appropriately low due to a mutation of the vasopressin receptor. There are many causes of SIADH and they can be broadly categorised into those related to malignant disease (e.g. pancreatic carcinoma and lymphoma), pulmonary disease (e.g. pneumonia and respiratory failure associated with positive pressure breathing), disorders of the central nervous system (e.g. subarachnoid haemorrhage) and drugs (e.g. MDMA and NSAIDs). Other causes outside those categories include pain, nausea, stress, general anaesthesia and endurance exercise. To make a diagnosis of SIADH the serum osmolality must be decreased in the presence of a relatively concentrated urine (osmolality usually >300 mOsm/kg of water) in a euvolaemic patient who has normal adrenal and thyroid function and has not taken recent diuretics. In terms of treatment the most important factors dictating the management of SIADH are the severity of the hyponatraemia, its duration and the presence or absence of symptoms. Syndrome of inappropriate antidiuretic hormone secretion may be difficult to distinguish from cerebral salt wasting, a syndrome of hyponatraemia and extracellular fluid volume depletion seen in patients with insults to the central nervous system, e.g. following traumatic brain injury.

Reference
Ellison DH, Berl T. Clinical practice. The syndrome of inappropriate antidiuresis. *New Engl J Med* 2007; **356**(20): 2064–72.

Question 186: Revised cardiac risk index

The five clinical risk factors that contribute to increased cardiac risk during major non-cardiac surgery, as proposed by Lee in 1999 and incorporated into the *ACC/AHA 2007 Guidelines on Perioperative Cardiovascular Evaluation*, are listed below. Indicate which one is INCORRECT.

a) History of ischaemic heart disease
b) History of pulmonary disease
c) History of cerebrovascular disease
d) Preoperative treatment with insulin
e) Preoperative serum creatinine >177 micromol/L

Answer: b

Explanation

There are a number of historical cardiac risk indices for evaluating cardiac risk in non-cardiac surgery. These have been superseded in recent years by the extensive reviews of the American College of Cardiologists and American Heart Association producing guidelines published most recently in September 2007.

These include a useful suggested algorithm for assessment of patients' cardiac risk before major surgery. Active cardiac conditions that should be investigated, optimised and potentially prompt deferment of elective surgery are: unstable coronary syndromes (unstable angina or recent myocardial infarction), decompensated heart failure, significant arrhythmias and severe valvular disease. The five clinical risk factors that indicate increased risk and influence management are: history of ischaemic heart disease, history of compensated or prior heart failure, history of cerebrovascular disease, diabetes mellitus and renal failure.

The Lee Revised Cardiac Risk Index and the Eagle Criteria are other terms used in this context.

Reference

Fleisher L, Beckman J, Brown K, *et al.* ACC/AHA 2007 Guidelines on perioperative cardiovascular evaluation and care for noncardiac surgery. *Circulation* 2007; **116**(17): 418–99.

Question 187: Patient-reported outcome measures

Hospitals are required to invite patients, who are undergoing certain operations, to undertake a number of questionnaires designed to look at patient-reported outcome measures (PROMs) related to that specific operation. Which of the following is NOT one of these operations?

a) Elective hip replacement
b) Laparoscopic cholecystectomy
c) Groin herniorrhaphy
d) Varicose vein surgery
e) Elective knee replacement

Answer: b

Explanation

Patient-reported outcome measures have been instituted by the Department of Health as a result of proposals set out in the report 'High quality care for all'. The mantra behind this report is putting quality at the heart of everything the NHS does. Particularly important is quality as assessed by patients themselves, and the report highlights PROMs as a means of assessing effectiveness of care from the patient's perspective. From April 2009, all licensed providers of NHS-funded unilateral hip replacements, unilateral knee replacements, groin hernia surgery or varicose vein surgery are expected to invite patients undergoing one of these procedures to complete a preoperative PROMs questionnaire. Patient-reported outcome measures are typically short, self-completed questionnaires, which measure the patients' health status or health-related quality of life at a single point in time. Furthermore, there is the intention to link payments to PROMs data as part of a range of quality measures covering safety (including cleanliness and infection rates) and clinical outcomes.

Reference

Department of Health. Guidance on the routine collection of Patient Reported Outcome Measures (PROMs). Online at www.dh.gov.uk/en/Publicationsandstatistics/Publicat ions/PublicationsPolicyAndGuidance/DH_092647 (Accessed 30 November 2009)

Question 188: Carbon monoxide poisoning

Regarding carbon monoxide poisoning, the following statements are true EXCEPT which one?

a) Carbon monoxide shifts the oxyhaemoglobin dissociation curve to the left
b) The main route of carbon monoxide excretion is pulmonary
c) Observable tissue hypoxia is greater than would be expected from the reduction in oxygen delivery alone
d) Arterial carboxyhaemoglobin (COHb) percentage at the time of admission does not grade the severity of the injury
e) COHb of >30% should prompt consideration of hyperbaric oxygen therapy

Answer: e

Explanation
Carbon monoxide poisoning is so deleterious to patient health because of its affinity for binding haemoglobin, which is 240 times greater than that of oxygen. Oxygen binding sites are therefore reduced but tissue hypoxia is worsened by the disruption of other haem-containing proteins such as myoglobin and cytochrome oxidase at mitochondrial level further impairing oxygen handling. Severity of injury is graded by the projected carboxyhaemoglobin percentage at time of exposure. It must take into account the inevitable delay (and thus decrement of percentage) between exposure and presentation in the emergency department. The mainstay of therapy is oxygen. This not only ameliorates the hypoxia by increasing the dissolved component of oxygen in plasma, but also shortens the half-life of COHb from 240min with the subject breathing air to 40min while breathing 100% oxygen. Historically, COHb of >40% would prompt hyperbaric oxygen therapy where available, but *Cochrane Review* suggests that there is no robust evidence for improvement in outcome with hyperbaric oxygen and often the sicker patients withstand transfer poorly. Recall that pulse oximetry will tend to overestimate arterial oxygen saturation, as COHb is interpreted as 90% saturated blood. Arterial blood gases should be analysed remembering that partial pressure of oxygen may well be high if the patient is breathing high-flow oxygen but this does not equate to adequate oxygen delivery. The co-oximetry oxygen saturation from those arterial blood gas machines that provide it will be informative.

Question 189: Postoperative complications

A 28-year-old woman has a retained placenta following uneventful vaginal delivery of her baby at term. She requires manual removal of the placenta for which subarachnoid anaesthesia is provided and the placenta is delivered. On arrival in the recovery room she suddenly becomes confused, agitated and clammy. She is noted to have a respiratory rate of 40breaths/min, a heart rate of 50bpm and a thready pulse volume. She then becomes unconscious. Her trachea is intubated and she is manually ventilated with 100% oxygen. Further examination reveals a blood pressure of 78/50 mmHg, SpO_2 of 88% and a loud murmur at the left sternal edge. She is unresponsive to painful stimuli despite no sedation, her pupils are small and gaze deviated to the right. Which one of the following is the MOST SUITABLE action to take next?

a) Arrange CT pulmonary angiogram
b) Insert a central venous catheter
c) Commence external cardiac massage
d) Place her in the left lateral position
e) Commence intravenous infusion of unfractionated heparin

Answer: d

Explanation

Manual removal of the placenta is high risk for venous air embolism. The pattern of cardiorespiratory collapse followed rapidly by cerebral dysfunction suggests para-doxical air embolism with arterial air embolism of the cerebral circulation. The mill-wheel murmur suggests a large-volume air embolism. This volume of air in the right heart is sufficient to cause an airlock in the pulmonary outflow tract, raising right-sided pressures to a point where they may exceed falling left-sided pressures. Now a right-to-left shunt arises if a patent foramen ovale is present. In fact, transpulmonary passage of air is also possible if the pressure gradient is adequate. Positioning the patient in the left lateral position (± head down) moves the air away from the pulmo-nary outflow tract and foramen ovale, preventing the situation deteriorating. Further management can then be planned. Cardiopulmonary resuscitation may well be required if the patient arrests, but not before. Systemic anticoagulation is not recom-mended. If a central venous catheter is *in situ* attempts may be made at aspirating the air but insertion of a new catheter is not the immediate priority at the stage described.

Reference

Webber S, Andrzejowski J, Francis G. Gas embolism in anaesthesia. *Contin Educ Anaesth Crit Care Pain* 2002; **2**(2): 53–7.

Question 190: Capnography

Regarding capnography, which one of the following statements is TRUE?

a) Capnography is a sensitive marker of endobronchial intubation
b) Certain capnography traces are pathognomonic of particular equipment failures
c) $PaCO_2$ is always equal to or greater than $P_{ET}CO_2$
d) Pulmonary air embolism will decrease the magnitude of the Pa-etCO$_2$ gradient
e) Capnography cannot be employed during high-frequency jet ventilation

Answer: e

Explanation

The capnograph, both the numerical values and the shape of the capnogram, provides a wealth of information of interest to the anaesthetist. It makes a good viva question to discuss the multiple clinical applications of carbon dioxide monitoring. Endobronchial intubation may produce a rise or fall in end-tidal carbon dioxide depending on the presence or absence of a cuff on the tube and the adoption of volume-control or pressure-control ventilation. Alternatively, the capnogram may be bi-phasic if the termination of the tube is just past the carina but the Murphy's eye may intermittently allow ventilation of the contralateral lung depending on the phase in the ventilatory cycle. Compliance and pulse oximetry are more sensitive markers of endobronchial intubation. Certain capnograms are strongly suggestive of particular equipment fail-ures; however, the capnogram trace is always considered in combination with the concurrent clinical features before an equipment-related issue is diagnosed. Pa-etCO$_2$ gradient is small and positive in healthy lungs where the phase III (alveolar plateau) phase of the capnogram is fairly horizontal. Classically the magnitude of the gradient was thought to reflect the degree of alveolar dead space caused by ventilation–perfusion mismatch (recall the terms in the Bohr equation). It is accepted that the determinants of the gradient are more complex than this. Pulmonary air embolism will increase the magnitude of the Pa-etCO$_2$ gradient by increasing the alveolar dead space. Pa-etCO$_2$ gradient can be negative if the upward slope of phase III is suffi-ciently steep that over the course of a slow expiration the end-tidal value will actually exceed the arterial value, resulting in a negative gradient. This also occurs physiolog-ically in infancy and pregnancy where dead space is low. Capnography can guide high-frequency jet ventilation (HFJV) but the ventilation mode must be paused and a single sigh-breath used to sample end-tidal carbon dioxide, before HFJV is resumed. This can be calibrated against an arterial sample as usual, so future sigh-breath values can guide ventilation adjustments.

Question 191: Thoracic anaesthesia emergencies

A 73-year-old, 68 kg male has a malignant intrathoracic tracheal stenosis. He needs a tracheal stent insertion on the thoracic surgery list for which your colleague is providing anaesthesia. The patient is considered at low risk of aspiration of gastric contents. He pre-oxygenates with the patient sitting up at 60°. He induces anaesthesia intravenously with 50 mcg of fentanyl and 80 mg of propofol, delivered very slowly until the patient is unresponsive and his eyelash reflex lost. His intention was to maintain spontaneous ventilation initially but on lying the patient supine and performing a chin lift he finds the patient coughs violently following which your colleague is unable to mask ventilate the patient. He performs direct laryngoscopy and finds a Cormack and Lehane Grade 4 view and is unable to intubate. He summons you to help and as you arrive the patient's SpO_2 is 82% and is showing no signs of regaining consciousness. In this 'can't intubate, can't ventilate' situation which one of the following is the MOST APPROPRIATE action?

a) Immediate cannula cricothyroidotomy and jet ventilation or tracheostomy by the surgeon, who is standing by
b) Insert a laryngeal mask airway and attempt to maintain ventilation and improve oxygenation
c) Give 100 mg suxamethonium intravenously to optimise the laryngoscopic view and intubate orally
d) Allow the patient to awaken from what was only a modest induction dose, and resume spontaneous ventilation sitting up
e) Give 100 mg of suxamethonium intravenously and request the surgeon perform rigid bronchoscopy

Answer: e

Explanation
Patients with a partial airway obstruction near the carina pose a serious challenge to the anaesthetist. The airway diameter can be positional and lying supine can precipitate occlusion. Equally, coughing must be avoided at all costs as it can induce complete airway obstruction as in this case. For this reason shallow planes of anaesthesia are best avoided. Beware of reverting to usual 'can't ventilate, can't intubate' solutions as tracheal ventilation may well not relieve the obstruction. The life-saving solution here is allowing the surgeon to perform rigid bronchoscopy, through which you may jet ventilate the patient with a Sander's jet ventilator. Soon after this is established you must address the issue of maintaining anaesthesia with a TIVA technique. Doing nothing while you hope that the patient will resume spontaneous ventilation before any hypoxaemic sequelae occur is not an option.

Reference
Conacher I. Anaesthesia and tracheobronchial stenting for central airway obstruction in adults. *Brit J Anaes* 2003; **90**(3): 367–74.

Question 192: Botulinum toxin

Regarding botulinum toxin, the following statements are true EXCEPT which one?

a) It is the most potent toxin found in nature
b) It produces non-competitive antagonism of post-synaptic acetylcholine receptors

c) It may cause a clinical condition in which the first parts of the body to be affected are often the cranial nerves

d) It is neutralised in canned food by heating the can to 121°C for three minutes

e) It has been demonstrated to be successful in the management of anal fissure

Answer: b

Explanation

The extremely potent botulinum toxin has an increasing number of clinical uses. One is in the management of anal fissure where the relaxation of the muscle allows for healing, breaking the cycle of spasm and injury. In poisoning, a flaccid paralysis is caused by the toxin affecting the peripheral nerve endings. The cranial nerves are usually the first to be affected with signs and symptoms such as ptosis and diplopia commonly recorded. The mechanism of action is that the toxin cleaves, with a heavy segment binding to pre-synaptic receptors, and a lighter part entering the neurone and through proteolytic cleavage of synaptobrevins produces an irreversible loss of the capacity to release acetylcholine by the neuron.

Reference

Wenham T, Cohen A. Botulism. *Contin Educ Anaesth Crit Care Pain* 2008; 8(1): 21.

Question 193: Autologous blood transfusion

Transfusion of allogeneic donated bank blood exposes a patient to a number of risks. To reduce this risk, the patient's own erythrocytes may be re-transfused. The following statements are true of autologous blood transfusion EXCEPT which one?

a) Acute normovolaemic haemodilution (ANH) is acceptable to some Jehovah's Witnesses

b) Preoperative autologous donation (PAD) negates the risk of transmission of infection

c) Postoperative cell salvage involves transfusing contents of wound drains once passed through an intrinsic filter in the reservoir – there is no further processing of transfusate

d) Cell salvage techniques may be used at caesarean section despite the presence of amniotic fluid

e) PAD involves collection of up to four units of blood over five weeks pre-operatively with concurrent iron supplementation

Answer: b

Explanation

Autologous blood transfusion consists of cell salvage, acute normovolaemic haemodilution (ANH) and preoperative autologous donation (PAD). Acute normovolaemic haemodilution involves collection of 20 mL/kg of a patient's blood immediately pre-operatively through a wide-bore cannula into a citrated blood collection bag available from the transfusion service. The patient is transfused crystalloid or colloid to restore euvolaemia. Blood loss intra-operatively is of a lower (diluted) haematocrit and once haemostasis is achieved the collected units (with the original, higher haematocrit) are transfused. The technique is sometimes acceptable to Jehovah's Witnesses if the collection system and reservoir remain in contact with the patient. Jehovah's Witnesses must not be assumed to accept or decline any technique – it is a matter of personal interpretation and must be explicitly discussed with the patient pre-operatively. Most hospitals have specific consent forms and liaison officers. Preoperative autologous donation involves collection of a patient's blood and storage in the main blood bank alongside allogeneic donor blood pending surgery. Clearly this cannot eliminate human error and if allogeneic blood is used in error, the risk of infection transmission is still present. Cell salvage has been used without event at caesarean section although a separate suction device is used for large volumes of amniotic fluid. Postoperative cell salvage uses a filter and citrated collection bag attached directly to the wound drains. The drain content that accumulates over up to 12 hours may be delivered directly intravenously.

Reference
Walunj A, Babb A, Sharpe R. Autologous blood transfusion. *Contin Educ Anaesth Crit Care Pain* 2006; **6**(5): 192–6.

Question 194: Clinical measurement

A ventilated patient is being monitored on the cardiac intensive care unit with a pulmonary artery flotation catheter. The values for some of the patient's parameters are as follows: Arterial blood pressure 115/70 mmHg; Pulmonary artery pressure 25/10 mmHg; Central venous pressure 10 mmHg; Pulmonary capillary wedge pressure 13 mmHg; Mean intrathoracic pressure 20 cmH$_2$0; Cardiac output 5 L/min. Measured in dyne.s.cm^{-5}, which one of the following options is his systemic vascular resistance?

a) 15
b) 18
c) 1080
d) 1200
e) 1680

Answer: d

Explanation
Darcy's law (analogous to Ohm's law applied to fluid dynamics) when crudely applied to tubular fluid flow gives Pressure = Flow × Resistance. Rearranged this gives Resistance = Pressure/Flow and when applied to the cardiovascular system:

Systemic Vascular Resistance (SVR) = Change in Systemic Pressure/Cardiac Output

Or: SVR = (MAP – RAP)/CO

where RAP is right atrial pressure (or CVP) and MAP is mean arterial pressure (diastolic plus one third of pulse pressure – in this case 85 mmHg).

If the pressure is measured in mmHg and the cardiac output in L/min, then the resultant SVR would be in mmHg/(L/min), or Woods units. By tradition SVR is expressed in dyne.s.cm^{-5}, which is a unit of fluid resistance measured in the cgs system of units (dyne is a unit of force – that required to accelerate one gram mass by one centimetre per second squared; 100 000 dyne = 1 newton). It can be simply shown that the conversion factor from Woods units to dyne.s.cm^{-5} is 80 giving:

SVR = 80 × (MAP – RAP)/CO

Question 195: Digital clubbing

The following conditions are associated with digital clubbing EXCEPT for which one?

a) Acromegaly
b) Pregnancy
c) Primary biliary cirrhosis
d) Infective endocarditis
e) Bronchitis

Answer: e

Explanation

First described by Hippocrates, digital clubbing is associated with a large number of clinical conditions. Its pathophysiology is unknown despite numerous theories but there is general acceptance that the common factor in most types of clubbing is distal digital vasodilation. Whether this vasodilatation results from a circulating or local vasodilator, is a response to hypoxia, is in some way genetically predisposed or a neural mechanism, is unknown. It is characterised by enlargement of the terminal segments of the fingers and/or toes that results from the proliferation of the connective tissue between the nail matrix and the distal phalanx giving the classic 'loss of nail bed angle' appearance. Clubbing is almost always painless unless in association with hypertrophic osteoarthropathy. Clubbing may be idiopathic or secondary to many underlying pathologies in various organ systems. Common conditions that give rise to clubbing include lung malignancy, inflammatory bowel disease, pregnancy, interstitial and suppurative lung disease, mesothelioma, cyanotic heart conditions and hyperthyroidism.

Reference

Myers KA, Farquhar DR. The rational clinical examination. Does this patient have clubbing? *JAMA* 2001; **286**(3): 341–7.

Question 196: AIDS-defining clinical conditions

In a patient known to be HIV positive, the following are all AIDS-defining clinical conditions EXCEPT which one?

a) Invasive cervical cancer
b) Pneumocystis jiroveci pneumonia
c) Pulmonary tuberculosis
d) Salmonella septicaemia
e) Toxoplasmosis of the brain

Answer: c

Explanation

In 2007, 33 million people across the world were living with the condition of AIDS. Tuberculosis is an AIDS-defining clinical condition if it is disseminated. Pneumocystis jiroveci pneumonia is the current term for the condition previously known as Pneumocystis carinii pneumonia.

Question 197: Standards of monitoring during anaesthesia and recovery

According to the Association of Anaesthetists of Great Britain and Ireland *Recommendations Regarding Monitoring* (4th edition, 2007) which one of the following statements is TRUE?

a) Monitoring airway pressure is essential to the safe conduct of anaesthesia
b) A vapour analyser to detect volatile anaesthetic agents is mandatory
c) Monitoring must be maintained between theatre and the recovery area as for any other intra-hospital transfer
d) Under no circumstances should an anaesthetist leave an anaesthetised patient for whom they are responsible
e) In the recovery area clinical observations must be supplemented by electrocardiograph, pulse oximetry and non-invasive blood pressure measurement

Answer: a

Explanation

The candidate should be familiar with the Association of Anaesthetists of Great Britain and Ireland 'glossies'. The publication mentioned in the question is sensible, pragmatic and intuitive. The following five devices are 'essential to the safe conduct of anaesthesia': pulse oximeter; non-invasive blood pressure monitor; electrocardiograph; airway gases (oxygen, carbon dioxide and vapour monitors); and an airway pressure monitor. The caveat to the fourth device is that vapour analysis is essential during anaesthesia whenever a volatile anaesthetic agent is in use. The popularity of total intravenous anaesthesia means that often only capnography and oxygen analysis is necessary. If the recovery area is immediately adjacent to the operating theatre then a brief interruption of monitoring is acceptable. There are circumstances in which an anaesthetist may leave an anaesthetised patient for whom they are responsible. A consultant anaesthetist may deputise a physician's assistant (anaesthesia) (sometimes called an anaesthetic practitioner). In exceptional circumstances an anaesthetist working alone may be called away to perform a brief, life-saving procedure. Surgery should stop while the anaesthetist is absent and the trained anaesthetic assistant should monitor the patient. In the recovery area, an electrocardiograph should be immediately available but is not a 'must'. Pulse oximetry and non-invasive blood pressure monitoring are mandatory.

Reference

Recommendations for standards of monitoring during anaesthesia and recovery, 4th edn. Association of Anaesthetists of Great Britain and Ireland, 2007. Online at www. aagbi.org/publications/guidelines.htm (Accessed 30 November 2009)

Question 198: Prolonging QT

All the following drugs may prolong the QT interval on a patient's electrocardiograph, EXCEPT which one?

a) Ketorolac
b) Haloperidol
c) Quinine
d) Tamoxifen
e) Ondansetron

Answer: a

Explanation

Long QT syndrome may be either congenital or acquired. The condition may present to anaesthetists either diagnosed or undiagnosed, coming for anaesthesia or following collapse and presentation to the emergency department. Some drugs used commonly in anaesthesia such as ondansetron are known to increase the QT interval, as do other commonly prescribed drugs such as quinine, haloperidol and tamoxifen. Ketorolac is not thought to prolong the QT interval, but may cause bradycardia in some patients following intravenous administration.

Question 199: Systemic absorption of local anaesthetic

Which one of the following sites would lead to the greatest plasma concentration of local anaesthetic if the same dose of the same agent was administered to the same patient (on separate occasions)?

a) Intercostal
b) Interscalene

c) Caudal extradural
d) Tranversus abdominis plane
e) Deep cervical plexus

Answer: a

Explanation
Systemic absorption of local anaesthetic depends on a number of physicochemical characteristics of the agent, whether or not a vasoconstrictor is co-administered and on the site of the injection. It is commonly quoted that sites of greater vascularity are associated with greater absorption. This seems intuitive but is probably over-simplistic. Intercostal nerves are in close proximity to the intercostal arteries and veins, and intrapleural and intercostal blocks carry the highest absorption rate. However, the quoted maximum safe dose for some local anaesthetic agents is increased if they are to be used for the purposes of plexus blocks despite the fact that, for example, the subclavian artery is extremely close to the brachial plexus at the level of a supraclavicular block. This perhaps suggests that the site-dependent variation in absorption of local anaesthetic is not solely due to proximity to vasculature.

Question 200: Cardiac pacing

Regarding cardiac pacing, which one of the following statements is TRUE?

a) Epicardial pacing wires emerge directly through the anterior chest wall
b) VVI pacemakers deliver pacing stimulation regardless of the intrinsic activity of the heart
c) Biventricular pacemakers require insertion of the left ventricular lead via the systemic arterial vasculature
d) Unipolar diathermy during a surgical procedure is absolutely contraindicated
e) AOO pacemakers provide synchronous stimulation in cases of sinus bradycardia

Answer: a

Explanation
Epicardial pacing wires are sited under direct vision at the end of cardiac surgery and are inserted through the anterior chest wall and sutured to the skin for use in the event of a malignant postoperative arrhythmia. They are removed at 24 hours by simple traction if no longer required. The five letters that code the function of a pacemaker refer (in order) to the chamber paced, the chamber sensed, the response to sensing, its programmability and any anti-tachycardia function. 'VVI' implies the ventricle will be paced, the ventricle will be sensed and, in the event of the unit sensing ventricular activity, it will inhibit itself (i.e. not deliver an impulse). Biventricular pacemakers do, as their name suggests, stimulate both ventricles, but access to the left ventricle does not involve wires resident in the arterial vasculature. The lead is sited via the standard venous approach and then, once in the right atrium, the coronary sinus is entered (as it terminates just to the left of the IVC termination) then the wire is advanced retro-gradely until in sufficient proximity to the left ventricular myocardium. Unipolar diathermy is acceptable if the grounding pad is >15 cm from all pacemaker compo-nents and the use of electrocautery is limited to short low-energy bursts, ideally for coagulation, not cutting (as the waveforms are different). AOO pacemakers have no sensing ability and pace the atrium in an asynchronous fashion in cases of sinus bradycardia.

Question 201: Subarachnoid anaesthesia in day case surgery

Regarding the use of spinal anaesthesia in the day case unit, the following statements are true EXCEPT which one?

a) Muscle tone is preserved with a low dose spinal, which may necessitate adaptation of arthroscope insertion
b) Stage one recovery time is reduced with a subarachnoid block
c) In the UK, levobupivacaine 2.5 mg/mL is now licensed for intrathecal administration
d) 5 mg of bupivacaine plus 10 mcg fentanyl is adequate for a variety of lower limb day case procedures including knee arthroscopy
e) Time to readiness for discharge increases with dose of intrathecal bupivacaine but is not affected by its volume or concentration

Answer: c

Explanation

Subarachnoid anaesthesia for day surgery is a popular, well established technique worldwide but in the UK it is less widely practised. Anaesthetists and surgeons are familiar with the method for in-patient procedures where doses in the region of 15 mg of bupivicaine are employed to produce a profound sensorimotor blockade. Using lower dose spinals with opioid supplementation adequate anaesthesia is achieved often without a motor block. Retained lower limb muscle tone may cause transient minor difficulties for the orthopaedic surgeon, but can be rapidly accommodated. The offset time of lower dose spinal anaesthesia is shorter than with the higher dose. Although time to readiness for discharge may, on average, be longer than with a general anaesthetic technique, in the population who would most benefit from regional anaesthesia, this time is rarely of significance and can be accommodated in the day case unit. Some resistance to wider adoption of the technique is logistical but simple measures may be incorporated into routine practice without disruption to regular service. Patients need spend little if any time at all in stage one recovery and pass rapidly through to stage two recovery. It is recommended that once the selected dose of bupivicaine and opioid is prepared, the injectate should be diluted to a volume of around 3 mL to minimise dose lost in needle dead space or spilt drops. Although widely used, intrathecal administration of plain bupivicaine is not licensed (whereas hyperbaric bupivicaine is).

Reference

Watson B, Allen J, Smith I. *Spinal Anaesthesia in Day Surgery*. British Association of Day Surgery Handbook. Norwich: Coleman Print, 2004. Online at: www.daysurgeryuk.net/bads (Accessed 30 November 2009)

Question 202: Eutectic mixture of local anaesthetics (EMLA) and amethocaine

A 5-year-old is assessed on the children's ward prior to anaesthesia for tonsillectomy. Some topical local anaesthetic is prescribed to reduce the pain associated with subsequent cannulation. Regarding the available agents, which one of the following statements is TRUE?

a) Application of amethocaine gel (Ametop) will make intravenous cannulation easier than application of a eutectic mixture of local anaesthetics (EMLA)
b) If the manufacturer's instructions are strictly followed there is no difference in the efficacy of Ametop compared with EMLA

c) Ametop reduces the pain associated with intravenous cannulation more than EMLA even when both have been applied for over 60 minutes
d) Ametop contains 2% amethocaine
e) A 5 g tube of EMLA will contain 150 mg of lidocaine and 150 mg of prilocaine

Answer: c

Explanation

Ametop (4% amethocaine) and EMLA (2.5% lidocaine and 2.5% prilocaine, hence 125 mg of each in a 5 g tube) are the two topical anaesthetic agents used in mainstream practice. A *Cochrane Review* in 2006 comparing the two concluded that although EMLA is an effective topical anaesthetic agent for children, Ametop is superior in preventing pain associated with needle procedures. This was true regardless of whether the manufacturer's instructions for each agent were strictly adhered to, or whether the drugs had been applied for 30 to 60 minutes or over 60 minutes. The latter two practices are more in keeping with actual clinical practice than the first. Skin erythema is associated with Ametop use and blanching with the use of EMLA. The erythema associated with Ametop use is thought to be related to peripheral vaso-dilatation, which may make cannulation theoretically easier but this has been refuted by the trial referenced below. EMLA is associated with a very small risk of methaemoglobinaemia.

References

Newbury C, Herd DW. Amethocaine versus EMLA for successful intravenous cannulation in a children's emergency department: a randomised controlled study. *Emerg Med J* 2009; **26**(7): 487–91.

Lander JA, Weltman BJ, So SS. EMLA and Amethocaine for reduction of children's pain associated with needle insertion. Cochrane Database of Systematic Reviews 2006, Issue 3. Online at www.cochrane.org/reviews/en/ab004236.html (Accessed 30 November 2009)

Question 203: Atlantoaxial instability

The following conditions are associated with atlantoaxial instability EXCEPT which one?

a) Rheumatoid arthritis
b) Neurofibromatosis
c) Hyperthyroidism
d) Down's syndrome
e) Ankylosing spondylitis

Answer: c

Explanation

Atlantoaxial instability (AAI) is important to anaesthetists as the act of rendering a patient unconscious and then moving their head and neck may prove hazardous in this condition. The correct answer here of hyperthyroidism may cause a certain amount of consternation among the better candidates who may think the slightly different endocrine disease is a bit obvious among the other four choices, but then start to find associations between Down's syndrome and thyroid disease. This may be further complicated by the knowledge that this tends to be hypothyroidism rather than hyperthyroidism. On the whole, try not to overinterpret questions. If you are convinced that four of the answers do cause AAI, and are unsure about the fifth, go for the one you are unsure about.

Question 204: Amiodarone

Amiodarone is contraindicated in the following cardiac conduction disturbances or arrhythmias EXCEPT which one?

a) The arrhythmias produced by digoxin toxicity
b) Wolff–Parkinson–White syndrome
c) Atrial fibrillation during thyrotoxicosis
d) Atrioventricular block
e) Torsades de pointes

Answer: b

Explanation
Amiodarone is a Class III anti-arrhythmic agent that prolongs phase 3 of the cardiac action potential. The list of side effects such as skin pigmentation, corneal deposits, thyroid disturbances (both hyper- and hypo-) and pulmonary fibrosis are essential knowledge. Amiodarone has been used for treating most tachyarrhythmias. It has increased in popularity and scope of use, despite its poor side-effect profile, because it produces minimal negative inotropy and is rarely arrhythmogenic. Amiodarone may be used to treat the tachycardia in patients with the ventricular pre-excitation syndrome, Wolff–Parkinson–White. The arrhythmias produced by digoxin toxicity may be treated by magnesium, phenytoin or lidocaine. Amiodarone increases the serum concentration of digoxin and can worsen toxicity. Amiodarone should be avoided in thyrotoxic patients. If the patient is symptomatic from their arrhythmia, they should have simultaneous anti-thyroid agents and rate control with digoxin or a beta-blocker. Atrioventricular block rarely needs treatment but may be worsened by amiodarone. The polymorphous ventricular tachycardia, torsades de pointes, may be induced or worsened by amiodarone. Initial treatment, if unstable, is DC cardioversion and further treatment is determined by the presence or absence of a prolonged QT interval.

Question 205: Intercostal chest drainage

Regarding the practicalities of intrapleural chest drainage, the following statements are true EXCEPT which one?

a) Obstructed inspiration can generate intrapleural pressures of negative $80 \, cmH_2O$
b) Maintaining the collection chamber below the level of the patient promotes a pressure gradient with the higher pressure at the patient end
c) The connection tubing has a length of 1800 mm and 12 mm internal diameter thus an internal volume of around 0.2 L
d) The suction system applied to a chest drain must be high flow and low pressure to meet potential high fluid flow rates from the pleural cavity
e) Tubing must be at least 2 cm under the surface of the water to minimise resistance to expulsion while ensuring the volume above the tip is less than the volume of the tubing

Answer: e

Explanation
There are only three components of a simple pleural drainage system: a pleural tube with conduit, a one-way valve and a collection chamber (and in certain circumstances even the third is optional). The system must allow evacuation of pleural contents with minimal resistance and prevent return of air or expulsed matter on reversal of pressure gradient along the pleural tube (for example on inspiration in a spontaneously

breathing patient). The standard method of ensuring egress only is the underwater seal. The principle is simple: given that a healthy individual may generate a negative intrathoracic pressure of $80 \, cmH_2O$ by attempting inspiration against a closed glottis, the system must accommodate this while maintaining its other functions. The internal diameter of intercostal chest drainage tubing is 12 mm and its length is 1800 mm – a simple calculation reveals its internal volume to be 204 mL. The collection reservoir with underwater seal is placed at least 100 cm below the chest of a spontaneously breathing patient such as to exceed the maximum height a healthy individual could 'suck' a column of water. When the system is set up, the end of the tubing is 2 cm beneath the surface of the water in the drainage bottle (commonly a 'rocket bucket'). This means that the resistance to the expulsion of pleural contents is only $2 \, cmH_2O$ but will increase as the bottle fills (with, for example, blood), progressively increasing the resistance to expulsion – care must be taken in this regard as the efficacy of the drainage will be reduced. As the internal diameter of the drainage bottle is 140 mm, another calculation reveals the volume of water above the end of the tubing is 309 mL hence even if the patient was able to suck water all the way up the tubing; the tip of the tube would still be submerged. The dimensions of the drainage bottle are important – it can be seen that the volume above the tip of the tubing could still exceed the volume of the tubing in a narrower reservoir but then the depth beneath the surface would have to be increased and resistance to expulsion would be increased.

Question 206: Acute renal failure

A 75-year-old male presents with a community-acquired pneumonia. He is oliguric and his admission blood biochemistry shows a creatinine of 309 micromol/L with previously normal renal function. Which one of the following would be consistent with a diagnosis of acute tubular necrosis and not pre-renal uraemia?

a) Urinalysis shows hyaline casts
b) Specific gravity of 1.020
c) Osmolality 500 mOsm/kg
d) Fractional excretion of sodium 2%
e) Urinary sodium 20 mmol/L

Answer: d

Explanation
Pre-renal uraemia and ischaemic acute tubular necrosis are on the same spectrum of pathophysiology (the former leading to the latter) and together account for 75% of cases of acute renal failure. While in pre-renal uraemia, tubular function is preserved. The urine produced will be very concentrated and low in volume, hence a high specific gravity (>1.020) and a high osmolality (>500 mOsm/kg). Sodium and water are preserved in pre-renal uraemia, therefore urinary sodium is <20 mmol/L and fractional excretion of sodium (as a proportion of that quantity filtered) is <1%. If pre-renal uraemia persists and acute tubular necrosis supervenes then the nephron loses its ability to concentrate urine (specific gravity <1.010 and osmolality <300 mOsm/kg) and no longer preserves sodium (urinary sodium >40 mmol/L, fractional excretion of sodium >2%). Other work has suggested that fractional excretion of urea may be a better distinguishing factor between pre-renal uraemia (<35%) and acute tubular necrosis (>35%).

Fractional excretion of urea = ((Urine urea × plasma creatinine)/(plasma urea × urine creatinine)) × 100

Reference
Lameire N, Van Biesen W, Vanholder R. Acute renal failure. *Lancet* 2005; **365**(9457): 417–30.

Question 207: Asthma

In a patient with asthma presenting with an exacerbation to the emergency department the following would be consistent with 'acute severe asthma' EXCEPT which one?

a) PEF 50% of predicted
b) $PaCO_2$ 5.2 kPa
c) Heart rate 110 bpm
d) Respiratory rate 27 breaths per minute
e) Unable to complete sentences in one breath

Answer: **b**

Explanation

It is important to be able to distinguish acute severe asthma from life-threatening or near-fatal exacerbation of asthma, although ultimately all may result in patient death (more likely when combined with a number of adverse psychological factors in the patient). In acute severe asthma the patient will be hyperventilating and a low $PaCO_2$ will be expected. A normal $PaCO_2$ indicates life-threatening asthma and if $PaCO_2$ is elevated this is near-fatal asthma. This is explained by the progressive exhaustion of the patient with subsequent inability to perform the increased work of breathing. Other features of life-threatening asthma can be categorised by systems as impairment of the respiratory system (SpO_2 <92%, PaO_2 <8 kPa, normal $PaCO_2$, PEF <33%, cyanosis, silent chest, feeble respiratory effort), impairment of the cardiovascular system (bradycardia, arrhythmias, hypotension) and impairment of the central nervous system (exhaustion, confusion, coma). According to the British Thoracic Society guidelines, any one of these features is sufficient to diagnose life-threatening asthma. Near-fatal asthma is diagnosed in the presence of elevated $PaCO_2$ and/or need for mechanical ventilation with elevated inflation pressures.

Reference

British Thoracic Society. British guideline on the management of asthma. Online at www.brit-thoracic.org.uk

Question 208: Total intravenous anaesthesia

An 84 kg patient is listed for urgent surgery but gives a suspicious family history and you decide to treat him as if he were malignant hyperthermia susceptible. There are no target control infusion pumps available – just 100 mL bottles of 2% propofol and infusion pumps. You decide to use the original Bristol model for manual total intravenous anaesthesia. Consistent with the original work, the patient is premedicated with 20 mg oral temazepam. At induction he receives 250 mcg of fentanyl and 85 mg of propofol. Using the model mentioned, what volume of propofol will the patient receive in the following ten minutes?

a) 5.6 mL
b) 7.0 mL
c) 8.4 mL
d) 11.2 mL
e) 14.0 mL

Answer: **b**

Explanation

The original regimen proposed for 'manual' total intravenous anaesthesia with propofol involved a premedication of 20 to 30 mg of temazepam, induction with 3 mcg/kg of fentanyl and 1 mg/kg of propofol followed by a '10–8–6' infusion algorithm: 10 mL/kg per hour for the first ten minutes, 8 mL/kg per hour for the next ten minutes then 6 mL/kg per hour thereafter. This is to allow for a three-compartment model of propofol pharmacokinetics. It has been rendered virtually obsolete by target controlled infusion pumps with programming built in that adjusts the infusion rate to accommodate this and provide a theoretical plasma concentration desired by the anaesthetist. The Bristol regime produces an average plasma concentration of 3.67 mcg/mL. It is worth remembering that they used a nitrous oxide and oxygen gas mixture to ventilate the patients. In our example 10 mL/kg per hour × 84 kg is 840 mg/h or 14 mg/min, which over ten minutes is 140 mg of propofol. This is contained in a volume of 7 mL of 2% propofol.

Reference
Roberts FL, Dixon J, Lewis GT, Tackley RM, Prys-Roberts C. Induction and maintenance of propofol anaesthesia. A manual infusion scheme. *Anaesthesia* 1988; **43**(Suppl): 14–17.

Question 209: Uterine tone

Which one of the following is LEAST LIKELY to reduce uterine tone?

a) Desflurane
b) Nifedipine
c) Diclofenac
d) Magnesium sulphate
e) Suxamethonium

Answer: e

Explanation
Excitation–contraction coupling in uterine smooth muscle is of relevance to the anaesthetist. When faced with post-partum haemorrhage, any reduction in uterine tone should be avoided (ideally). During intra-uterine foetal resuscitation, immediate and effective tocolysis (uterine relaxation) prior to emergency caesarean section can buy time and improve foetal outcome. As with all muscular contraction, the final common pathway is an increase in cytoplasmic ionised calcium concentration with associated cascade of events resulting in contraction. Trigger pathways are different from other muscles however. Oxytocin and prostaglandins are pivotal and L-type voltage-gated calcium channels are also involved. Substances that increase uterine tone are oxytocin, ergometrine, ergonovine and prostaglandins (E_1, E_2 and $F_{2\alpha}$). Ketamine increases uterine tone. Volatile anaesthetic agents and all other intravenous anaesthetic agents (to some extent) decrease uterine tone. Other classes of drugs to decrease uterine tone are β-adrenoceptor agonists (terbutaline and salbutamol are used clinically), calcium channel antagonists, inhibitors of prostaglandin synthesis (e.g. NSAIDs) and magnesium. Suxamethonium does not interfere with any element of the pathways and has no effect on uterine tone.

Question 210: Pulmonary artery flotation catheters

Pulmonary artery flotation catheters can be used to measure the following variables EXCEPT which one?

a) Core temperature
b) Cardiac index
c) Mixed venous oxygen saturation

d) Pulmonary capillary wedge pressure

e) Mean pulmonary artery pressure

Answer: b

Explanation

Variables yielded by a pulmonary artery flotation catheter may be either measured or derived. Derived variables rely on calculations or assumptions and therefore may be less representative of the true value. Measured values include cardiac output, systolic, diastolic and mean pulmonary artery pressure, pulmonary capillary wedge pressure, mixed venous oxygen saturation and core temperature. Derived variables include cardiac index, systemic and pulmonary vascular resistance, stroke volume, oxygen flux, oxygen consumption and venous admixture.

Question 211: Hydrogen electrode

Regarding the operation of a hydrogen electrode in order to measure pH, which one of the following statements is CORRECT?

a) A special membrane is selectively permeable to H^+ ions

b) A calomel reference electrode describes a silver electrode in direct contact with silver chloride

c) The 'salt-bridge' is potassium chloride

d) A highly sensitive ammeter is required

e) A unit difference in pH will produce a voltage of 6V

Answer: c

Explanation

The basic components of any electrochemical electrode set-up are a reference electrode (with salt-bridge), a working electrode (with an abundant supply of ions), a sensitive electronic measurement device (ammeter if a current is generated, voltmeter if a potential difference is generated), and a solution to be analysed (the analyte). The reference electrode is commonly either silver/silver chloride or calomel, which is made from mercury and mercurous chloride (Hg_2Cl_2). With these, a 'salt-bridge' of saturated potassium chloride solution completes the electrochemical contact between sample and reference electrode. The design of the working electrode depends upon which is the ion (or gas) of interest. With the hydrogen electrode the working electrode has a H^+ ion sensitive glass membrane, which is only microns thick but not permeable to H^+ ions – the internal pH of the working electrode must remain constant and is carefully buffered. It can be shown that the voltage difference is given by:

$E = (RT/F).(pH_a - pH_i)$

where pH_a is the pH of the analyte and pH_i is the inner reference pH. As all the terms except pH_a and E are fixed, it may be seen that E is directly proportional to pH_a. For every unit change in pH a 60 mV potential difference is expected, so to detect a 0.1 pH change the measurement device must be a high impedance voltmeter ($\sim 10^{12}\Omega$) sensitive to changes in the order of 6 mV and smaller. Ammeters are used to measure current and are employed in the oxygen electrode.

Question 212: Obstetric anaesthesia

A 26-year-old woman with a history of syncope requires spinal anaesthesia for lower segment caesarean section. The subarachnoid injection is performed with the patient sitting on the operating table, whereupon she is assisted in lying supine with a 15° left lateral tilt on the table. Four minutes later, the patient becomes drowsy and confused and her monitor shows a heart rate of 49 bpm and a non-invasive blood pressure of

78/35 mmHg. Rapid infusion of intravenous fluid is commenced, the left lateral tilt of the operating table is increased and an assistant manually displaces the gravid uterus. Given the mechanism of the evolving phenomenon, which one of the following agents should BEST treat this patient?

a) Ephedrine
b) Atropine
c) Glycopyrrolate
d) Phenylephrine
e) Adrenaline

Answer: a

Explanation

In this case there are a number of factors contributing to the developing clinical situation. Patients prone to syncope need a careful history taken to assess the severity of the complaint, identify any known precipitants and if necessary seek an underlying cause. A lateral patient position for subarachnoid injection is suggested. The combination of the sympatholysis caused by spinal anaesthesia and aortocaval compression by the gravid uterus conspire to produce a bradycardic hypotension (or at worst asystole) via a number of mechanisms. Progressive sympathetic block reduces systemic vascular resistance (SVR) via vasodilation and increases peripheral venous capacitance causing a reduction in venous return (worsened by inferior vena cava compression) with consequent fall in cardiac output. The compensatory reflex increase in heart rate may be inhibited by a high spinal block directly preventing sympathetic action on the heart or by concurrent vagal overactivity as seen in subjects with vasovagal syncope. The reflex vasoconstriction to increase SVR is limited to those regions unaffected by sympathetic block (i.e. upper limbs only) and is inadequate to compensate. Priority is to restore venous return, counteract the vasodilation causing reduced SVR, and increase the heart rate and cardiac output. Based on these requirements it has been argued that the indirectly acting sympathomimetic ephedrine is the 'most logical choice' for this scenario. An anticholinergic such as atropine would eliminate the vagal component here but would do nothing to increase SVR or cause the venoconstriction that would return pooled peripheral venous blood. Adrenaline would have a similar effect but is reserved for if cardiac arrest occurs. Phenylephrine would raise SVR but could worsen the bradycardia. Pharmacological treatments should accompany intravenous fluid and physical measures to restore venous return.

Reference

Kinsella S, Tuckey J. Perioperative bradycardia and asystole: relationship to vasovagal syncope and the Bezold–Jarisch reflex. *Br J Anaes* 2001; **86**(6): 859–68.

Question 213: Guillain–Barré syndrome

Which of the following would you find MOST SURPRISING in a patient presenting to an intensive care unit with Guillain–Barré syndrome?

a) An elevated cerebrospinal fluid cell count
b) A recent history of a respiratory tract illness
c) Delayed F waves on nerve conduction studies
d) The presence of a bulbar palsy
e) No response to high dose oral corticosteroid therapy

Answer: a

Explanation

Guillain–Barré syndrome (GBS) is a peripheral neuropathy that causes acute neuro-muscular failure. It is more common in men and has an incidence of 1.6 per 100 000 Europeans, which rises with age but is bimodal in some studies, with a minor peak in young adults. It consists of a number of pathological and aetiological subtypes. The acute inflammatory demyelinating polyneuropathy (AIDP) subtype is the most commonly identified form in Europe and North America comprising over 90% of cases, with the other 10% made up of acute axonal motor disorders and acute sensory and motor axonal neuropathies. The AIDP subtype is usually preceded by a bacterial or viral infection with up to 40% of patients being seropositive for *Campylobacter jejuni*. Other infections linked to GBS include HIV, Epstein Barr virus, cytomegalovirus (CMV) and *Mycoplasma*. Limb weakness is usually mild and anti-GQ1b antibodies are common. All major types of GBS present with acute neuropathy, with limb weakness usually being global, i.e. both proximal and distal limb involvement. Symptoms suggestive of respiratory tract or gastrointestinal tract infection are common at presentation. Sensory loss is variable in the AIDP subtype though typically there are sensory symptoms but few sensory signs. Reflexes are usually lost early in the illness, although the acute motor axonal neuropathy subtype can be associated with retained or even brisk reflexes. Autonomic involvement is common with signs such as tachycardia, hypertension or absence of sinus arrhythmia. Nerve conduction studies are abnormal in 85% of patients even early on in the disease. Typically they show signs of conduction block, prolonged distal latencies, delayed F waves and sometimes the paradox of a small median sensory action potential with retained sural responses. Initial motor conduction velocities are usually normal but may slow later. Characteristic CSF findings consist of elevated protein (higher than 5.5 g/L) without pleocytosis (abnormal number of cells in the CSF). Cerebrospinal fluid findings may be normal when symptoms have been present for less than 48 hours. Treatments include plasma exchange and intravenous immunoglobulin and a Cochrane analysis has shown both to be of similar efficacy in reducing the time to recovery. Another *Cochrane Review* has shown that oral corticosteroids may actually delay recovery from GBS whereas intravenous corticosteroids may hasten recovery when given with intravenous immunoglobulin but do not affect the long-term outcome. Overall there is a mortality of around 10% with a further 20% being left with a residual disability.

Question 214: Thiopentone

A 30-year-old obese male presents with an incarcerated femoral hernia. A rapid sequence induction of general anaesthesia is planned. He has a cannula *in situ* in his left antecubital fossa through which doses of thiopentone and suxamethonium are delivered and eventually the patient's trachea is intubated with a certain amount of difficulty, which is ascribed to the patient's body habitus. During the operation it is noticed that his fingers on the left hand are white and cold and that blood is pulsating up the tubing of the intravenous fluid giving set. Which one of the following statements describes the MOST APPROPRIATE action to take next?

a) Remove cannula and commence immediate heparinisation via a new intravenous cannula
b) While under anaesthesia perform brachial plexus block
c) Infuse pressurised 0.9% saline through the existing cannula
d) Inject 10 mg of diluted papaverine into the existing cannula
e) Inject 10 mg of diluted bupivicaine into the existing cannula

Answer: c

Explanation

Inadvertent intra-arterial injection of thiopentone is a recognised complication of the use of the drug. The antecubital fossa is eschewed for placement of cannulae for rapid sequence induction. Intra-arterial placement is more likely in the antecubital fossa than on the dorsum of the hand. Also if an intravenous cannula has been displaced and thiopentone is injected extravascularly, then a greater volume may be delivered to the antecubital fossa before detection, whereas on the dorsum of the hand it will be immediately obvious. The dorsum of the hand does not entirely avoid intra-arterial cannula placement – the literature is peppered with case reports of cannulation of aberrant arteries at this site. Thiopentone in solution has a pH of 10.8. Unless it is rapidly diluted by collateral venous blood flow returning to the heart, it precipitates at physiological pH. This occurs if thiopentone is injected intra-arterially and thiopentone crystals wedge in arterioles of diminishing diameter. Management involves leaving the cannula *in situ*, immediate dilution with saline (necessarily under pressure to infuse into an artery), systemic heparinisation and injection of papaverine (40 to 80 mg) to aid vasospasm and procaine (10 mL of 1%) for analgesia. Sympathetic blockade via stellate ganglion block or brachial plexus block may well be indicated for analgesia and vaso-dilation, but this would not be performed without consent.

Question 215: Prolonged QT interval

A patient's electrocardiogram is reviewed prior to surgery for suspected ischaemic bowel. The patient is unwell and it is noted they have a prolonged QT interval. Due to which of the following would you LEAST expect this to be?

a) Beta blocker therapy
b) A history of breast carcinoma with known bone metastases
c) Jervell–Lange–Nielsen syndrome
d) A history of ischaemic heart disease with daily angina
e) Hypothermia

Answer: b

Explanation

The QT interval is measured from the first deflection of the QRS complex (positive or negative) to the end of the T wave. It then needs to be corrected for different heart rates by dividing the QT interval by the square root of the cardiac cycle length. This is to eliminate the effect of a variation in heart rate on the measured QT interval. Hence without this correction anything that causes a relative bradycardia will lengthen the QT interval (e.g. beta blockade). Non-physiological causes of a prolonged QT interval include hypocalcaemia, hypothermia, ischaemic heart disease (independent of under-lying cause), myocarditis and two rare syndromes: Jervell–Lange–Nielsen and Romano–Ward. Breast carcinoma with bony metastases is more likely to cause hyper- rather than hypocalcaemia so is the least likely option in this situation.

Question 216: Marfan's syndrome

An 18-year-old man with Marfan's syndrome requires anaesthesia for knee arthro-scopy and medial meniscal repair. He is tall, with very long arms and a thoracolumbar scoliosis. His father looks similar. Which of the following would be LEAST LIKELY to be noted in this patient?

a) An ejection systolic murmur radiating to the carotids
b) A pansystolic murmur loudest at the apex

c) High arched palate
d) Pectus excavatum
e) Needing to use glasses to see to sign the consent form

Answer: a

Explanation

Marfan's syndrome is a connective tissue disorder resulting from mutations in the fibrillin-1 gene on chromosome 15, which encodes for the glycoprotein fibrillin. Fibrillin is a major building block of microfibrils, which constitute the structural components of the suspensory ligament of the lens and also serve as substrates for elastin in the aorta and other connective tissues. It is inherited in an autosomal dominant manner and an incidence of approximately 1 in 10 000 making it one of the commonest single-gene mutations. It is equally common in men and women and has a high (approximately 30%) incidence of new mutation. Clinical presentation is variable and the diagnosis is made on clinical grounds based upon typical abnormalities and various criteria classifications may be used (e.g. the Berlin or Ghent criteria). Classic features include limbs that are disproportionately long compared with the trunk, arachnodactyly, tall stature, ectopia lentis, mitral valve prolapse, aortic root dilatation, lumbosacral scoliosis and aortic dissection. Cardiovascular disease is the major cause of morbidity and mortality. Progression from mitral valve prolapse to mitral regurgitation, often in conjunction with tricuspid prolapse and regurgitation is the most common cause of infant morbidity. If untreated, Marfan's syndrome is associated with reduced life expectancy. An ejection systolic murmur radiating to the carotids is suggestive of aortic stenosis, which is not a recognised feature of Marfan's syndrome.

Question 217: Apgar score

While on-call for the obstetric unit you are urgently bleeped to a delivery room where a mother has delivered her baby. She is well but the baby has a heart rate of 90 bpm, cries weakly and flexes when stimulated, has poor muscle tone, blue hands and feet, but has a pink trunk. Which of the following is the CORRECT Apgar score for this baby?

a) Six
b) Five
c) Four
d) Three
e) Two

Answer: b

Explanation

The Apgar score was initially developed by Virginia Apgar (an American obstetric anaesthetist) as a way of ascertaining the effects of obstetric anaesthesia on the newborn baby. It uses five easily identifiable characteristics: heart rate, respiratory effort, muscle tone, reflex irritability and colour – each of which is assigned a score of zero, one or two, dependent on findings. Heart rate is divided into absent, less than 100 bpm and greater than 100 bpm, scoring zero, one and two respectively. Respiratory effort may be absent, a weak cry or a strong cry, scoring zero, one or two respectively. Reflex irritability refers to the response to some form of stimulation, e.g. suctioning with an oropharyngeal suction catheter, with no response, some movement and strong withdrawal, scoring zero, one and two respectively. For colour, blue or pale scores zero, a pink body with blue extremities scores one, and pink all over scores two. Finally muscle tone may be limp, poor or good, again scoring zero, one or two respectively. Apgar scores are usually done at one and five minutes post delivery with the five-minute score being regarded as a better predictor of survival in infancy. Scoring is then generally repeated after this in infants with low initial scores. An Apgar score at five minutes of seven or more usually indicates the infant's condition to be good. Apgar scoring has not been validated as a predictor of neurological development of the infant but remains as relevant for the prediction of neonatal survival today as it was over 50 years ago.

References

Apgar V. A proposal for a new method of evaluation of the newborn infant. *Anesth Analg* 1953; **32**: 260–7.
Casey B, McIntire D, Leveno K. The continuing value of the Apgar score for the assessment of newborn infants. *N Engl J Med* 2001; **344**(7): 467–71.

Question 218: Chronic low back pain

A 50-year-old woman presents to the pain clinic with a three-year history of low back pain with occasional radiation down the left leg. The severity and impact on her functional ability is increasing and her general practitioner feels he has explored all the options open to him. Careful history-taking eliminates the 'red flags' of chronic back pain. Which one of the following options is NOT a 'yellow flag' of chronic back pain?

a) A negative attitude that back pain is harmful or potentially severely disabling
b) Fear avoidance behaviour and reduced activity levels
c) An expectation that passive, rather than active, treatment will be beneficial
d) A comorbid psychiatric diagnosis or history of substance misuse
e) A tendency to depression, low morale and social withdrawal

Answer: d

Explanation

In the UK, chronic back pain is responsible for a greater proportion of days absent from employment than any other diagnosis. The Royal College of General Practitioners publishes guidelines on its management and the National Institute for Health and Clinical Excellence published guidelines in May 2009. A proportion of these patients will present to pain clinicians and hence familiarity with the widely accepted red and yellow flags of chronic back pain is important. Red flags are those that may signify serious spinal pathology and may prompt further investigation. Yellow flags are those psychosocial factors that influence long-term outcome in patients with chronic back pain and suggest those patients in whom the greatest 'life-impact' will be felt. There are five yellow flags, which are listed above, with the exception of Option (d), 'A comorbid psychiatric diagnosis or history of substance misuse', which should read 'social or financial problems'. This option may seem familiar because it is a risk factor for addiction to prescribed opioids – another list with which the pain clinician will be familiar.

Reference

Samanta J, Kendall J, Samanta A. 10-minute consultation: chronic low back pain. *Brit Med J* 2003; **326**(7388): 535.

Question 219: Properties of local anaesthetics

Regarding the properties of some local anaesthetics, with respect to levobupivacaine, which one of the following statements is CORRECT?

a) It has the same potency as ropivacaine, and at equipotent doses has the same onset of action as racemic bupivacaine and the same duration of action as lidocaine

b) It has greater potency than lidocaine, and at equipotent doses has the same onset of action as racemic bupivacaine and the same duration of action as ropivacaine

c) It has greater potency than ropivacaine, and at equipotent doses has a slower onset of action than lidocaine and a longer duration of action than racemic bupivacaine

d) It has greater potency than racemic bupivacaine, and at equipotent doses has a slower onset of action than ropivacaine and a longer duration of action than lidocaine

e) It has greater potency than lidocaine, and at equipotent doses has a slower onset of action than ropivacaine and a longer duration of action than racemic bupivacaine

Answer: b

Explanation

Levobupivacaine and ropivacaine are s-enantiomers that are currently being marketed to compete with the long-established drugs, lidocaine and bupivacaine. They both have less cardiac toxicity and preferentially block sensory nerves more than motor nerves. When making a choice between these agents it is useful to understand the advantages offered by each drug. Potency of a local anaesthetic is usually related to the lipid solubility of the drug. Bupivacaine is marginally more potent than levobupivacaine and ropivacaine, although not to the point of being clinically important. Lidocaine is less potent than the others. The degree of ionisation determines the speed of onset of a local anaesthetic, and lidocaine is faster than the other drugs. Duration of action of local anaesthetics is related to the degree of protein binding. The more highly bound, the longer their duration of action. In most trials, levobupivacaine, racemic bupivacaine and ropivacaine have the same duration of action, with a few trials demonstrating a longer duration for bupivacaine, and some a longer duration for levobupivacaine. All three last longer than lidocaine.

Question 220: Pharmacodynamics

The classical approach to the study of pharmacodynamics involves analysis of dose–response curves and application of various equations. Log(dose)–response curves can theoretically distinguish between competitive and non-competitive antagonists at a particular receptor. However, given that experiments are limited by dose ranges and responses that must be safe, data at the extremes are often incomplete. Via what transformation may 'mid-range' data be manipulated to reveal linear graphs that demonstrate whether an antagonist is competitive or non-competitive?

a) Gaussian distribution
b) Lineweaver–Burke plot
c) Bland–Altman plot
d) Michaelis–Menton equation
e) Conductance ratio application

Answer: b

Explanation

The Michaelis–Menton equation serves to describe the relationship between drug concentration and observed clinical effect (as a proportion of maximal clinical effect) by considering that effect as a function of proportional receptor occupancy. If the Michaelis–Menton equation is inverted and manipulated the equation of a straight line may be produced. When plotted on suitably chosen axes, the straight lines produced are called a Lineweaver–Burke plot. Simple analysis of their gradients and intercepts tells us whether the antagonist present in the experiment is competitive or non-competitive. Gaussian distribution is another term for normal distribution. The Bland–Altman plot is a statistical test applied to data collected from two different devices to establish if there is acceptable agreement between the measurements made by the novel device when compared to those from the established one. Conductance ratios is a term applied to the pharmacokinetics of drug diffusion rates between body compartments.

Question 221: Carbon dioxide carriage in the blood

Regarding carbon dioxide transport, which one of the following statements is CORRECT?

a) Between arterial and venous blood, the mechanism with the greatest proportional change in carbon dioxide carriage is the bicarbonate component
b) Dissolved carbon dioxide component contributes $0.0225\,mL/dL/kPa$ to the carriage of the gas
c) Deoxygenated blood has greater carbon dioxide carrying capacity than oxygenated blood – the Bohr effect
d) Carbamino compounds are generated by the combination of carbon dioxide with blood proteins
e) Plotted with the same scales, the carbon dioxide dissociation curve is much shallower than the oxyhaemoglobin dissociation curve

Answer: d

Explanation

Carbon dioxide is transported in the blood, dissolved as bicarbonate and as carbamino compounds. The latter are the combination of carbon dioxide with the terminal amine group of a variety of blood proteins, the most significant of which is the globin of haemoglobin. This reaction occurs three times more readily in deoxygenated haemoglobin thus explaining the superior carbon dioxide carriage capacity of deoxygenated haemoglobin – the Haldane effect. The Haldane effect is also explained by the fact that deoxygenated haemoglobin is a better acid buffer, which facilitates the bicarbonate carriage sequence. The solubility of carbon dioxide at $37\,°C$ is $0.5\,mL/dL$ per kPa. $0.0225\,mL/dL$ per kPa is the solubility of oxygen. Although the largest amount of carbon dioxide carriage in arterial blood is bicarbonate (90%), the greatest proportional change is in the carbamino component. This accounts for 5% of carbon dioxide in arterial blood but 30% of the a–v difference (i.e. that gas liberated at the lungs). This is a six-fold change. Arterial carbon dioxide content is in the region of $50\,mL/dL$, significantly more than the $20\,mL/dL$ of oxygen and when plotted on the same scales the carbon dioxide dissociation curve is much steeper than the oxyhaemoglobin dissociation curve.

Reference

West JB. Gas transport by the blood. In: *Respiratory Physiology: The Essentials*, 7th edn. Baltimore: Lippincott Williams and Wilkins, 2005; pp. 75–92.

Question 222: Cyanosis

Which one of the following statements regarding cyanosis is TRUE?

a) Central cyanosis is always a manifestation of hypoxaemia
b) Central cyanosis is always accompanied by a reduced arterial PaO_2
c) Central cyanosis is detectable at a concentration of arterial reduced haemoglobin of $2.5\,g/dL$
d) Peripheral cyanosis is detectable at a concentration of arterial reduced haemoglobin of $1.5\,g/dL$
e) Methaemoglobinaemia will cause a drop in arterial oxygen saturations without clinically apparent cyanosis

Answer: a

Explanation

Cyanosis is the visible bluish tinge of skin or mucous membranes that may represent hypoxaemia. It is caused by the presence of defined concentrations of reduced (deoxygenated) haemoglobin in the *capillaries* of superficial tissues. It is widely accepted that central cyanosis is detectable at a reduced haemoglobin concentration *in the capillaries* of $5\,g/dL$ (±1), which corresponds to a reduced haemoglobin concentration of $3.4\,g/dL$ in arterial blood. Debate of this figure sometimes confuses arterial and capillary values. Peripheral cyanosis is detectable at $1.5\,g/dL$ of reduced haemoglobin in the capillaries but this can be secondary to peripheral vasoconstriction and not be a sign of arterial hypoxaemia. Hypoxaemia is defined as a deficit in arterial blood oxygen content and central cyanosis cannot be present without it. In cases of methaemoglobinaemia, unbound haemoglobin is in its ferric (Fe^{3+}) not ferrous (Fe^{2+}) form and is unavailable to bind oxygen. Arterial oxygen saturation falls by the same percentage that MetHb is present; however, unless there is concurrent lung pathology, pulmonary transfer of oxygen is normal and thus PaO_2 is unaffected – hence cyanosis with a normal PaO_2. Sulphaemoglobinaemia, where sulphur binds haemoglobin preventing oxygen from doing so, produces a similar phenomenon. Beware confusing carboxyhaemoglobinaemia (COHb), where despite low oxygen saturations the patient does not appear cyanosed (and may appear cherry red). Pulse oximeters also tend to read 90% in the presence of COHb.

Reference

Martin L, Khalil H. How much reduced hemoglobin is necessary to generate central cyanosis? *Chest* 1990; **97**(1):182–5.

Question 223: Metabolic stress response

Which one of the following would NOT be consistent with the initial neurohumoural response following major trauma in a previously well patient?

a) Serum cortisol concentration 1250 nanomol/L
b) An increase in serum tri-iodothyronine concentration
c) A release of arginine vasopressin from the posterior pituitary
d) A surge of interleukin-1 and interleukin-6
e) A small rise in glucagon secretion

Answer: b

Explanation

The metabolic stress response is an area of current research in critical care. The evolutionary benefit is thought to be the mobilisation of energy and repair substrates from existing body stores. The historical terms of the 'ebb' and 'flow' stages are perpetuated but are redefined from their original descriptions, which were based on historical animal experiments. With all the therapeutic options of modern medicine, there is debate as to whether the intense physiological changes are of benefit or detriment to a patient following major trauma or surgery. The three components of the inducible reaction are the sympathetic adrenal response, the endocrine response (pituitary hormones and insulin resistance), and the haematological and immunological response. Thyroxine (T_4) and tri-iodothyronine (T_3) increase metabolic rate, oxygen consumption and sensitivity of the cardiovascular system to the actions of catecholamines. It would be intuitive therefore to assume an increase in thyroid hormone activity following a major physiological insult. However, the reverse is true and levels decrease after surgery returning to normal over several days. This may be due to hypercortisolaemia depressing T_3 concentrations. Baseline serum cortisol is 400 nanomol/L and the rise to 1250 nanomol/L (as in the question) would be expected if the hypothalamo–pituitary–adrenal axis is intact.

Reference
Desborough J. The stress response to trauma and surgery. *Brit J Anaesth* 2000; **85**(1): 109–17.

Question 224: Trauma management

A 29-year-old male is involved in a road traffic collision on his motorbike. He suffers blunt trauma to his head, chest and abdomen. His Glasgow Coma Score (GCS) is 5 at the scene (abnormal flexion to pain). In the emergency department (ED), his GCS is 4 and his ventilation is inadequate. His cervical spine is already immobilised with a hard collar, sand bags and tape. His trachea is intubated by the ED registrar and mechanical ventilation commenced. Plain radiographs of the cervical spine, chest and pelvis are taken in ED. The cervical spine radiograph looks normal. The ED registrar escorts the patient to CT where the patient undergoes CT of head, chest and abdomen. Immediate surgery is not indicated so the ED registrar escorts the patient to the intensive care unit where the ICU trainee has been busy to this point. With respect to this patient's spinal clearance, which one of the following actions is MOST APPROPRIATE once the patient has been stabilised?

a) Return to the imaging department for thin-slice cervical spine CT
b) Leave hard collar in place, but elevate the head of the bed 30° because the patient's intracranial pressure must be minimised
c) Given a normal plain film of the c-spine, an MRI of the spine to identify unstable ligamentous injury should be arranged urgently
d) Arrange thoracolumbar spine plain X-rays
e) Remove hard collar to reduce sequelae of long-term immobilisation but continue to log-roll the patient

Answer: a

Explanation
The usual criteria for removal of hard collar cervical spine (c-spine) immobilisation cannot apply to those patients who are unable to participate in a clinical examination and are unlikely to be able to do so in the 48 hours following presentation. Radiological clearance of the c-spine must be based on thin-slice (2 to 3 mm) CT reconstructed in sagittal and coronal planes and interpreted by a senior radiologist. It is recommended that this is performed at the time of the first brain scan in trauma patients so unfortunately this patient must return to CT. Plain films are not adequate if the patient cannot participate in assessment. Plain films of the thoracolumbar spine are not necessary here as it is acceptable to reconstruct images from the chest and abdominal CT. While in CT the patient could have had a pelvic CT also. The intracranial pressure is an issue so, pending clearance, the whole bed may be tilted head-up and full spinal precautions continued. MRI has high sensitivity but only moderate specificity and is a logistical challenge with new ICU trauma patients. Remember that 50% of spinal injuries are thoracolumbar and 20% are at two levels of the vertebral column.

Reference
British Orthopaedic Association Standards for Trauma. BOAST 2: Spinal clearance in the trauma patient. November 2008. Online at www.boa.ac.uk/default.aspx?ID=280 (Accessed 30 November 2009)

Question 225: Macrocytic anaemia

A 36-year-old female patient presents to the pre-assessment clinic prior to undergoing surgery for removal of metalwork. Her full blood count shows haemoglobin 9 g/dL and mean cell volume 107.3 fL. Which of the following investigations or observations would be the LEAST LIKELY to be helpful in elucidating the cause of her macrocytic anaemia?

a) A positive β-HCG
b) A raised TSH and low T4
c) That the patient has end-stage renal failure and is on haemodialysis
d) A history of excess alcohol intake
e) Abnormal liver function tests

Answer: e

Explanation

Macrocytic red blood cells have an MCV of greater than 100 fL. Causes may be divided into megaloblastic anaemia (the result of impaired DNA synthesis) and normoblastic anaemia. A megaloblastic anaemia is secondary to folate or vitamin B_{12} deficiency and may be associated with both a low white cell count and thrombocytopaenia. Causes of vitamin B_{12} deficiency can be divided up into reduced intake (e.g. veganism), reduced absorption (Crohn's, previous gastrectomy, pernicious anaemia, etc.), increased utilisation (blind loop syndrome), abnormal metabolism (transcobalamin II deficiency) or may be caused by some drugs, e.g. metformin. Causes of folate deficiency can be categorised into reduced intake (poor diet), reduced absorption (coeliac disease, Crohn's disease), increased utilisation (pregnancy, malignancy, chronic inflammation, dialysis) and may also be caused by some drugs, e.g. trimethoprim, methotrexate and a number of anticonvulsants. A normoblastic macrocytic anaemia may be secondary to excessive alcohol intake, liver disease, pregnancy, hypothyroidism, chronic obstructive pulmonary disease and any condition leading to a reticulocytosis, e.g. haemolytic anaemia or post-haemorrhagic anaemia. Investigation of a megaloblastic anaemia following the findings of an abnormal blood film, elevated lactate dehydrogenase and bilirubin includes direct measurement of serum vitamin B_{12} and then more specific tests for a cause of vitamin B_{12} deficiency (e.g. gastric parietal antibodies positive in 90% of patients with pernicious anaemia). If the vitamin B_{12} levels are normal, RBC folate levels are performed (more reliable than serum folate) to identify a folate deficiency. Option (e) is the most unhelpful as abnormal liver function tests (usually raised bilirubin) may be either a cause or effect of the anaemia and are non-specific.

Paper D

Question 226: Neuromuscular blockade

With regard to the monitoring of neuromuscular blockade, the following statements are true EXCEPT which one?

a) An acceptable level of neuromuscular function for extubation is present if a patient has a train-of-four ratio of >0.90
b) The gold standard for accurately assessing train-of-four ratio is mechanomyography
c) Post-tetanic count is most useful for assessing deep neuromuscular blockade
d) The presence of a single twitch on train-of-four indicates a 90% reduction in muscle tone following electrical stimulation
e) At the wrist, the negative electrode should be placed proximally

Answer: e

Explanation
Despite the finding in a survey in the UK in 2007 that the majority of anaesthetists omit neuromuscular blockade (NMB) monitoring from their routine practice, the ability to make a formal assessment of NMB remains a core skill for an anaesthetist. Neuromuscular blockade may be monitored for deep or moderate block and there are now monitors such as the acceleromyograph that can make a good quantitative assessment of block. The gold standard for accurate quantitative assessment of moderate block remains the mechanomyograph, but this bulky piece of equipment is not used in clinical practice and remains a research tool. When measuring the train-of-four (TOF) ratio, the size of the fourth twitch is divided by the size of the first twitch. This gives more information for moderate block than straightforward TOF. For straightforward TOF, the presence of three twitches represents a 75% reduction in muscle tone following electrical stimulation. Two twitches indicates an 85% reduction in tone, one twitch a 90% reduction and no twitches a 98 to 100% reduction. Post-tetanic count is used when the patient has a deep block and a count of five to seven twitches indicates that the TOF will reappear shortly. It has been demonstrated that neuromuscular response to stimulation is greater if the negative electrode is placed distally. Remember 'Positive is Proximal, Negative to Nerve'

References
Fuchs-Buder T, Schreiber J, Meistelman C. Monitoring neuromuscular block: an update. *Anaesthesia* 2009; **64**(S1): 82–9.

Brull S, Silverman D. Pulse width, stimulus intensity, electrode placement, and polarity during assessment of neuromuscular block. *Anesthesiology* 1995; **83**(4): 702–9.

Question 227: Clonidine

Regarding clonidine, which one of the following statements is CORRECT?

a) Clonidine produces vasodilation and a compensatory tachycardia is observed
b) Clonidine is an agonist at α_1 and α_2 adrenoreceptors
c) Reduction of minimum alveolar concentration (MAC) of volatile anaesthetic agents is limited to 20%
d) With higher therapeutic doses, respiratory depression is observed
e) Clonidine may increase small bowel motility and cause diarrhoea

Answer: b

Explanation

Clonidine has wide-ranging applications including an adjuvant in neuraxial anaesthesia, regional anaesthesia, oral premedication and intravenous sedation on the ITU. It can also be used as an antihypertensive, in chronic pain and in the treatment of drug and alcohol withdrawal. It acts at α_1 and α_2 adrenoreceptors although it has 200 times greater affinity for α_2 receptors. The distribution of these receptors, especially in the central nervous system, explains its multisystem effects and many of the useful properties of the drug. In the lateral reticular nucleus, sympathetic efferent activity is reduced while augmentation of endogenous opioid release in the spinal cord is responsible for the analgesic properties. Noradrenaline-mediated descending inhibition of pain pathways is also augmented. Despite a transient rise in blood pressure due to the α_1 effect this is rapidly dominated by the α_2 effects and a drop in blood pressure is expected. Baroreceptors' sensitivity is altered and a mild bradycardia is seen. Minimum alveolar concentration (MAC) of volatile anaesthetic agents may be reduced by up to 50% and as an analgesic it has an opioid-sparing effect when administered intravenously, epidurally or intrathecally. It does not produce respiratory depression. Among its many other effects, it reduces gut motility and may cause constipation.

Question 228: Delirium in the critically ill

It is suspected that a patient on an intensive care unit has become delirious following recent surgery for a perforated diverticular abscess and consequent peritonitis. Which of the following statements regarding their management is INCORRECT?

a) The CAM-ICU screening tool may be a valuable aid to diagnosis in this situation
b) Drugs with central antimuscarinic or dopaminergic activity should be avoided wherever possible in critically ill patients with or at risk of delirium
c) Once the diagnosis has been established treatment with haloperidol is useful
d) Benzodiazepines should, generally, be avoided in the management of patients with delirium
e) Opioids, noradrenaline and corticosteroids all reduce rapid eye movement (REM) sleep, which contributes to an increased risk of delirium

Answer: a

Explanation

Delirium in the critically ill patient is common with some studies suggesting an incidence of up to 80%. Three delirium subtypes have been identified: hyperactive, hypoactive and mixed, with the hypoactive subtype being particularly difficult to diagnose. There are many predisposing factors for the development of delirium including pain, hypoxia, acidosis, advancing age, immobilisation, drugs (interactions, treatment and withdrawal), pre-existing memory impairment and interruption of the sleep–wake cycle. The confusion assessment method for the intensive care unit (CAM-ICU) uses a four-feature checklist to screen for delirium and is one of a number of validated specific screening tools. Others include the intensive care delirium screening checklist (ICDSC) and the delirium detection score (DDS). These tools all screen for the presence of delirium, they do not help to diagnose the underlying cause. Prevention of delirium involves provision of a supportive, unambiguous environment with an effort made to maintain competence by encouraging self-care and participation in treatment and attempting to allow the maximum amount of uninterrupted sleep as possible. Prompt identification of potential delirium precipitants and close attention paid to the drug chart is also important. In general drugs that exhibit antimuscarinic or dopaminergic activity are particularly associated with the development of delirium. A number of drugs including benzodiazepines, opioids, noradrenaline, adrenaline and corticosteroids all affect the sleep–wake cycle by a reduction in REM sleep. For the drug treatment of delirium, haloperidol is the agent of choice. Benzodiazepines should, in general, be avoided unless used to manage specific delirium syndromes such as alcohol or benzodiazepine withdrawal.

Reference

Borthwick M, Bourne R, Craig M, Egan A, Oxley J. Detection, prevention and treatment of delirium in critically ill patients. United Kingdom Clinical Pharmacy Association. 2006. Online at www.ukcpa.org/ukcpadocuments/6.pdf (Accessed 30 November 2009)

Question 229: Serum troponin

Which of the following is NOT associated with a significantly raised serum troponin I?

a) Elective DC cardioversion
b) Meningococcal septicaemia
c) Subarachnoid haemorrhage
d) Acute renal failure
e) Pulmonary embolus

Answer: a

Explanation

Cardiac troponins are regulatory contractile proteins that control the calcium-mediated interaction of actin and myosin and are not normally found in blood. There are three subunits found in a troponin complex: troponin I, troponin T and troponin C, which bind to actin, tropomyosin and calcium ions respectively. Detection in the circulation of troponin I and T (the cardiac troponins) have been shown to be both sensitive and specific markers for myocardial cell damage. Troponin C is not used because both cardiac and smooth muscle share troponin C isoforms. 'Cardiac specific' troponin has been shown to be elevated in a number of conditions, other than acute coronary syndromes, including sepsis, hypovolaemia, cardiac failure, myocarditis, myocardial contusion, renal failure and even strenuous exercise. This makes the interpretation of a raised serum troponin in the setting of the critically ill patient difficult. It is therefore unwise to make a diagnosis of myocardial infarction in the critically ill based on a raised troponin alone in the absence of ischaemic ECG changes or new wall motion abnormalities on echocardiography. Of interest, several studies examining troponin levels in the critical care patient population have shown raised troponin levels occurring in up to 70% of studied patients. In a population (n = 84 872) presenting with acute decompensated heart failure a positive cardiac troponin test (troponin I or T) was associated with an adjusted odds ratio of death of 2.55 (95% CI 2.24–2.89; P <0.001). Surprisingly, elective DC cardioversion is associated with a minimally elevated cardiac troponin at worst.

Reference
Jeremias A, Gibson C M. Narrative review: alternative causes for elevated cardiac troponin levels when acute coronary syndromes are excluded. *Ann Int Med* 2005; **142** (9): 786–91.

Question 230: Prone position

Regarding positioning a patient prone under anaesthesia, which one of the following statements is TRUE?

a) In one configuration, shoulder and abdominal rolls allow adequate chest excursion
b) The pleural pressure gradient is considerably increased when prone, compared with supine
c) When optimally positioned, the prone patient will virtually always have an increased cardiac index
d) One of the few advantages of partial inferior vena cava obstruction is reduced blood loss during lumbar spinal surgery
e) Pancreatitis is a recognised complication of positioning patients prone for scoliosis surgery

Answer: e

Explanation
The prone position is commonly used for spinal surgery, posterior fossa intracranial surgery and to improve ventilation-perfusion matching and thus oxygenation indices in the critically hypoxaemic intensive care patient (usually with acute respiratory distress syndrome). There are numerous other indications and the anaesthetist should be familiar with the physiological changes to be expected while the patient is prone and also aware of the potential complications such that they might be avoided.

There are many described and eponymous prone positions. They all attempt to avoid abdominal compression as partial obstruction of the inferior vena cava increases venous pressure in the valveless alternative routes of blood return to the heart, including the venous plexuses of Batson, which will cause increased bleeding and obscuration of the surgical field. Decreased venous return is one of the explanations for a consistently reduced cardiac index in the prone position. Of note is that haemodynamic compensation masks this change (largely by increased systemic vascular resistance) and commonly monitored measurands such as heart rate and arterial blood pressure may remain unchanged. The other main reason abdominal compression must be avoided is related to adequacy of ventilation. Reduced abdominal excursion restricts diaphragmatic displacement thus causing raised peak airway pressures during positive pressure ventilation, decreased total compliance, hypoventilation and hypercapnia. A simple prone position involves placement of foam rolls under the chest and pelvis (with caution to avoid compression of the breasts or external genitalia) with the abdomen hanging free.

Aside from physiological sequelae, complications may be categorised as: injuries to the central nervous system, peripheral nerve injuries, direct pressure effects, indirect pressure effects (macroglossia, oropharyngeal oedema, etc.) and always consider venous air embolism. Consider too the challenges of practical procedures with limited access to the patient.

Pancreatitis is a well recognised complication of scoliosis surgery. Suggested causes include hypotension, blood loss, drug effects and cell salvage. The review below cites a report of pancreatitis in the absence of other causes where the prone position was thought to be responsible.

Reference
Edgecombe H, Carter K, Yarrow S. Anaesthesia in the prone position. *Brit J Anaesth* 2008; **100**(2): 165–83.

Question 231: Acute severe asthma

A patient with known brittle asthma is admitted with a serious acute exacerbation. They have a respiratory rate of 30 with saturations of 93% on 15 L/min of oxygen via a non-rebreathing mask. In the management of this patient, which of the following treatments is the LEAST LIKELY to be of benefit?

a) Regular oral prednisolone
b) Heliox
c) A single dose of intravenous magnesium sulphate
d) Intravenous aminophylline
e) Nebulised ipratropium bromide

Answer: b

Explanation
Patients at greatest risk of near-fatal or fatal exacerbations of asthma usually have a combination of known poorly controlled asthma and adverse behavioural or psycho-social features, e.g. denial, excessive alcohol intake, drug abuse or non-compliance with treatment. Signs of life-threatening asthma include altered conscious level, exhaustion, hypotension, cyanosis, poor respiratory effort, arrhythmia, peak expira-tory flow less than a third of predicted, hypoxia and a normal $PaCO_2$. A raised $PaCO_2$ shows near-fatal asthma. Treatment of acute severe asthma is well documented in guidelines (see reference below) that have been ratified by a number of organisations. In addition to oxygen and multiple nebulised β_2 agonist bronchodilators (salbutamol 2.5 to 5.0 mg), a number of drug therapies have been tried in these patients. There is no evidence that nebulised epinephrine is more effective than a selective β_2 agonist and intravenous β_2 agonists (salbutamol 250 mcg over ten minutes) should be reserved for those patients in whom inhaled therapy cannot be used reliably. Oral steroid (prednisolone 40 to 50 mg daily), provided it can be swallowed and main-tained, is as effective as intravenous hydrocortisone (100 mg four times per day). Combining nebulised ipratropium bromide (0.5 mg every four to six hours) with nebulised salbutamol produces significantly greater bronchodilation than salbutamol alone. A single dose of intravenous magnesium sulphate (1.2 to 2.0 g over 20 minutes) is safe and may improve acute severe asthma. There is some evidence for a benefit from nebulised magnesium sulphate and more trials on the safety and efficacy of repeated intravenous doses is needed. The use of intravenous aminophylline has been the subject of two *Cochrane Reviews* in 2000 and 2007, which failed to show an overall benefit. However, some patients with near-fatal asthma or life-threatening asthma with a poor response to initial therapy may gain additional benefit from intravenous aminophylline (5 mg/kg loading dose over 20 minutes unless on maintenance oral therapy, then infusion of 0.5 to 0.7 mg/kg per hour). The use of heliox, (helium: oxygen mixture in a ratio of 80:20 or 70:30) has again been the subject of a 2006 *Cochrane Review*. Its use either as a driving gas for nebulisers, as a breathing gas or for artificial ventilation in adults with acute asthma was not supported. Non-invasive ventilation, nebulised furosemide and leucotriene receptor antagonists may have a place in acute management of asthma but at the moment there is insufficient evidence to recommend them.

Reference

British Thoracic Society. British guideline on the management of asthma. Online at www.brit-thoracic.org.uk (Accessed 30 November 2009)

Question 232: WHO Surgical Safety Checklist

Which of the following is NOT a question asked during the 'Time out' section of the WHO Surgical Safety Checklist?

a) Has the sterility of the instruments been confirmed?
b) Have all team members introduced themselves by name and role?
c) Has antibiotic prophylaxis been given within the last 60 minutes?
d) Does the patient have a known allergy?
e) Is essential imaging displayed?

Answer: d

Explanation

There is evidence that up to half of all surgical complications are avoidable and a growing body of evidence linking good teamwork in surgery to improved outcomes. Recently the WHO launched their Safe Surgery Saves Lives campaign, part of which involved the publication of the Surgical Safety Checklist. This is a simple 19-point checklist carried out before induction of anaesthesia (the 'sign in'), before skin incision (the 'time out') and before the patient leaves the operating room (the 'sign out'). This was designed to reduce surgical complications by addressing important safety issues, including inadequate anaesthetic practices, avoidable surgical infection and poor communication among team members. Perhaps somewhat surprisingly a recent multinational study has shown that, even in 'developed world' hospitals, implementation of this checklist has resulted in a significant reduction in both rates of death and surgical complications. The reasons for improvement post checklist implementation are unclear and likely to be multifactorial. It is also possible that the improvement is contributed to by the Hawthorne effect – i.e. an improvement in performance due to subjects' knowledge of being observed. However, whatever the reasons the results are impressive and it would appear that some form of this checklist is becoming part of everyday operative practice. Allergies should be confirmed, during the 'sign-in' phase.

References

Haynes A. Weiser TG, Berry WR, *et al.*; Safe Surgery Saves Lives Study Group. A surgical safety checklist to reduce morbidity and mortality in a global population. *New Engl J Med* 2009; **360**(5): 491–9.

Advice available online at www.who. int/patientsafety/safesurgery/en/ (Accessed 30 November 2009)

Question 233: Nasal surgery

In order to achieve topical analgesia and vasoconstriction of the nasal mucosa prior to surgery, Moffett's solution is sometimes used. According to the original description, which one of the following describes the constituents of Moffett's solution?

a) 1 mL 10% cocaine, 2 mL 8.4% sodium bicarbonate, 1 mL 1:1000 adrenaline
b) 2 mL 8% cocaine, 2 mL 1% sodium bicarbonate, 1 mL 1:1000 adrenaline
c) 2 mL 10% cocaine, 2 mL 8.4% sodium bicarbonate, 1 mL 1:1000 adrenaline
d) 1 mL 8% cocaine, 2 mL 8.4% sodium bicarbonate, 2 mL 1:10 000 adrenaline
e) 2 mL 10% cocaine, 1 mL 8.4% sodium bicarbonate, 2 mL 1:1000 adrenaline

Answer: b

Explanation

Moffett was an ENT surgeon in the Birmingham Children's Hospital in 1947. He described the combination of the agents in the question for direct application to the nasal mucosa with a specially designed needle:

'An adult patient is given a hypodermic injection of morphia gr. ¼ and hyoscine gr. 1/100 one hour and fifteen minutes before the anæsthetic is begun . . . . After cleansing the nares with spirit, three positions are assumed by the patient during the induction of the analgesic and each is maintained for 10 minutes by the clock.'

His technique was popular and his name has been incorporated into anaesthetic practice and the constituents of the mixture have been modified from the original description over the years. The combination in Option (a) is sometimes used. It is argued by some that the desired result of topical anaesthesia and vasoconstriction are equally achievable without the use of agents that are stimulant, sympathomimetic and arrhythmogenic. The maximum recommended dose of cocaine is 1.5 mg/kg, which for a 70 kg patient is only 1 mL of a 10% solution. This maximum dose can still be found quoted as 2 to 3 mg/kg, which should be avoided. Proponents of the use of cocaine in otolaryngology argue that its unique combination of characteristics make it ideally suited to the task, and using the lower safe dose toxicity is not seen. Some anaesthetists omit the adrenaline as cocaine is sufficiently vasoconstrictive alone and co-administered adrenaline may increase the risk of arrhythmias.

Reference

Moffett A. Nasal analgesia by postural instillation. *Anaesthesia* 1947; **2**(1): 31–9.

Question 234: Malignant hyperthermia

The laboratory diagnosis of malignant hyperthermia involves exposure of a muscle biopsy of standardised dimensions to various chemicals while being electrically stimulated. Which one of the following chemicals is used with the greatest quantity in these tests?

a) Ryanodine
b) Caffeine
c) Enflurane
d) Dantrolene
e) Suxamethonium

Answer: b

Explanation

In over 25 years the protocol for diagnosis of malignant hyperthermia (MH) using the in vitro contracture test has remained largely unchanged. A biopsy of quadriceps muscle 15 to 25 mm by 2 to 3 mm is suspended at room temperature in carboxygenated Krebs–Ringer solution of specified electrolyte constituents. The muscle is electrically stimulated with a supramaximal current of 1 ms duration and 0.2 Hz frequency. Three tests are performed on three separate biopsies: the static caffeine test, the static halothane test and the dynamic halothane test. The muscle is preloaded to give optimal twitch height upon stimulation. It is then exposed to sequentially increasing concentrations of caffeine or halothane and its contractile behaviour noted. From observing the threshold concentration at which a given response is seen, a patient can be diagnosed as MHS (susceptible), MHN (normal – but reserved for individuals *with* a family history of MH) or MHE (equivocal – where specified thresholds are not met – these patients are sometimes regarded clinically as MH susceptible). There is a protocol for an optional contracture test involving ryanodine, and various genetic tests are in development.

References

European Malignant Hyperthermia Group. Guidelines for the halothane and caffeine in vitro contracture test (2006). Online at www.emhg.org (Accessed 30 November 2009)

European Malignant Hyperpyrexia Group. A protocol for the investigation of malignant hyperpyrexia (MH) susceptibility. *Brit J Anaes* 1984; **56**: 1267–9.

Question 235: 0.9% saline

Regarding intravenous fluid administration with 0.9% saline solution to an adult surgical patient, the following statements are true EXCEPT which one?

a) May produce abdominal discomfort
b) May reduce glomerular filtration rate principally due to the sodium load affecting the renin–angiotensin system
c) Involves infusing a solution with a higher calculated osmolality compared to plasma
d) Every litre infused provides 1½ times the guideline daily allowance for dietary salt (NaCl) intake
e) Will produce a greater immediate rise in chloride concentration than sodium concentration

Answer: b

Explanation

The 2008 GIFTASUP report has come out strongly against the routine use of 0.9% saline, principally because of the risk of developing hyperchloraemic metabolic acidosis. This starts with the greater contribution of adding 154 mmol/L of chloride to a plasma concentration of around 100 mmol/L compared to adding 154 mmol/L sodium to a plasma concentration of 140 mmol/L. The relative increase in chloride concentration provides a disproportionate rise in strong anions reducing the bicarbonate concentration as predicted by the Stewart equations. In addition to the acidosis, saline produces a number of other problems. Abdominal discomfort is occasionally experienced and there is some research evidence that saline produces reduced gastrointestinal perfusion compared to balanced solutions. Hyperchloraemia produces an increase in renal eicosanoid release leading to renal vasoconstriction and reduced glomerular filtration rate. With a calculated osmolality of 308 mOsm/kg, saline is slightly hyperosmolar compared to plasma but this is probably not clinically significant. The measured osmolality using a micro-osmometer is 286 mOsm/kg, implying that saline is not fully ionised at 0.9% concentration. The GDA for dietary salt is 6 g per day for an adult, so a litre of saline with 9 g/L is 1½ times the GDA.

Reference

Powell-Tuck J, Gosling P, Lobo DN, *et al*. British consensus guidelines on intravenous fluid therapy for adult surgical patients (GIFTASUP). 2008. Online at www.ics.ac.uk/icmprof/standards.asp?menuid=7 (Accessed 30 October 2009)
GDAs from Somerfield Healthy Choice Bran Flakes

Question 236: Awareness

Prior to elective surgery a 47-year-old female patient wants to discuss the risk of awareness under anaesthesia. This is her first anaesthetic and she is American Society of Anesthesiologists (ASA) grade I. The following statements are true EXCEPT which one?

a) A risk of awareness of 1 to 2 per 1000 general anaesthetics should be quoted to her
b) If she were ASA grade III her chance of awareness would be higher
c) If she were male her chance of awareness would be higher
d) If she were older, but still ASA grade I, her chance of awareness would be similar
e) Roughly 5% of patients will dream while under general anaesthesia

Answer: c

Explanation
Several studies have looked at the incidence of awareness under anaesthesia and a quoted figure in the region of 1 to 2 per 1000 general anaesthetics for genuine awareness is not unreasonable. When figures for possible awareness are included, the rate approximately doubles. Awareness is associated with higher ASA grades but not with either age or sex. It is most likely during endotracheal intubation or skin incision. The former is probably most likely due to the administration of a 'lighter' anaesthetic. Hypertension and tachycardia are generally not associated with reports of awareness. Dreaming during anaesthesia occurs in roughly 5% of cases and is more common in younger patients, those with lower ASA grade and patients undergoing anaesthesia for day surgery procedures. The significance of dreaming is currently unclear, as is the effect of bispectral index monitoring (BIS) on the incidence of awareness. Post-traumatic stress disorder is, not surprisingly, common in patients who were aware under anaesthesia.

Reference
Sebel PS, Bowdle TA, Ghoneim MM, *et al*. The incidence of awareness during anaesthesia: a multicenter United States study. *Anesth Analg* 2004; **99**(3): 833–9.

Question 237: Creutzfeldt–Jacob disease

Regarding clinical practice relevant to the potential transmission of Creutzfeldt–Jacob disease (CJD) the following statements are true EXCEPT which one?

a) For tonsillectomy surgeons routinely use traceable re-usable instruments
b) Use of disposable laryngoscope blades for tonsil and adenoid surgery is strongly recommended
c) In a known case of CJD, high-infectivity tissues are brain, spinal cord and posterior eye
d) In the UK, in order to reduce the risk of transmission of variant CJD a donor may not give blood if they have received a blood transfusion since 1 January 1990
e) If a laryngeal mask airway is used for tonsillectomy, it must be disposable

Answer: b

Explanation
In CJD, high-infectivity tissues are the brain, spinal cord and posterior eye. In variant CJD, medium-infectivity tissues are the anterior eye, olfactory epithelium and lymphoid tissue such as that found in the appendix and tonsils. Theoretically, during tonsillectomy, surgical instruments or laryngoscopes used at the end of the procedure could be contaminated. Single-use surgical instruments cause excessive bleeding, and risk of transfer is low. The AAGBI Working Party concluded that transmission risk is 'extremely small' with laryngoscopes, and not as dangerous as a poorer performing disposable laryngoscope blade might be in an emergency. Batch cleaning of laryngeal mask airways (LMAs) potentially disseminates the prions to the other devices – all airway devices should be destroyed after use for tonsillectomy or adenoidectomy. Bovine spongiform encephalitis prions entered the UK food chain around 1980. If a donor has received blood since 1 January 1980 they may not give

blood, in order to eliminate this route of transmission. The pedantic nature of single best answer questions operates here: the statement in Option (d) is correct, as the period stated is within the actual period set by the blood transfusion service, which is from 1 January 1980.

Reference
Association of Anaesthetists of Great Britain and Ireland. Infection control in anaesthesia. *Anaesthesia* 2008; **63**: 1027–36.

Question 238: Gram stain

A 70-year-old man is admitted to the intensive care unit with severe sepsis needing multiorgan support. Blood cultures have come back positive for Gram-negative bacilli. Which of the following is LEAST LIKELY to be the infecting organism?

a) *Neisseria meningitidis*
b) *Klebsiella pneumoniae*
c) *Pseudomonas aeruginosa*
d) *Escherichia coli*
e) *Enterobacter cloacae*

Answer: a

Explanation
The Gram stain is the most important staining procedure in microbiology. Gram-positive organisms retain the purple of crystal violet after iodine fixation and alcohol washing. Gram-negative organisms lose the purple colour with alcohol and need counterstaining with a pink dye. This difference in staining is due to the different composition of Gram-positive and Gram-negative organisms' cell walls. The cell wall of Gram-positive organisms consists mainly of multiple layers of peptidoglycan, a complex polymer of long glycan chains of alternating N-acetylglucosamine and N-acetyl muramic acid, cross-linked to each other by peptide bonds giving a rigid polar wall. The cell wall of Gram-negative organisms has a thinner layer of the same peptidoglycan found in Gram-positive organisms but the cross-linking occurs in different areas. Further differentiation of organisms into bacilli and cocci may be done on initial staining and microscopy as well as differentiation into aerobic or anaerobic dependent on the blood culture bottle that has become positive. Aerobic Gram-negative bacilli can be divided into three broad groups: the coliforms (e.g. *E. coli*, *Shigella*, *Enterobacter* and *Klebsiella*), the parvobacteria (e.g. *Haemophilus* and *Brucella*) and the pseudomonads (e.g. *Pseudomonas aeruginosa*). There are rare exceptions to these groups including *Stenotrophomonas maltophilia* an opportunistic pathogen that has developed difficult resistance patterns. Anaerobic Gram-negative bacilli include the *Bacteroides* and *Fusobacteria* species. *Neisseria meningitidis* is a Gram-negative coccus as is *Branhamella* (formerly known as *Moraxella*) *catarrhalis*. Common Gram-positive rods include *Clostridium difficile*, *Clostridium perfringens* and *Clostridium tetani*. Gram-positive cocci are easy to remember as they all end in coccus (*Staphylococcus*, *Enterococcus* and *Streptococcus*).

Question 239: Aspiration

Anaesthesia is provided for a 23-year-old, ASA grade I male undergoing an elective orthopaedic procedure. The airway is managed with a Laryngeal Mask Airway ProSeal™ (LMA ProSeal™). Shortly after entering theatre, the patient coughs and a small volume of gastric contents is noticed in the drain tube of the LMA ProSeal™. Of the following sequences of actions, which one would be MOST APPROPRIATE?

a) Place the patient in the left lateral position; remove the LMA ProSeal™ and wake the patient up
b) Keep the patient supine; remove the LMA ProSeal™; give suxamethonium with cricoid pressure applied by a trained assistant; intubate the trachea and perform endobronchial suction prior to insufflations of the lungs
c) Place the patient in the left lateral position; remove the LMA ProSeal™; give suxamethonium with cricoid pressure applied by a trained assistant; intubate the trachea and perform endobronchial suction prior to insufflations of the lungs
d) Deepen your anaesthetic and observe the patient for any problems while cautiously proceeding with surgery
e) Suction down the drain tube with an endobronchial suction catheter, suction around the back of the oropharynx and proceed if there is no obvious gastric content contamination

Answer: b

Explanation

This question is more subjective than some as there are a number of possible options that could be considered in this situation. One answer is 'this might be what I would do in everyday clinical practice' and another 'this is what I would do in an exam'. Considering these options our advice would be to play it safe and to go for the 'under exam conditions' answer every time. Hence Options (d) and (e) are not advisable. Option (a) would probably be excessive, which leaves Options (b) and (c). The difference with these is clearly positioning for intubation. There may be an argument, in terms of airway protection, for placing the patient in the left lateral position, but if you have ever tried to intubate someone in this situation you will know that the safe but practical answer is Option (b).

Reference

Rawlinson E, Minchom A. Pulmonary aspiration *Anaes Intens Care* 2007; **8**(9): 365–7.

Question 240: Management of tracheostomy

A 42-year-old male is diagnosed with Guillain–Barré syndrome of a severe nature requiring mechanical ventilation. Early in his intensive care unit admission, a percutaneous tracheostomy is sited and his sedation is ceased. Twelve hours after this procedure you are called to his bedside. The patient is agitated and cyanosed. The flange of the tracheostomy tube is 3 cm proud of the front of his neck. His pulse oximeter shows arterial oxygen saturation of 82%. The ventilator alarm is sounding indicating high airway pressures and low minute volume. Insertion of a suction catheter into the tracheostomy tube meets with resistance immediately beyond the tube.

Which one of the following is the MOST APPROPRIATE action?

a) Manually ventilate with 100% oxygen via the tracheostomy tube
b) Remove existing tracheostomy tube and reinsert one of a smaller size
c) Induce anaesthesia and perform orotracheal intubation
d) Insert an Aintree exchange catheter into the stoma and insufflate oxygen
e) Cover the stoma and perform facial mask ventilation

Answer: c

Explanation

This situation represents critical hypoxaemia secondary to hypoventilation with a partially or fully obstructed airway. The existing tracheostomy tube is clearly no longer in the trachea. The tracheotomy stoma is recent and a fistula will not have granulated therefore blind passage of a smaller tube or an Aintree catheter will risk formation of a false passage. Manual ventilation via the existing tracheostomy tube will not improve the situation and will likely result in subcutaneous emphysema or a pneumomediastinum. In some circumstances covering the stoma and mask ventilation may serve as a temporising measure, but in this case the tracheotomy is fresh and the patient agitated. It is likely therefore that mask ventilation will not be tolerated and if a successful facial seal is achieved it would result in subcutaneous emphysema and hypoventilation of the trachea. The indication for this patient's tracheostomy did not involve distortion of his upper airway anatomy, thus he can be assumed to be a straightforward oral intubation. This is the life-saving course of action here. Of course the cuff of the endotracheal tube must be beyond the iatrogenic hole in his trachea. His tracheostomy tube may be replaced later, in more controlled circumstances.

Question 241: Ankylosing spondylitis

Regarding ankylosing spondylitis, which one of the following statements is CORRECT?

a) Disease prevalence in men and women is approximately the same
b) In over 90% of cases the patient is positive for the type I HLA antigen, HLA-B37
c) A presenting feature of the condition is reduced range of movement of the cervical spine
d) The anaesthetic technique of choice, where suited to the proposed operation, is central neuraxial anaesthesia
e) Providing the cervical spine has a normal range of movement, patients with ankylosing spondylitis do not pose challenges to intubation greater than normal controls

Answer: a

Explanation

Ankylosing spondylitis is an example of a seronegative spondarthritis, so called because, despite the histological similarity to the inflammation seen in rheumatoid arthritis, there is absence of rheumatoid factors in the serum. There is a significant association with the immunotype HLA-B27 – found in over 90% of patients with the condition. Although the condition is demonstrable in equal numbers of men and women, women often have mild symptoms such that the ratio of men to women in patients who present with the disease is 4:1. The disease causes an enthesitis (inflammation at the insertion of ligaments into bone) initially at the sacroiliac and thoracolumbar intervertebral ligament insertions. Patients present in their twenties with episodic low back pain and uni- or bilateral buttock pain. Enthesitis progresses to form syndesmophytes (akin to vertical osteophytes) and eventual fusion of these causes the characteristic bamboo spine in advanced disease where all vertebral levels become involved. Implications for anaesthesia are typically considered as articular and non-articular. Even if the cervical spine movement is normal, intubation may be inhibited by reduced temporomandibular joint movement (causing reduced mouth opening) in 10% of patients or >30% of patients with advanced spondylitis. Crico-arytenoid arthritis is a theoretical (although rare) challenge also. Cervical spine fractures associated with intubation have been reported. Advanced calcified change of the intervertebral ligaments may make central neuraxial anaesthesia impossible, and epidural haematomas are more common, but the technique is not contraindicated. Non-articular manifestations can have cardiovascular, pulmonary, neurological and renal sequelae.

Question 242: Cerebrospinal fluid

When compared to mean plasma values, which one of the following statements regarding mean cerebrospinal fluid (CSF) values is TRUE?

a) CSF potassium concentration is 2.9 mmol/L when plasma is 4.6 mmol/L
b) CSF protein concentration is approximately one fifth of the plasma value
c) CSF glucose concentration is slightly less than plasma glucose concentration
d) The pH of CSF is marginally alkaline
e) The partial pressure of carbon dioxide is lower in CSF than in plasma

Answer: a

Explanation

Although sodium concentration in plasma and CSF are equal, CSF potassium is lower as stated. Plasma protein is of the order of 70 g/L whereas CSF protein is less than 0.5% of this value at 0.3 g/L. Cerebrospinal fluid glucose is two thirds of the plasma glucose concentration. Cerebrospinal fluid has a pH of 7.3 and a $PaCO_2$ of 6.7 kPa.

Question 243: Trigeminal neuralgia

The following are considered therapeutic options for the treatment of trigeminal neuralgia EXCEPT which one?

a) Stereotactic radiosurgery
b) Percutaneous radiofrequency thermoablation
c) Topical capsaicin
d) Oral lamotrigine
e) Microvascular decompression

Answer: c

Explanation

Trigeminal neuralgia is the archetypal neuropathic pain, i.e. pain caused by a primary lesion or dysfunction of the nervous system, in this case the trigeminal nerve. The clinical features are of intermittent brief episodes of severe lancinating pain unilaterally in the distribution of the maxillary or mandibular branch of the trigeminal nerve. The ophthalmic branch is exceedingly rarely affected. As for all pain conditions, the four Ps of intervention must be considered: physical, psychological, pharmacological and procedural. The pharmaceutical choices are compared to the performance of carbamazepine, long established in the treatment of trigeminal neuralgia. Most antidepressants and anticonvulsants have been tried. Topical capsaicin (a substance P depletor derived from chillies) is used in the treatment of post-herpetic neuralgia where the pain is a constant and relentless burning, but not in trigeminal neuralgia where the pain is episodic. In addition, it is highly unlikely that capsaicin cream would be used on the face or near the eyes. The procedural options involve: (i) ablating the nerve such that impulses are not generated (and numbness results); or (ii) relieving any mechanical deformation of the nerve that might be the origin of the neuropathic pain. A needle can be passed through the cheek into close proximity of the gasserion ganglion whereupon alcohol or glycerol may be applied, radiofrequency thermoablation performed or a balloon inflated repeatedly to crush the nerve. Alternatively, high-energy photons may be focused on the nerve causing selective destruction ('gamma-knife'). A technique gaining popularity due to its high success rate is microvascular decompression, which involves minimally invasive neurosurgery in the mastoid region where the trigeminal nerve is physically isolated from the nearby vasculature preventing the latter compressing the nerve.

Question 244: Procalcitonin

A patient with severe pancreatitis and CT-proven pancreatic necrosis becomes pyrexial, tachycardic and hypotensive two days after admission. Regarding the use of serum procalcitonin (PCT) as a marker of sepsis, which of the following statements is TRUE?

a) PCT is less sensitive than CRP in the diagnosis of severe sepsis
b) PCT is less specific than CRP in the diagnosis of severe sepsis
c) PCT is undetectable in the bloodstream in the absence of sepsis
d) PCT has a bloodstream half-life of approximately six hours
e) For severe bacterial infection to be likely, the serum PCT level is greater than 20 ng/mL

Answer: c

Explanation

The host response to bacterial infection involves the activation of complex immune mechanisms and the release of a wide array of inflammatory mediators, several of which (e.g. CRP, IL-6 and TNF-α) have been both studied and used as markers of both infection and its severity. The common problem for these mediators is their non-specific nature and in particular the correlation between CRP and the severity of disease is not always clear. Procalcitonin (PCT) is a 116-amino-acid peptide precursor of the hormone calcitonin which is produced by the C-cells of the thyroid gland and cleaved into calcitonin, katacalcin and a protein residue. It has been proposed as a marker of bacterial infection in the critically ill patient. It is not released into the bloodstream of healthy individuals. During an episode of severe bacterial infection with an associated systemic response the blood levels of PCT may rise to as much as 100 ng/mL but a level >2 ng/mL may be considered diagnostic. Levels greater than 2 ng/mL are not seen in viral infection, chronic inflammatory processes, autoimmune diseases, localised mild to moderate bacterial infection or in isolated systemic inflammatory response syndrome (SIRS) without bacterial infection. Levels rise faster than CRP levels, which may make the decision whether or not to initiate antibiotic therapy easier, particularly in cases like severe pancreatitis and burns where there is often already a pronounced inflammatory response making diagnosis of super-added infection difficult.

Question 245: Definitions in pain

Of the following definitions regarding pain, which one is CORRECT?

a) Allodynia: increased response to spontaneous or evoked pain
b) Hyperalgesia: stimulus and response mode are the same but response is exaggerated
c) Hyperpathia: intermittent, repetitive spontaneous pain sensation
d) Neuralgia: pain caused by primary lesion or dysfunction of the nervous system
e) Causalgia: properly known as complex regional pain syndrome type I

Answer: b

Explanation

Allodynia describes where pain is perceived at the site of a normally non-painful stimulus. It is evoked rather than spontaneous. The mode refers to the nature of the stimulus or response, e.g. painful vs. non-painful or burning, shooting, aching, etc. In allodynia the mode of stimulus and response differ. The stimulus is non-painful whereas the response is one of pain. Hyperalgesia describes increased response to a stimulus that is normally painful, i.e. the modes are the same but a disproportionate response is elicited. Hyperpathia is the abnormally painful reaction to a repetitive stimulus. It is evoked, not spontaneous. The definition: pain caused by primary lesion or dysfunction of the nervous system, is that of neuropathic pain. Neuralgia is simply pain in the distribution of a nerve. Causalgia is a syndrome of sustained burning pain and allodynia following a traumatic nerve lesion associated with vasomotor, sudomotor and trophic changes. It is more correctly known as complex regional pain syndrome type II.

Reference

H Merskey, N Bogduk. *Classification of Chronic Pain: Descriptions of Chronic Pain Syndromes and Definitions of Pain Terms*, 2nd edn. IASP Task Force on Taxonomy. Seattle: IASP Press, 1994. Online summary at www.iasp-pain.org (Accessed 30 November 2009)

Question 246: Preoperative cardiovascular drugs

A 68-year-old male patient with a history of well controlled hypertension, stable angina and hypercholesterolaemia is scheduled for lumbar microdiscectomy as the second case on the following morning's operating list. He normally takes simvastatin, losartan, bisoprolol, bendroflumethiazide and nicorandil. In addition, the aspirin he normally takes was stopped nine days previously. On your preoperative visit the evening before, the ward nurse asks you which drugs to give and which to omit between now and his anaesthetic, tomorrow morning. Which of the following combinations is MOST APPROPRIATE?

a) Give the bisoprolol, the bendroflumethiazide and the nicorandil. Omit the simvastatin and the losartan
b) Give the nicorandil. Omit the bisoprolol, the bendroflumethiazide, the simvastatin and the losartan
c) Give the simvastatin, the bisoprolol and the nicorandil. Omit the bendroflumethiazide and the losartan
d) Give the losartan, the bisoprolol, the bendroflumethiazide and the nicorandil. Omit the simvastatin
e) Give all the drugs

Answer: c

Explanation

The answer advocates omitting the diuretic and the angiotensin-2 antagonist (AT2). AT2 antagonists may cause significant hypotension during an anaesthetic and should be omitted. The omission of the diuretic is more debatable, but as there was no option with just the losartan, then Option (c) must be the correct answer. The statin should be continued for its plaque stabilisation properties and would normally be given at night because the LDL reduction effect is greater when no dietary cholesterol has been recently ingested. The anti-anginal anti-hypertensive drugs should also be given.

Question 247: Community-acquired pneumonia

A patient has been admitted with suspected community-acquired pneumonia and has been referred to critical care outreach by the medical team for consideration of ventilatory support. A CURB65 score is completed. The following variables score one point EXCEPT for which one?

a) Mental test score 7/10
b) Urea 9 mmol/L
c) Age 73 years
d) Diastolic blood pressure 55 mmHg
e) Respiratory rate 25 breaths per minute

Answer: e

Explanation

It is vital to be able to identify those patients at highest risk when considering who to admit to critical care. The CURB65 score has been developed by the British Thoracic

Society and uses five features (mental confusion, respiratory rate, systolic or diastolic blood pressure, blood urea and age) to separate patients presenting with community-acquired pneumonia (CAP) into three risk groups. A score of three or more points places a patient in the highest risk group. Confusion is defined as a mental test score of less than 8/10 or new confusion in time or place. A urea level of >7 mmol/L scores a point as does a respiratory rate of ≥30 breaths per minute. Age >65 and systolic BP <90 mmHg or diastolic <60 mmHg also both score a point. *Streptococcus pneumoniae* is the most frequently identified cause of severe CAP, but up to a third of all cases have no identifiable organism. Other common causes of severe CAP include *Legionella* and *Staphylococcus aureus* with the latter being of particular concern due to the emergence of strains producing the Panton–Valentine leucocidin toxin, which may be methicillin resistant.

Reference
Information online at www.brit-thoracic.org.uk/Portals/0/Clinical%20Information/Pneumonia/Guidelines/MACAP2001gline.pdf (Accessed 30 November 2009)

Question 248: Volatile anaesthesia

Which one of the following statements regarding volatile anaesthesia is CORRECT?

a) End tidal agent monitoring on most anaesthetic machines allows display of minimum alveolar concentration (MAC) for the patient
b) The MAC of desflurane is 6%
c) The oil:gas solubility coefficient of halothane is among the lowest of the volatile anaesthetic agents
d) Female gender decreases MAC
e) Hyponatraemia decreases MAC

Answer: e

Explanation
Minimum alveolar concentration is a representation of the potency of a volatile agent. It is the percentage concentration of volatile in a stated carrier gas, at steady state (for at least 15 minutes) and at sea level that will obtund response to a standard surgical stimulus in 50% of patients. The patients are unpremedicated, unparalysed 40-year-olds; the stimulus is a groin incision and a response is spontaneous physical movement by the patient. This will not obtund autonomic response necessarily, but by this effect-site concentration it is usually assumed that the chance of awareness is negligible. Most anaesthetic machines do not require input of patient demographical data so the 'MAC' value displayed is not for the patient attached to the anaesthetic machine, but for the very unlikely combination of pre-conditions described above. Unpremedicated, for example, would preclude use of opioids at induction of anaesthesia as this reduces 'MAC'. It is for this reason that the author believes that the display of 'MAC' by the anaesthetic machine is pointless or even misleading. Absolute end-tidal concentration of agent with use of knowledge of population MAC values and combined individual circumstances and patient characteristics would more accurately direct administration of volatile anaesthesia. Lists of factors that increase and decrease MAC should be learned for this reason. Gender does not influence MAC. The MAC of desflurane in 70% nitrous oxide is 2.5% and in 100% oxygen is quoted as 6%. The question does not specify the carrier gas. Also, the range of desflurane MAC values across patient ages and in the presence or absence of benzodiazepines or opioids is so wide as to make nonsense of the statement 'the MAC of desflurane is 6%'.

Question 249: Suxamethonium

The following are unwanted effects of suxamethonium EXCEPT which one?

a) Masseter spasm
b) Tachycardia
c) Hyperkalaemia
d) Malignant hyperpyrexia
e) Prolonged muscle relaxation

Answer: b

Explanation

Administration of suxamethonium is often accompanied by a rise in heart rate but this may be attributable to the use of thiopentone (which directly causes a tachycardia) or during induction of anaesthesia in the absence of concurrent opioid use in which the tachycardia represents an adrenergic response to laryngoscopy. In fact, suxamethonium itself is likely to exert a bradycardic effect especially when used in repeated doses. For this reason an anti-cholinergic agent such as atropine should be immediately available if a second dose of suxamethonium is to be given.

The side effects and complications of suxamethonium are legion and should be well known to the candidate, as well as its cautions and contraindications. Masseter spasm may be isolated and self-limiting or prolonged and problematic. It may or may not represent the onset of malignant hyperpyrexia. During global muscle depolarisation, potassium efflux from cells may increase serum potassium concentration by 0.5 mmol/ L, in a normal individual. In cases of denervation injuries or burns, extra-junctional acetylcholine receptors may underlie the exaggerated efflux with catastrophic consequences. Suxamethonium apnoea, which may cause prolonged muscle relaxation, is an example of pharmacogenetics in action, of which there are a number of examples in anaesthesia.

Question 250: Gas embolism

Concerning the presentation and treatment of a patient with suspected gas embolism the following statements are true EXCEPT which one?

a) The reason hyperbaric therapy reduces the volume of a gas bubble is because volume is inversely proportional to pressure at a constant temperature, which is explained by Boyle's law
b) The reason hyperbaric oxygen therapy also reduces the size of the gas bubble is due to the alteration of diffusion gradients of both nitrogen and oxygen
c) The commonest reason for a paradoxical gas embolus is due to the presence of a patent foramen ovale that occurs in upto 30% of the adult population
d) The 'mill wheel murmur' sometimes heard over the praecordium is due to blood and air mixing within the left ventricle
e) A patient in the 'deckchair' position is at increased risk of gas embolism

Answer: d

Explanation

There are two broad categories of gas embolism – venous and arterial. Paradoxical gas embolism, when gas enters the venous circulation then moves into the arterial circulation, occurs most commonly when there is a patent foramen ovale. This occurs in up to 30% of the population. Gas embolism occurs more often into non-collapsing veins, e.g. the epiploic veins, emissary veins and the dural venous sinus. Hence neurosurgical patients, especially those being operated on in the 'deckchair' position (a semi-recumbent position), are at particular risk. Signs and symptoms are, in the main, related to the volume of gas entering the circulation. The mill wheel murmur is secondary to blood and air mixing in the right ventricle. The presence of a mill wheel murmur is a late sign indicating large-volume embolus and absence of it does not exclude the diagnosis of gas embolism. Option (a) is true – the gas laws are happy hunting grounds for examiners as these laws are easily confused. Hyperbaric oxygen works by producing a steep oxygen diffusion gradient into the bubble and a nitrogen gradient out. It may also reduce the embolic insult to the microvasculature by improving oxygen delivery. There is also evidence to suggest an attenuation of the endothelial insult.

Reference
Muth C, Shank E. Gas embolism. *New Engl J Med* 2000; **342**(26): 476–82.

Question 251: Pyloric stenosis

A 6-week-old term infant presents for surgery to treat hypertrophic pyloric stenosis (HPS). Which of the following statements regarding this child and its treatment is LEAST CORRECT?

a) Both acid and alkaline urine occur
b) Attempts by the surgeon to take the patient straight to theatre should be resisted until attempts have been made to correct the biochemical abnormalities
c) If the infant has acid urine they are likely to have a significant potassium deficit
d) The infant is more likely to be female than male and to have a parent who also had HPS
e) In HPS, potassium and hydrogen ion excretion by the kidneys is designed to maintain a normal pH

Answer: d

Explanation
Hypertrophic pyloric stenosis is a common cause of vomiting in infants, with an incidence of 3 cases per 1000 live births in Whites. It is less prevalent among Blacks and Asians and is four times as common in male infants as in female infants. It also appears to occur more frequently in first-born males. A family history has been reported in approximately 10% of cases. Diagnosis is often made by history and physical examination. An 'olive' shaped mass is sometimes palpated in the epigastrium just to the right of the midline in addition to visible gastric peristaltic waves. Ultrasound may be used to confirm the diagnosis. Hypertrophic pyloric stenosis is characterised by projectile vomiting, failure to thrive, dehydration and electrolyte abnormalities. Hypochloraemic hypokalaemic metabolic alkalosis is the classic electrolyte abnormality seen. This is due to the persistent (acidic) vomiting leading to loss of sodium, potassium and chloride ions. This leads to two renal responses. The first is designed to restore pH by the excretion of bicarbonate (which is combined with sodium ions). The second is the excretion of potassium and hydrogen ions and the retention of sodium ions in an attempt to preserve extracellular fluid volume. The first response tends to produce alkaline urine, the second an acid urine. This acid urine tends to increase the metabolic alkalosis, hence resulting in worsening hypokalaemia.

Question 252: Revised cardiac risk index

Regarding Lee's revised cardiac risk index, which one of the following would score one point?

a) Serum creatinine 120 micromol/L
b) Open hemicolectomy
c) On insulin sliding scale to manage hyperkalaemia
d) Poorly controlled hypertension
e) Hypercholesterolaemia

Answer: b

Explanation

Lee investigated 4315 patients aged over 50 years having major, non-cardiac surgery. In 1999 he published a simple revised cardiac risk index (RCRI), listing six factors, which scored one point each. This was meant to simplify the Goldman and Detsky scores with their high number of variables and weighted scores for each variable. The components of the RCRI are high-risk surgery (such as intraperitoneal or intrathoracic), evidence of ischaemic heart disease (such as previous myocardial infarction or on nitrate therapy), evidence of congestive heart failure (such as radiographic appearance of outer-zone blood diversion or S3 gallop), history of cerebrovascular disease (such as stroke or transient ischaemic attack), diabetics on preoperative insulin therapy, and renal insufficiency determined by a serum creatinine >2.0 mg/dL (177 micromol/L). If you scored zero points, your risk of major cardiac complication was 0.4%, one point gave a 0.9% risk, two points a 6.6% risk and three or more points an 11% risk.

Reference

Lee TH, Marcantonio ER, Mangione CM, *et al.* Derivation and prospective validation of a simple index for prediction of cardiac risk of major noncardiac surgery. *Circulation* 1999;**100**(10): 1043–9.

Question 253: Complex regional pain syndromes

A patient presents to your chronic pain clinic with a two-month history of severe pain in the right forearm. Of the following features, which is LEAST CONSISTENT with a diagnosis of a complex regional pain syndrome type I?

a) Pain that is in an ulnar nerve distribution
b) A history of a fractured ulna occurring 24 months previously that required reduction and immobilisation
c) Worsening of the pain when the arm is placed in a dependent position
d) Loss of hair on the right forearm but preservation of hair on the left forearm
e) The presence of a tremor in the right arm

Answer: a

Explanation

Complex regional pain syndrome (CRPS) is a chronic, progressive disease with a number of characteristic features. It may be divided into two categories: CRPS type I and CRPS type II. The former (which is also known as reflex sympathetic dystrophy) tends to develop after a minor injury to or fracture of a limb; the latter (also known as causalgia) develops after injury to a major peripheral nerve. Symptoms and signs associated with CRPS include pain disproportionate to the intensity of the inciting event, pain that usually worsens when the extremity is in a dependent position, mechanical and thermal allodynia and/or hyperalgesia. Typically in CRPS type I, sensory abnormalities have no consistent spatial relationship to individual nerve territories. There are also a number of common autonomic abnormalities associated with CRPS including swelling of the distal extremity, hyper- or hypohidrosis, vasodilatation or vasoconstriction, and changes in skin temperature. Trophic changes include thin, glossy skin, fibrosis and changes in hair growth. Finally, there may be a number of motor changes including weakness, coordination defects and tremor. Treatment of CRPS type I or II is often multidisciplinary and includes a number of different drug therapies, e.g. antidepressants, anti-inflammatory agents, GABA analogues and beta blockers. Physiotherapy and occupational therapy as part of pain management programmes are helpful, as well as injection of local anaesthetic. In severe cases there are promising results from neurostimulation techniques, e.g. spinal cord stimulators.

Question 254: Paediatric fluid management

Regarding the administration of intravenous infusions to children, the following statements are correct EXCEPT which one?

a) Sodium chloride 0.45% + glucose 2.5% may be safely administered to the majority of children
b) Sodium chloride 0.18% + glucose 4% should not be available in areas that treat children
c) Sodium chloride 0.45% + glucose 5% is hyperosmolar with respect to plasma and hypotonic with reference to the cell membrane
d) On going losses may be replaced by, for example, compound sodium lactate solution
e) Severe acute hyponatraemia is defined as a decrease in plasma sodium from normal to less than 130 mmol/L in less than 24 hours

Answer: e

Explanation
This question tests understanding of physics (distinguishing osmolality from tonicity), physiology (electrolyte and fluid disorders) and current practice of anaesthesia (2007 National Patient Safety Alert regarding paediatric fluid administration). Option (e) would be a correct statement if the time quoted was 48 hours. An osmole is the molecular weight of a substance divided by the number of independent moieties into which it dissociates in a solution. Osmolality is an expression of the concentration of osmoles per kilogram of specified solvent. This is a property of a solution, without reference to semi-permeable membranes. Tonicity refers to the sum of osmotic pressures due to active particles exerted by a solution at a specified cell membrane. At cell membranes solutes may be either permeant (the membrane is permeable to them) or non-permeant (they can not cross). This clearly influences their tonicity as if a solute may freely cross a cell membrane then it exerts no osmotic pressure at that cell membrane. This is the case with glucose contained in intravenous infusions as, in the presence of insulin, glucose is permeant so although a 5% solution is isosmolar and will not cause haemolysis, once the glucose has equilibrated across cell membranes or been metabolised by erythrocytes, effectively free water is left. This can cause rapid and catastrophic hyponatraemic encephalopathy – especially in children. Free water passage into neurones can cause cerebral oedema, fits and death. For this reason significantly hypotonic solutions (i.e. glucose solutions with no or low sodium) have virtually no place in paediatric fluid prescription (with some specialist exceptions).

Reference
National Patient Safety Agency. Reducing the risk of hyponatraemia when administering intravenous infusions to children. Patient safety alert 22. NPSA, 28 March 2007. Online at www.npsa.nhs.uk/nrls/alerts-and-directives/alerts/intravenous-infu sions/ (Accessed 30 November 2009)

Question 255: Common paediatric surgical conditions

Regarding paediatric surgical conditions, the following statements are true EXCEPT which one?

a) The commonest type of tracheo-oesophageal fistula is oesophageal atresia with a distal fistula
b) Pyloric stenosis classically presents with bilious projectile vomiting at six weeks of age
c) Gastroschisis involves a defect in the anterior abdominal wall, usually on the right
d) In >50% of cases of intussusception, the patient is less than one year of age
e) Inguinal hernias are almost exclusively of the indirect type

Answer: b

Explanation

In pyloric stenosis, hypertrophy of the pyloric musculature causes gastric outflow obstruction and prevents duodenal reflux therefore vomiting, although classically projectile, is non-bilious. The incidence is 3:1000 infants (male to female ratio, 4:1). The candidate should be familiar with the metabolic derangements encountered and the preoperative resuscitation and intraoperative considerations.

In tracheo-oesophageal fistula (TOF), 85% are Gross type C (of A–E) as described in the question. The incidence is quoted, depending on source, as between 1:2500 and 1:3500 live births. Beware of the VACTERL association (vertebral abnormalities, anal atresia, cardiac defects, tracheo-oesophageal fistula, oesophageal atresia, renal and limb anomalies; also known as VATER syndrome).

Peak incidence of intussusception is at four to ten months. Around 70 to 90% of cases (depending on series) are resolved with radiologically guided pneumatic reduction. Direct infantile inguinal hernias are rare and virtually always associated with previous surgery.

Question 256: Pancreatitis

Regarding the management of acute pancreatitis, which one of the following has been most universally ABANDONED?

a) Maintaining the patient nil-by-mouth
b) Use of pethidine, rather than morphine, for analgesia
c) Administration of prophylactic antibiotics
d) Laparotomy
e) Early computerised tomography

Answer: a

Explanation

Acute pancreatitis is inflammation of the pancreas secondary to autodigestion by the digestive enzymes that it produces. Common precipitants are excessive alcohol consumption and cholelithiasis but the list of potential aetiologies is long. The pancreas is not encapsulated, so inflammation is poorly confined and generalised peritonitis is a common sequela. Progression to haemorrhagic pancreatitis or necrosis and superinfection with enteral organisms increases the severity of the condition and worsens the prognosis. A frustrating diagnosis in some respects, patients may be extremely unwell and yet no definitive management strategy exists. Treatment is often supportive rather than specific. Early computerised tomography is widely used to define the extent of inflammation in the organ and the presence of developing complications such as pseudocysts. Laparotomy is indicated if there is pancreatic abscess or haemorrhage and is sometimes indicated if there is extensive necrosis. Regarding antibiotics, *Cochrane Review* could not demonstrate clear-cut benefit, but the evidence was not strong enough to propose their withdrawal and they are still used in moderate or severe pancreatitis, often based on the judgement of the responsible clinician. Pancreatitis patients are in a catabolic state and nutrition is paramount. When the risks and benefits of enteral vs. parenteral nutrition are considered, enteral feeding is favoured. Although its clinical significance is unclear, pethidine does cause less spasm in the sphincter of Oddi than morphine, and where cholelithiasis is the cause, pethidine could theoretically be the superior analgesic. Whatever the reader's opinion on this, pethidine does still appear on many current pancreatitis management protocols, whereas nil-by-mouth does not.

Question 257: Oesophageal Doppler interpretation

Following emergency surgery for a ruptured abdominal aortic aneurysm a 76-year-old patient is on noradrenaline 0.35 mcg/kg/min. They remain hypotensive (80/35) with a decreased urine output despite being warmed since returning from theatre (34.5 °C to 37.1 °C) and having received 500 mL of intravenous colloid. An oesophageal Doppler probe is inserted, which gives a corrected flow time (FT_C) of 290 ms (normal range = 330 to 360 ms) and a peak velocity (PV) of 40 cm/s (normal range = 50 to 80 cm/s). Which of the following represents the MOST APPROPRIATE immediate management plan?

a) Cautious introduction of low dose dobutamine with the aim to slowly escalate dose
b) Fluid challenge with boluses of 250 mL of Gelofusine® titrated to response
c) Aim to slowly reduce noradrenaline dose and give fluid challenges based on response
d) Further, cautious escalation of noradrenaline dose
e) Introduce nitrate infusion combined with cautious fluid challenges

Answer: c

Explanation

Following insertion of an oesophageal Doppler probe approximately 40 cm from the incisors, a waveform is displayed on a screen that gives a beat-to-beat picture allowing real-time assessment of a number of haemodynamic variables. This probe produces an ultrasonic Doppler measurement of blood velocity in the descending thoracic aorta. This then allows calculation of a number of cardiac output and haemodynamic variables by integration of this velocity with respect to time using an assumption of the aortic diameter by entering the patient's height, weight and sex. Its use is contraindicated in patients following oesophagectomy and in those with known or suspected oesophageal varices. Care should be taken in patients with severe coagulopathy and it is difficult to use in the conscious patient. Measured values include heart rate, stroke distance, peak velocity (PV), mean acceleration and corrected flow time (FT_C). Derived values include cardiac output and index, stroke volume and stroke volume index, and systemic vascular resistance. Of all these, PV and FT_C provide most information about a patient's haemodynamic status. In this patient the FT_C and the PV are both low. Causes of the former include low left ventricular filling, e.g. secondary to hypovolaemia or a high afterload secondary to vasoconstriction or an obstructed circulation. Causes of the latter include decreased left ventricular contractility and increased afterload. In this patient the most likely reason for these results and the consequent hypotension is overconstriction secondary to the noradrenaline with probable hypovolaemia, hence Option (c) represents the best management plan.

Question 258: Accidental hypothermia

A patient with alcohol dependency was found unconscious in the community and transferred to the emergency department in your hospital. His admission temperature is 32 °C. Which one of the following list is the MOST IMMEDIATE threat to his outcome?

a) This severe hypothermia will result in malignant arrhythmias
b) Hypokalaemia causing myocardial depression

c) Acidaemia
d) Progressive reduction in ionised calcium with reduction in pH
e) Spontaneous central apnoea

Answer: c

Explanation

The classification of hypothermia is mild (32 to 35°C), moderate (28 to 32 °C) and severe (<28 °c) so this case is in fact mild hypothermia. Patients become acidotic, hyper-magnesaemic and hyperkalaemic (as intracellular magnesium and potassium exit the cells). Ionised calcium tends to increase with decreasing pH, but changes in ionised calcium are not always entirely pH dependent. Parathyroid hormone influences calcium, even acutely, mediated by interleukin-6. Below 32 °C, acidosis does not improve with re-warming, but rapidly improves with re-warming above this temperature. At 32 °C atrial fibrillation is common and J-waves may be seen but these are not malignant and maintain a spontaneous circulation. Fortunately, central apnoea would not be expected until around 24 °C.

Reference

McInerney JJ, Breakell A, Madira W, Davies TG, Evans PA. Accidental hypothermia and active rewarming: the metabolic and inflammatory changes observed above and below 32 °C. *Emerg Med J* 2002; **19**(3): 219–23.

Question 259: Hyponatraemia

A patient is admitted to the intensive care unit with a reduced GCS and a serum sodium of 120 mmol/L. Which of the following potential causes of this hyponatraemia is MOST LIKELY to result in a decreased extracellular fluid compartment volume?

a) Pancreatitis
b) Bronchopneumonia
c) Severe cirrhosis
d) Congestive cardiac failure
e) Nephrotic syndrome

Answer: a

Explanation

Hyponatraemia is defined as a decrease in serum sodium concentration to below 136 mmol/L. Normally the extracellular fluid (ECF) and intracellular fluid (ICF) compartments make up one third and two thirds of total body water respectively, and depending on the cause of the hyponatraemia these volumes will change. Unlike hypernatraemia, which is always associated with hypertonicity, hyponatraemia may be associated with either low, normal or high tonicity, so measurement of a serum osmolality in patients presenting with hyponatraemia may be extremely useful. Causes of hypotonic hyponatraemia may be divided into those associated with a decreased, increased or essentially normal extracellular fluid volume. Causes of hypotonic hyponatraemia and low ECF volume include renal sodium loss (e.g. diuretics, adrenal insufficiency), extrarenal sodium loss (e.g. diarrhoea, vomiting, blood loss, sweating) and third-space fluid sequestration (e.g. secondary to pancreatitis, burns or peritonitis). Causes of hypotonic hyponatraemia with increased ECF volume include congestive cardiac failure, cirrhosis, nephrotic syndrome, acute or chronic renal failure and pregnancy. Causes of hyponatraemia with essentially normal ECF fluid volume include hypothyroidism, syndrome of inappropriate ADH secretion (SIADH), a number of drugs (e.g. desmopressin, nicotine and opiate derivatives), pulmonary conditions (e.g. ARDS and pneumonia) and others including pain and HIV infection.

Reference
Adrogue H, Madias N. Hyponatraemia. *N Eng J Med* 2000; **342**(21): 1581–9.

Question 260: Latex allergy

During their preoperative assessment, a patient volunteers the information that they are allergic to a number of fruit and vegetables. Which of the following would be the LEAST LIKELY to be associated with a potential latex allergy?

a) Avocado
b) Strawberry
c) Kiwifruit
d) Banana
e) Cauliflower

Answer: e

Explanation

Natural rubber latex (NRL) is a milky fluid obtained from the *Hevea brasiliensis* tree. The introduction of universal precautions in the late 1980s led to a huge increase in the use of NRL gloves and this, combined with the increase in atopic allergic disease in recent decades, has led to a significant rise in latex allergy. Groups at greatest risk include healthcare workers, individuals undergoing multiple surgical procedures, individuals with a history of atopy, individuals exposed to NRL on a regular basis (e.g. car mechanics) and finally, individuals with a history of certain food allergies. These include apple, avocado, banana, chestnut, fig, grape, kiwifruit, mango, passionfruit, peach, nectarine, pear, strawberry and tomato. Latex exposure is associated with three clinical syndromes. The first and most common is irritant dermatitis which occurs as a result of the mechanical disruption of the skin due to rubbing by the gloves. It is not immune mediated. The second is a delayed (type IV) hypersensitivity reaction resulting in a typical contact dermatitis. Symptoms usually develop within 24 to 48 hours of exposure and this is usually secondary to the accelerators and antioxidants used in the manufacturing process. The third and most serious is an immediate (or type I) hypersensitivity reaction. This is IgE mediated and may develop into a full-blown anaphylactic reaction. The vast majority of anaesthetic and surgical equipment is now latex free and the vast majority of individuals with a latex allergy will not develop a type I hypersensitivity reaction. However, avoidance of any potential reaction is clearly the correct strategy and this may be aided by knowledge of food allergy to fruit and vegetables known to contain similar proteins to those in NRL.

Question 261: Central venous access devices

With regard to central venous catheters (CVCs), which one of the following statements is TRUE?

a) Approximately one third of all hospital-acquired bloodstream infections are CVC related
b) *Staphylococcus aureus* is the commonest organism implicated in CVC infection
c) Both CVCs that are externally coated and CVCs that are internally AND externally coated with antimicrobial substances significantly lower the risk of CVC-related infection
d) The administration of antibiotics at the time of CVC insertion is recommended as it reduces the risk of CVC-related bloodstream infection
e) 1% chlorhexidine in 70% isopropyl alcohol should be used to clean the skin at the site of the CVC

Answer: a

Explanation

Approximately 3 in 1000 patients admitted to hospital in the United Kingdom acquire a bloodstream infection, and approximately one third of these are related to CVCs. In an attempt to reduce the rate of CVC-related bloodstream infection (CR-BSI), national guidelines endorsed by the Department of Health have attempted to identify best practice for the insertion and maintenance of CVCs. Coagulase-negative staphylococci, particularly *Staphylococcus epidermidis*, are the most frequently implicated microorganisms. CVC-related bloodstream infection is usually caused by skin microorganisms at the insertion site that contaminate the catheter during insertion, or microorganisms from the hands of healthcare workers that contaminate and colonise the catheter during care interventions. Seeding from other sites of infection is rare. Only CVCs both internally and externally coated with antibiotic, silver or silver/chlorhexidine have been statistically proven to reduce the rate of CR-BSI and these CVCs are recommended in patients requiring access for greater than one week or who are thought to be at high risk of CR-BSI. The skin disinfectant of choice is 2% chlorhexidine in 70% isopropyl alcohol. Antibiotic administration at the time of insertion is not recommended due to the potential risk of increased microbial resistance.

Reference

Pratt RJ, Pellowe CM, Wilson JA, *et al.* epic2: National evidence-based guidelines for preventing healthcare-associated infections in NHS hospitals in England. *J Hosp Infect* 2007; **65**(Suppl 1): S1–S64.

Question 262: Rhabdomyolysis

Twenty-four hours after a road traffic accident and prolonged extraction a 27-year-old woman is found to have a creatine kinase (CK) of 57 000 units/L. You suspect rhabdomyolysis. Which of the following does NOT support your diagnosis?

a) Raised troponin I (TnI)
b) Urine microscopy showing red blood cells
c) Myoglobinuria
d) Urine dipstick positive for blood
e) Hypocalcaemia

Answer: b

Explanation

There are a number of causes of rhabdomyolysis and these may be conveniently categorised into several groups as follows. Post trauma (the so-called 'crush syndrome'), post exertion (e.g. following strenuous exercise), post infection (e.g. influenza A or B), secondary to genetic defects (e.g. disorders of glycolysis or lipid metabolism), body temperature changes (e.g. malignant hyperpyrexia), metabolic and electrolyte disorders (e.g. diabetic ketoacidosis), secondary to drugs and toxins (e.g. statins), muscle hypoxia (e.g. tourniquet use) and idiopathic causes. Rhabdomyolysis is characterised by leakage of muscle cell contents into the circulation. One of these, creatine kinase (CK), is used to aid diagnosis with levels commonly in the tens of thousands in severe cases. Acute renal failure (ARF) is one of the more severe consequences of rhabdomyolysis, though compared to other causes of ARF chances of recovery of renal function are good. Myoglobinuria occurs only in the context of rhabdomyolysis, and will cause a false-positive urine dipstick for blood even though urine microscopy will be negative for red blood cells. Myoglobin appears in the urine only when the renal threshold of 0.5 to 1.5 mg/dL of myoglobin is exceeded, so not all cases of rhabdomyolysis are associated with myoglobinuria. The exact mechanism of ARF secondary to rhabdomyolysis is unclear, but probably involves a combination of intrarenal vasoconstriction, both direct and indirect tubular injury and tubular obstruction. Due to fluid sequestration in muscle, the majority of patients with rhabdomyolysis need fluid replacement, which should be given both early and in large volumes if the patient's condition allows. Alkalinisation of fluid replacement and/or the use of mannitol both have theoretical advantages but neither has ever been shown to improve outcome in good-quality clinical trials. Hypocalcaemia is common early in the course of rhabdomyolysis and usually results from calcium entering the ischaemic and damaged muscle cells and from the precipitation of calcium phosphate with calcification in necrotic muscle. Rebound hypercalcaemia may occur with recovery of renal function and is unique to rhabdomyolysis-induced ARF.

Reference
Bosch X, Poch E, Grau JM. Rhabdomyolysis and acute kidney injury. *N Engl J Med* 2009; **361**(1): 62–72.

Question 263: Myasthenia gravis

Regarding a patient presenting with myasthenia gravis (MG), the following statements are true EXCEPT which one?

a) MG is an autoimmune condition in which IgG autoantibodies interact with acetylcholine receptors at the neuromuscular junction
b) MG is most common in young men and older women
c) Reflexes in a patient with MG are normal
d) There is no association with malignant disease
e) Diagnosis of MG is, in part, made by assessment of the response to administration of a reversible acetylcholinesterase inhibitor

Answer: b

Explanation
Myasthenia gravis predominantly affects older men (60 to 70 years old) and younger women (20 to 30 years old). Symptoms and signs are exclusively limited to the motor system, with no changes in sensation, coordination or reflexes. In some patients (approximately 15%) the features of MG are confined to the eyes with diplopia and ptosis being common presenting symptoms. MG is an autoimmune condition in which IgG anti-acetylcholine receptor antibodies (anti-AChR antibodies), present in 80 to 90% of sufferers, interact with postsynaptic acetylcholine receptors at the neuromuscular junction. Patients with MG but without anti-AChR antibodies often have antibodies against muscle-specific kinases, which play a role in postsynaptic differentiation and clustering of acetylcholine receptors. Like many other autoimmune conditions MG is associated with other autoimmune conditions including, rheumatoid arthritis, thyroid abnormalities and systemic lupus erythematosis. Diagnosis is made on the basis of history, examination, electromyography, detection of the IgG autoantibodies and assessment of response to the reversible acetylcholinesterase inhibitor, edrophonium (the so-called 'Tensilon test'). MG should not be confused with the condition myasthenic syndrome (also known as the Eaton–Lambert syndrome). The latter is a pre rather than post synaptic disorder in which voltage-gated calcium channels on the presynaptic motor nerve terminal are damaged. This results in decreased acetylcholine release (unlike in MG in which acetylcholine release is normal). In addition in the myasthenic syndrome tendon reflexes are

depressed and, unlike MG, 50 to 70% of cases are associated with malignancy, with the overwhelming majority of these being small-cell lung carcinoma.

Reference

Thavasothy M, Hirsch N. Myasthenia gravis. *Cont Educ Anaes Crit Care Pain* 2002; **2**: 88–90.

Question 264: Anaesthesia for strabismus surgery

For satisfactory progression of surgery involving transposition and shortening of muscles of the eye, it may be preferable to use a non-depolarising muscle relaxant for which one of the following reasons?

a) Depth of anaesthesia can interfere with the forced duction test
b) Bell's phenomenon interferes with the position of the eye and thus surgical field
c) The incidence of the occulocardiac reflex is diminished with muscle relaxation
d) The incidence of postoperative nausea and vomiting is diminished if muscle relaxation has been used
e) Postoperative pain scores are reduced if muscles have been relaxed during traction or manipulation

Answer: a

Explanation

Bell's phenomenon is the natural rolling backwards of the globe in the orbit upon closure of the eyelids. Specific work has looked at the angles of deviation with different anaesthetic agents and in the presence and absence of muscle relaxation and no statistically significant association was shown. The occulocardiac reflex may be reduced by prophylactic anti-cholinergics, local anaesthesia of the surgical site and avoiding hypercapnia. Muscle relaxants have no effect on the reflex. Furthermore, they do not decrease pain or nausea. Indeed if neostigmine is used to reverse non-depolarising muscle relaxation this can be emetogenic. The forced duction test is performed by the surgeon, where forceps are used to grasp the sclera near the limbus and the globe manipulated through its range of movement allowing the surgeon to distinguish between paretic muscle and mechanical restriction to eye movement. This guides the nature and extent of surgery. If, due to anaesthetic technique, the eye is less than immobile or muscular tone is changing, an inaccurate forced duction test can necessitate a prolonged procedure or even repeat surgery.

References

Hartwig, P. Anaesthesia for correction of strabismus. *Update in Anaesthesia*. Online at www.nda.ox.ac.uk/wfsa/html/u17/u1709_01.htm (Accessed 30 November 2009)
Paez J, Isenberg S, Apt L. Torsion and elevation under general anesthesia and during voluntary eyelid closure (Bell phenomenon). *J Pediatr Ophthalmol Strabismus*. 1984; **21** (1): 22–4.

Question 265: Breastfeeding

Eight weeks post-partum, a 30-year-old woman requires an emergency appendicectomy. She is currently breastfeeding and wishes to continue as soon as possible after her operation. Which one of the following drugs should be avoided to allow her to return safely to breastfeeding in the shortest possible time?

a) Oxycodone
b) Atracurium
c) Propofol
d) Suxamethonium
e) Diclofenac sodium

Answer: a

Explanation

There have, for obvious reasons, been few human clinical trials looking at prescribing in pregnancy and there is a consequent dearth of epidemiologic data on the probability of adverse effects in breastfed infants. In addition, few drug companies will be happy to say that drugs they manufacture are completely safe for the infant. General advice is to express and discard milk for the first 24 hours after an anaesthetic, to use as few different types of drug as possible and to avoid drugs in the British National Formulary listed as 'ones to avoid'. There is no data on the use of suxamethonium but thousands of breastfeeding mothers have received it without any apparent untoward effect on their children. All analgesic drugs appear to be safe with the exception of oxycodone and pethidine. Breastfed infants whose mothers have received pethidine have a higher risk of neurobehavioural depression than breastfed infants whose mothers are administered morphine. Oxycodone is concentrated in human breast milk for up to 72 hours post-partum. Breastfed infants may receive >10% of a therapeutic infant dose. For potent analgesia, single dose morphine is unlikely to cause harm to the infant. For longer term use the infant should be observed for adverse effects, in particular depression of the central nervous system. Paracetamol (including intravenous preparations) and non-steroidal anti-inflammatory drugs are safe. Of the non-depolarising muscle relaxants manufacturers advise avoiding rocuronium and there is no avoidance advice given for the others. Both propofol and thiopentone will be present in the breast milk following their use in an anaesthetic. Thiopentone manufacturers advise avoidance if breastfeeding. Short-term administration of benzodiazepines is probably safe, but for the vast majority of situations their use is avoidable.

Reference

Ito S. Drug therapy for breast-feeding women. *N Eng J Med* 2000; **343**(2): 118–26.
Further information online at www.bnf.org (Appendix 5 Breast-feeding).

Question 266: Oxygen requirements in ventilated patients

A patient needs transferring from one hospital to another. He is ventilated with a minute volume of 14 L/min. The journey will take 90 minutes in total. Assume he is transferred with an FiO_2 of 1.0 on a 100% efficient ventilator that uses a minute volume's worth of oxygen every minute. You want to carry enough oxygen to last for twice the anticipated journey time. Which of the following oxygen volumes (in cylinders) is the nearest to the ideal calculated amount?

a) 1C + 1D + 1E + 1F
b) 2F
c) 2E + 5C
d) 1F + 3E
e) 5D + 1E

Answer: a

Explanation

The approximate volume of oxygen needed for this journey is 2520 litres (14 × 90 × 2). 1C + 1D + 1E +1F cylinders would give 2550 litres of oxygen if all were full. Most frontline ambulances carry one F-sized oxygen cylinder containing 1360 litres of oxygen, as well as a number of portable (and hence much smaller volume) ones. A useful rule of thumb is every time you go up or down a cylinder size you can calculate the oxygen content by doubling or halving the volume. Thus an E-size cylinder (the size on the back of most anaesthetic machines) contains 680 litres, and a D-size contains 340 litres. Of note, not all oxygen cylinders have the same fill pressure. For those used in everyday anaesthetic practice this is 137bar, but some of the larger ones (BOC sizes W, X and Y) have a fill pressure of 230bar. Oxygen cylinders are made of molybdenum steel and are regularly tested (including tensile strength, endoscopic examination and impact testing).

Reference

Lutman D, Petros AJ. How many oxygen cylinders do you need to take on transport? A nomogram for cylinder size and duration. *Emerg Med J* 2006; **23**(9): 703–4.

Question 267: Down's syndrome

Regarding Down's syndrome (DS), the following statements are true EXCEPT for which one?

a) The commonest cardiac abnormality in a patient with DS is an atrial septal defect
b) There is an increased incidence of subglottic and tracheal stenosis in patients with DIS
c) The incidence of non-haematological solid tumours is lower in patients with DIS than in a matched non-DS population
d) Patients with DS have a higher incidence of hypothyroidism than the normal population
e) The incidence of Alzheimer's dementia is increased in patients with DS

Answer: a

Explanation

Regarding patients with DS: 95% have trisomy 21, the remainder either have a chromosomal translocation (the long arm of chromosome 21 is translocated onto another chromosome, usually chromosome 14) or have mosaic trisomy 21 (when some of the cells are normal and some have trisomy 21). Up to 60% of patients with DS have a cardiac abnormality, with atrioventricular canal defects being the most common followed by atrial and ventricular septal defects, patent ductus arteriosus and tetrad of Fallot. They are also prone to the development of aortic regurgitation and mitral valve prolapse in later life. The extent of cardiac disease strongly correlates with life expectancy in this population. Many of the cardiac abnormalities place DS patients at risk of pulmonary hypertension due to the left-to-right shunt. There is a well documented link between DS and leukaemia (particularly acute myeloid leukaemia) – but interestingly studies have shown the risk of solid non-haematological tumours to be lower in the DS population. Subglottic or tracheal stenosis is seen in up to 6% of patients with DS, and there is a high incidence of atlanto-axial instability. What to do about the latter is controversial as only a small proportion of documented radiographic instability develops into symptomatic neurological disease. There is an increased incidence of both hypo- and hyperthyroidism. There is an increased incidence of Alzheimer's dementia and interesting research has suggested a gene dosing effect of amyloid coding genes located on chromosome 21.

Question 268: Statistics – distribution of data

Regarding skewness and kurtosis, which one of the following statements is TRUE?

a) With negatively skewed data, the mean > median > mode
b) Positive kurtosis indicates a tall peaked distribution with shorter tails than a normal distribution
c) The standard normal distribution has a kurtosis of zero
d) Power transformations may not be applied to positively skewed data
e) When compared to other transformers, logarithmic transformation has least impact on skew

Answer: c

Explanation

The advantage of a standard normal distribution is that it obeys certain rules with respect to its parameters and distribution of data. The same does not apply when data is distorted by kurtosis or skew. Here, transformations may be employed to normalise the distribution.

Skewness refers to a situation where the bulk of the data is concentrated off centre, giving rise to the characteristic graphs. Positive skew has the tail off to the right (towards the positive numbers) and mean > median > mode; negative skew has the tail to the left (towards the negative numbers) and mean < median < mode.

Kurtosis, from the Greek for 'bulging', describes how peaked the data distribution is: positive kurtosis indicating tall central peak with long tails stretching out to the extremes; negative kurtosis is a low rounded peak with short thin tails.

Transformations applied in order to normalise skewed data may involve logarithms, inverse or power manipulations (including square or cube root). Logarithmic transformations tend to work for grossly positively skewed data but they are a powerful transformer and can render the distribution skewed the other way. Power distributions may be applied to positively or negatively skewed data.

Question 269: Pharmacogenetics

A previously healthy 68-year-old female presents with an acute abdomen with clinical and radiological features of small bowel obstruction. The general surgeons propose an urgent laparotomy. She reports she has had one previous anaesthetic – 12 years ago for a hysterectomy – and considers that she had no problems with the anaesthetic. A rapid sequence induction is performed with thiopentone and suxamethonium, and a peripheral nerve stimulator is used to establish return of neuromuscular function. Unexpectedly it is 40 minutes post-induction that one twitch is first detected on a train-of-four stimulation. Having excluded other causes, which one of the following is the MOST LIKELY pseudocholinesterase genotype she carries?

a) $E_1{}^s E_1{}^u$
b) $E_1{}^a E_1{}^a$
c) $E_1{}^u E_1{}^a$
d) $E_1{}^f E_1{}^a$
e) $E_1{}^s E_1{}^s$

Answer: c

Explanation

Pseudocholinesterase deficiency is compatible with an entirely normal health and life expectancy as the enzyme pseudocholinesterase serves no physiological function. It specifically hydrolyses exogenous choline esters. Of relevance to anaesthesia is the prolonged metabolism of drugs such as suxamethonium, mivacurium, procaine and cocaine. Note that offset of esmolol and remifentanil are not prolonged in pseudocholinesterase deficiency. Of the population, 96% are homozygous for the usual gene ($E_1{}^u E_1{}^u$) and normal muscle function can be expected approximately five minutes after a paralysing dose of suxamethonium. The $E_1{}^a E_1{}^u$ heterozygous genotype ('a' for atypical) is the single most common mutation accounting for 2.5% of individuals – a greater proportion than all the other mutations summed. In these patients, following a paralysing dose of suxamethonium, neuromuscular relaxation of duration greater than five minutes but less than one hour will be observed. The fluoride-resistant allele produces clinically insignificant prolongation of block if heterozygous ($E_1{}^f E_1{}^u$). If combined with another atypical allele, the fluoride-resistant allele will cause a prolonged paralysis potentially of similar duration to that in the question but it is statistically far less likely. The silent allele, if homozygous ($E_1^sE_1^s$), results in complete absence of pseudocholinesterase and an eight-hour loss of neuromuscular function if suxamethonium is used. In fact, only 0.1% of the population carry a genotype that would result in a block duration of greater than one hour and the prevalence of the eight-hour $E_1^sE_1^s$ genotype is 1:100 000.

Reference
Alexander DR. Pseudocholinesterase deficiency. *eMedicine* 2006. Online at emedicine. medscape.com/article/247019-overview (Accessed 30 November 2009)

Question 270: Chronic renal failure

Patients with chronic renal failure tend to have a coagulopathy prompting careful consideration of the use of regional anaesthetic techniques. Which one of the following tests is MOST LIKELY to demonstrate the presence of a coagulopathy in a patient with end-stage renal failure?

a) Platelet count
b) Prothrombin time
c) Activated partial thromboplastin time
d) Serum fibrinogen concentration
e) Bleeding time

Answer: e

Explanation
The coagulopathy of chronic renal failure is unfortunately not quantifiable by the standard laboratory investigations of clotting. If the bedside test of bleeding time is performed this may be prolonged. Where available, thromboelastography would demonstrate the deficit. It is the defective adhesion, activation and aggregation of platelets that is responsible for the impaired clotting mechanism secondary to reduced endothelial production of von Willebrand factor/factor VIII complex. Other mechanisms of inhibition may be platelet release of β-thromboglobulin, endothelial prostaglandin I_2 or increased production of nitric oxide. Platelet transfusion does not ameliorate the situation but dialysis does. Acutely, cryoprecipitate or DDAVP should confer a benefit by increasing plasma concentration of von Willebrand factor.

Reference
McDonald C, Milner Q. Chronic renal failure and anaesthesia. *Update in Anaesthesia* 2004. Online at www.nda.ox.ac.uk/wfsa/html/u18/u1804_01.htm#haem (Accessed 30 November 2009)

Question 271: Postural cardiovascular homeostasis

On rising from the supine to the erect position and remaining still, the following physiological responses would be expected EXCEPT which one?

a) 20% decrease in cerebral blood flow
b) A rise in venous pressure at the foot to 90 mmHg
c) 40% fall in stroke volume
d) An increase in plasma concentration of renin and aldosterone
e) Minimal change in cardiac output

Answer: e

Explanation

When a subject moves from supine to erect the gravitational effects on the hydrostatic pressure in vessels must be compensated for in order to maintain adequate pressure and flow in all body regions. Because 90 mmHg is around 120 cmH$_2$O, even disregarding the increased density of blood over water, it is plausible that venous pressure at the foot rises to 90 mmHg – the pressure at the bottom of a 120 cm column of blood between the foot and the right heart. It is understandable how remaining stationary while erect can lead to dependent interstitial oedema if consideration is given to the Starling forces involved. Fortunately the muscle pump mechanism in the legs in the presence of intact venous valves maintains venous return and the venous pressure rise at the foot is limited to around 30 mmHg. Despite this, reduction of return and venous pooling in capacitance vessels results in a 40% decrease in stroke volume. Heart rate will rise to compensate to some extent but cardiac output will fall by up to 25%. A corresponding rise in total peripheral resistance will render arterial blood pressure at the level of the heart virtually unchanged. Intracerebral arterial pressure drops, offset somewhat by a reduction in jugular venous pressure, such that cerebral perfusion pressure fall is minimised. Although intact autoregulation prevents too great a drop; nevertheless a 20% decrease in cerebral blood flow is expected. Cerebral oxygen extraction ratio increases, thus cerebral oxygen consumption remains unchanged and hypoxia does not ensue. Postural increases in renin, aldosterone and antidiuretic hormone serve to conserve water to preserve venous return. Sensitivity to these reflexes is required by the anaesthetist, as general anaesthesia, and particularly regional anaesthesia, inhibits effective responses such that rapid postural change in the recovery period may lead to unpleasant sequelae including syncope, hypotension and vomiting.

Reference

Ganong W. Cardiovascular homeostasis in health and disease. In: *Review of Medical Physiology*, 18th edn. Connecticut: Appleton and Lange, 1997; pp. 586–602.

Question 272: Anticoagulants

Which one of the following statements regarding anticoagulant agents is correct?

a) Low molecular weight heparins have a greater ability to inhibit thrombin than to inhibit Factor Xa
b) Fondaparinux is contraindicated for thromboprophylaxis in major joint replacement surgery
c) Unfractionated heparin inhibits platelet activation by fibrin and also binds reversibly to antithrombin III
d) Neuraxial blockade is acceptable 12 hours after ceasing an infusion of abciximab (ReoPro®)
e) In heparin-induced thrombocytopenia, danaparoid (a heparinoid) should be avoided as an alternative agent

Answer: c

Explanation

Anaesthetists must understand the implications of anticoagulation in the perioperative period. Low molecular weight heparins (LMWH) are so called because they comprise those fractions of unfractionated heparin with smaller molecular size. They have a lower tendency to cause bleeding due to their lesser platelet effect, and their longer half-life lends convenience of administration. They interact with factor Xa more than thrombin and do not alter the activated thromboplastin time such that if their activity is to be monitored, specific factor Xa assays must be measured. Factor Xa assays also indicate the activity of danaparoid, a suitable alternative anticoagulant agent in cases of heparin-induced thrombocytopenia. For example, this may be used on the intensive care unit for a patient receiving continuous veno-venous haemo(dia) filtration where heparin and epoprostenol have proved unsuitable. Of note, the ratio of anti-Xa to anti-thrombin activity is 28:1 for danaparoid compared to 3:1 for LMWH.

Fondaparinux is a synthetic pentasaccharide with anti-Xa properties that appears in national guidelines for the prevention of thromboprophylaxis in hip replacement surgery.

Glycoprotein IIb/IIIa is involved in the interaction of platelets and fibrin in the process of coagulation. Glycoprotein IIb/IIIa inhibitors prevent this interaction exerting a potent anticoagulant effect. Abciximab, a monoclonal antibody to the receptor, is an example and is employed after percutaneous transluminal coronary intervention. Its duration of action is 48 hours during which neuraxial blockade should not be attempted. Other glycoprotein IIb/IIIa inhibitors have shorter duration of action.

Unfractionated heparin inhibits platelet activation by fibrin and also binds reversibly to antithrombin III augmenting its inhibition of factors II (thrombin), IX, X, XI, XII and plasmin (to use out-dated terminology, it effects the intrinsic pathway). Average molecular weight is around 16 kDa (as opposed to 2 to 10 kDa of LMWH). It can be used for therapeutic and prophylactic anticoagulation subcutaneously or intravenously by infusion. Large intravenous boluses are used to ensure full anticoagulation during cardiac surgery with or without cardiopulmonary bypass. A near patient test of its effects is the activated clotting time (ACT) and thromboelastography (TEG) may also demonstrate its presence. The formal laboratory test is the activated thromboplastin time, which will be prolonged in a dose-dependent manner. If required, its anticoagulant properties may be reversed acutely with the administration of protamine but heparin's short duration of action and thus spontaneous reversal over about an hour means protamine is usually reserved for particular circumstances.

References
Oranmore-Brown C, Griffiths R. Anticoagulants in the perioperative period. *Contin Educ Anaesth Crit Care Pain* 2006; **6**(4): 156–9.
NICE Clinical Guideline 46: Reducing the risk of venous thromboembolism in inpatients. April 2007. Online at http://guidance.nice.org.uk/CG46 (Accessed 30 November 2009)

Question 273: Hangover

A 37-year-old female accidentally transected her dominant hand radial artery on a broken wine glass while washing-up at midnight after an evening of alcohol excess. It is now 09.00 hours and she has been transferred to the regional plastic surgery unit for urgent surgery. She describes herself as fit and well apart from having one of the worst hangovers she can ever remember suffering. Compared to normal values, all of the following are likely to be found EXCEPT which one?

a) A low total body glutathione level
b) A low plasma magnesium level
c) A low level of the neurotransmitter glutamine in the brain
d) A high plasma acetaldehyde level
e) A low gastric pH

Answer: c

Explanation
Alcohol is metabolised by alcohol dehydrogenase to produce acetaldehyde; this is then degraded by acetaldehyde dehydrogenase to produce non-toxic acetate. The second reaction requires glutathione to contribute cysteine to the reaction. This works well for a small amount of alcohol, but if a large amount is ingested, the glutathione stores

quickly become exhausted and accumulation of acetaldehyde may occur producing headaches and nausea. Alcohol initially inhibits the effects of the stimulatory neuro-transmitter glutamine in the brain. When consumption of alcohol drops and blood alcohol starts to fall, the brain starts to produce high levels of glutamine. This may result in a rebound state with an inability to achieve restful deep sleep, anxiety and subsequent fatigue. Alcohol is a potent inhibitor of anti-diuretic hormone (ADH) secretion. Despite taking on extra enteral fluids with the alcohol, the net result of fluid balance is usually reduced total body water. A 300 mL glass of 16% alcohol in water has been shown to produce a diuresis of between 600 to 1000 mL. Sweating and vomiting may also contribute to this dehydration which may produce headache. Following the diuresis, hypomagnesaemia and hypokalaemia may also occur, produc-ing further neurological symptoms such as headache and fatigue. Alcohol directly promotes secretion of excess hydrochloric acid by the gastric mucosa, producing a lower gastric pH than normal. Hypoglycaemia is also a feature of hangovers, although this is most common following binge drinking in someone suffering from a poor nutritional state.

Question 274: Paediatric dental surgery

Regarding the options for facilitating dental procedures in children, which one of the following statements is TRUE?

a) A general anaesthetic may be used in a community setting if administered by a consultant paediatric anaesthetist
b) Orthodontic extraction of sound permanent pre-molar teeth in a healthy child rarely justifies a general anaesthetic
c) Conscious sedation or behavioural techniques (including hypnosis) should not be attempted in a child
d) Physical, emotional or learning impairment is not a justification for general anaesthesia in circumstances that do not otherwise justify general anaesthesia
e) The primary objective of comprehensive treatment planning is to ensure that follow-up general anaesthetic procedures are of minimal duration

Answer: b

Explanation

General anaesthesia *must* be administered in a hospital setting with critical care facilities. On the spectrum of patient management, in paediatric dentistry general anaesthesia represents maximum physiological intrusion and other options such as behavioural techniques, local anaesthesia and conscious sedation should be explored if possible. This is possible in the large majority of cases. The guideline below lists those indications that justify general anaesthesia and, importantly, those that do not. Consistent with common sense, it is acknowledged that physical, emotional or learning impairment may mean that general anaesthesia is required to facilitate treatment that would otherwise not indicate it. Comprehensive treat-ment planning is the responsibility primarily of the dentist, but also of the whole team, to ensure that all treatment is carried out under a single general anaesthetic with no need for repeat procedures (under local or general anaesthesia). Planned follow-up procedures under local anaesthesia frequently result in repeat general anaesthesia.

Reference
Davies C, Harrison M, Roberts G. Guideline for the use of general anaesthesia (GA) in paediatric dentistry (2008). Online at www.rcseng.ac.uk/fds/clinical_guidelines/ (Accessed 30 November 2009)

Question 275: Management of the acutely unwell

A 77-year-old female was admitted three days ago with diabetic hyperosmolar non-ketotic acidosis (HONK). This had been treated appropriately. The patient now requires urgent assessment because her heart rate of 160 beats per minute has triggered the medical early warning score system. The patient is found to be drowsy, spontaneously breathing oxygen via a facemask with a respiratory rate of 24 breaths per minute and an SpO_2 of 91%. She has some basal crepitations on chest auscultation. Her blood pressure is 92/50 mmHg – less than her recorded baseline of 154/88 mmHg. Her arterial blood gases show pH 7.35 and glucose 14 mmol/L. Her ECG shows a heart rate of 160 beats per minute, QRS duration of 160 ms and occasional capture and fusion beats.

Which one of the following is the HIGHEST PRIORITY action to take?

a) Adjust her intravenous sliding scale insulin to address recurrence of her metabolic disorder
b) Initiate infusion of intravenous amiodarone – 300 mg over one hour
c) Arrange for synchronised DC cardioversion
d) Introduce continuous positive airway pressure non-invasive ventilation
e) If vagal manoeuvres fail, try incremental boluses of adenosine intravenously

Answer: c

Explanation

This patient has a peri-arrest arrhythmia and is unstable with impaired consciousness, relative hypotension and evidence of incipient pulmonary oedema. Many diabetics with autonomic neuropathy have asymptomatic or silent myocardial ischaemia so the absence of chest pain is not reassuring. The presence of capture and fusion beats indicates independent atrial activity and identifies this broad complex arrhythmia as ventricular tachycardia. Immediate DC cardioversion is indicated. Distinguishing ventricular tachycardia from a supraventricular tachycardia with aberrant conduction (e.g. a bundle branch block) is not always easy but may not be relevant (as in this case) where DC cardioversion would be indicated wherever the origin of the arrhythmia.

Reference

Nolan, J. Peri-arrest arrhythmias. Resuscitation guidelines 2005. Resuscitation Council (UK). Online at www.resus.org.uk (Accessed 30 November 2009)

Question 276: Increased cardiac silhouette

A 55-year-old man requires elective formation of a vascular access graft to allow commencement of renal replacement therapy. His chest radiograph is reviewed. This shows an enlarged heart with a cardiac/thoracic diameter ratio of 0.65. Which of the following investigations would demonstrate the risk factor most COMMONLY associated with this abnormal chest X-ray finding in this patient group?

a) Thyroid function tests
b) Coronary angiogram
c) Echocardiogram
d) 24-hour ambulatory blood pressure monitor and access to previous blood pressure measurements
e) A full blood count and access to copies of previous full blood counts

Answer: d

Explanation

An enlarged heart on a chest X-ray is a common preoperative finding. Remember it is very difficult to comment on heart size based on the cardiac silhouette seen on an anteroposterior (AP) film. Heart failure is highly prevalent in a population with chronic kidney disease with up to 40% of patients, at commencement of dialysis, having had an episode of heart failure. In this subgroup the mortality risk is doubled. Both systolic and diastolic dysfunction may be impaired. Up to 75% of patients starting dialysis will have echocardiographic evidence of left ventricular hypertrophy. Hypertension and coronary artery disease are both extremely common in this population with the prevalence of the latter approaching 40% among patients commencing dialysis. The increased incidence of cardiovascular disease is due to both an increased incidence of 'traditional' risk factors (e.g. age, male gender, hypertension, lipid abnormalities, diabetes, smoking, etc.) and 'non-traditional' risk factors (e.g. anaemia, abnormal calcium/phosphate metabolism, volume overload, sustained inflammatory response). Up to 80% of patients approaching dialysis have hypertension, with the prevalence increasing as the glomerular filtration rate declines. The investigation plan in Option (d) will reveal this. Anaemia contributes to cardiomyopathy in this population, with up to 50% of end-stage renal failure patients with a severe cardiomyopathy having a haemoglobin below 12 g/dL. Thyroid disease is a rare cause of cardiomyopathy in this population and an echocardiogram in the majority of cases makes the diagnosis rather than giving an underlying cause.

Question 277: Fluid content

Regarding the content of intravenous fluids, the following statements are correct EXCEPT which one?

a) 1000 mL of Gelofusine® contains 60 mmol of chloride ions
b) 200 mL of sodium bicarbonate 8.4% contains approximately 200 mmol of sodium ions
c) 500 mL of 20% mannitol contains approximately 100 g of mannitol
d) 500 mL of 6% hydroxyethyl starch (Voluven®) contains approximately 77 mmol of sodium ions and 77 mmol of chloride ions
e) 500 mL of 10% hydroxyethyl starch contains approximately 77 mmol of sodium ions and 77 mmol of chloride ions

Answer: a

Explanation
Remember to read the question carefully to check the volume of fluid you are being asked about. 8.4% sodium bicarbonate contains 16.8 g of sodium bicarbonate per 200 mL giving approximately 200 mmol of sodium and bicarbonate respectively. 500 mL of Gelofusine® contains 20 g of succinylated gelatine with a mean molecular weight (MMW) of 30 000, 77 mmol of sodium ions and 60 mmol of chloride. Gelofusine® has a pH of 7.4 and an osmolarity of 274 mOsm/L. 6% hydroxyethyl starch (Voluven®) has an osmolarity of 308 mOsm/L, a pH of 4.0 to 5.5 and contains 154 mmol/L of sodium ions and 154 mmol/L chloride ions. Its MMW is 130 000. 10% hydroxyethyl starch has the same osmolarity, sodium ion and chloride ion content as Voluven® but an MMW of 200 000. Each mL of 20% mannitol contains 200 mg (remember one mL of any 1% solution contains 10 mg of the given substance) so there is approximately 100 g of mannitol in 500 mL of a 20% mannitol solution. We leave you to make sure you know the electrolyte content of the common crystalloids!

Question 278: Electrocardiogram monitoring

Regarding intraoperative monitoring of the electrocardiogram, which one of the following statements is TRUE?

a) Lead II is most sensitive for detecting ischaemia
b) The CM$_5$ configuration requires four wires/electrodes
c) The CH$_5$ configuration involves sticking an electrode on the patient's head
d) To achieve alternative monitoring configurations once the leads are arranged appropriately, lead III is selected on the monitor display
e) Intraoperative manipulation of electrode placement and lead display selection is not recommended

Answer: c

Explanation

During an operation it is not practical to monitor a 12-lead electrocardiogram (ECG) but it is mandatory that early detection of, in particular, ischaemia and arrhythmias is facilitated. There are many configurations of three ECG electrodes and wires that have variable sensitivity to ischaemia, arrhythmias or both. Keep in mind when considering all these configurations that with only three leads, at any one time only two can be active and one be passive (ground), so the resulting vector between the two active leads will be the axis on which the heart is monitored. Lead II (60° axis) is traditionally used as it gives a familiar 'textbook' ECG morphology. It shows progression of electrical activity across the heart very well as it commonly coincides with the axis of the heart. This makes it sensitive to detection of arrhythmias. In cases of myocardial ischaemia, over 90% are detectable in chest lead V$_5$, but lead II performs poorly. To address this there are a number of three-lead configurations, all of which involve the positive/left arm/yellow electrode in the V$_5$ position (5th intercostal space, left anterior axillary line). (Note that black = negative, red = positive does NOT apply here). The indifferent/left leg/green electrode remains on the left hip or leg. It is the negative/right arm/red electrode that has variable placement as follows: manubrium (CM$_5$), right shoulder (CS$_5$), middle of right scapula on the back (CB$_5$), head (CH$_5$), etc. As we are using the right arm and left arm electrodes in the position of interest we must ensure that these are the active electrodes and the left leg electrode is ground. We therefore select lead I, once the electrodes are appropriately sited. In order to maximise sensitivity to ischaemia and arrhythmias intra-operatively, a vigilant anaesthetist will, if necessary, manipulate ECG electrode placement and lead selection as circumstances dictate.

Question 279: Intraoperative cell salvage

A patient presents for surgery during which blood loss of more than 1000 mL is anticipated. The theatre team suggests using intraoperative cell salvage (ICS). Regarding the use of ICS the following statements are correct EXCEPT which one?

a) If the scheduled surgery is radical prostatectomy for carcinoma of the prostate then ICS should be avoided
b) If the patient is presenting for surgery to control a significant post-partum haemorrhage then ICS can be used safely
c) If the rinse fluid from the swabs is not collected, usable yield is limited to 50 to 70% of total blood loss
d) The vast majority of Jehovah's Witnesses will agree to the use of blood obtained via ICS
e) The cost of the consumables for ICS in one case is approximately equal to the cost of one unit of transfused packed red cells

Answer: a

Explanation

It is well recognised that there is both a morbidity and mortality associated with allogenic blood transfusion. Combined with the increasing cost of allogenic blood this makes a compelling argument for the use of ICS. At present the consumables per case cost roughly the equivalent of one unit of allogenic blood. However, this does not include the cost of purchasing and maintaining the ICS machine and the cost of a staff member to operate it. The financial equation becomes even more complex when one tries to include the risks associated with ICS and allogenic blood transfusion. Intraoperative cell salvage is indicated in surgery with anticipated blood loss of >1000 mL or >20% estimated blood volume, for patients with anaemia or increased risk factors for bleeding, patients with multiple antibodies or rare blood types and patients with objections to receiving allogenic blood (e.g. Jehovah's Witnesses). Two publications from the National Institute of Health and Clinical Excellence have declared that ICS may be used safely both in urological malignancies and obstetric haemorrhage. With the latter there is a potential concern regarding re-infusion of foetal red blood cells from the operative field. If the mother is rhesus negative and the foetus rhesus positive, the extent of maternal exposure should be determined by Kleihauer testing and where appropriate Anti D given. A study in hepatocellular carcinoma and ICS use has also shown no difference in recurrence rates between those who did and did not receive cell salvaged blood. Intraoperative cell salvage use in contaminated bowel surgery is contraindicated by manufacturers of ICS systems, but further work is needed in this area as there is evolving evidence that with precautions there may be a role for ICS in this area.

Reference

AAGBI Safety Guideline. Blood transfusion and the anaesthetist. Intraoperative cell salvage. September 2009. Online at www.aagbi.org (Accessed 1 December 2009)

Question 280: Levosimendan

Regarding levosimendan, which one of the following statements is TRUE?

a) It elevates intracellular calcium concentration
b) It decreases afterload but not preload
c) It binds to troponin T thus increasing the force of myocardial contractility
d) It works throughout the cardiac cycle
e) It has an effect on adenosine triphosphate (ATP) sensitive potassium channels

Answer: e

Explanation

Levosimendan is currently licensed for the treatment of acute heart failure and is recommended by the European Society of Cardiology for patients with symptomatic low output cardiac failure secondary to cardiac systolic dysfunction without severe hypotension. It exerts its positive inotropic action by sensitising the myocardium to the effect of calcium rather than increasing the calcium concentration per se. It does this by binding to cardiac troponin C thus facilitating and prolonging actin–myosin filament protein cross-bridge formation. This increase in contractility comes without a signifi-cant increase in total myocardial energy demand and oxygen consumption. This bind-ing to troponin C only occurs in systole, hence the duration of diastole is not altered. This is important as there is consequently little effect on ventricular filling and coronary perfusion. Levosimendan also has an action on ATP-sensitive potassium channels, causing their activation in cardiac myocytes, coronary arteries and peripheral blood vessels. This action reduces both preload and afterload, which may help the failing heart and also improves coronary and renal blood flow. It is 98% bound to plasma proteins and completely metabolised prior to excretion. Evidence for its use is still considered equivocal as several large-scale trials (e.g. SURVIVE, LIDO and REVIVE) have given conflicting results. Trials of oral levosimendan in the treatment of chronic heart failure are currently in progress, and the role of the drug in the treatment of severe sepsis is under investigation.

Reference
De Luca L, Colucci WS, Nieminen MS, Massie BM, Gheorghiade M. Evidence-based use of levosimendan in different clinical settings. *Eur Heart J* 2006; **27**(16): 1908–20.

Question 281: Severe malaria

Concerning severe infection with malaria, the following statements are true EXCEPT for which one?

a) The commonest laboratory finding in severe malaria is thrombocytopenia
b) Females contracting severe malaria have a higher mortality rate than males
c) A thin smear is more sensitive than a thick smear in the diagnosis of *Plasmodium falciparum* malaria
d) Only female mosquitoes are capable of haematophagy (drinking blood)
e) 'Blackwater fever' is usually not associated with acute renal failure

Answer: c

Explanation
Worldwide an estimated 300 million to 500 million people contract malaria annually, of whom approximately 1.5 million to 2.7 million die. Worryingly the spread of drug-resistant *P. falciparum* malaria continues to increase. Humans can be infected by any one of four species of the genus *Plasmodium* (an obligate intra-erythrocytic protozoan); *P. falciparum*, *P. vivax*, *P. ovale* and *P. malariae*. Of these, *P. falciparum* is responsible for the vast majority of the severe malaria cases, though *P. vivax* and *P. ovale* carries a mortality following infection. Transmission is via a female mosquito of the *Anopheles* genus (male mosquitoes feed exclusively on nectar!). The World Health Organization (WHO) has developed criteria for the diagnosis of severe malaria which include hyperparasitaemia, hyperbilirubinaemia, renal failure, severe anaemia, acidosis and reduced conscious level. The commonest presenting symptoms are fever, chills and headache. Thrombocytopenia is the commonest laboratory finding in severe malaria, followed by hyperbilirubinaemia, anaemia and elevated hepatic aminotransferase levels. While there is usually a marked neutrophilia the total leucocyte count is usually normal or low. Thick smears are much more sensitive at diagnosing *P. falciparum* than thin smears, the latter being better for quantifying the degree of parasitaemia. Cerebral malaria is exclusively caused by *P. falciparum*. The term blackwater fever refers to the passage of dark red/brown urine secondary to intravascular haemorrhage and the resulting haemoglobinuria. This is usually transient and not associated with acute renal failure. Drug treatment of severe malaria depends on drug resistance patterns and on local protocols, but may involve quinine, quinidine, artemisinin derivatives, doxycycline or mefloquine; alone or in combination.

Reference
Trampuz A, Jereb M, Muzlovic I, Prabhu RM. Clinical review: severe malaria. *Crit Care* 2003; **7**(4): 315–23. Online at http://ccforum.com/content/7/4/315 (Accessed 1 December 2009)

Question 282: Statistics – measures of spread

Regarding the standard error of the mean (SEM), the following statements are true EXCEPT which one?

a) Calculation of the SEM is the product of the standard deviation and the reciprocal of the square root of the sample size

b) The SEM can be regarded as a measure of spread of multiple means about the mean-of-means
c) The SEM is necessary for calculating the 95% confidence intervals
d) The SEM gives a better representation of spread of actual sample data than standard deviation
e) The SEM gives an impression of how precisely a sample mean corresponds to the true population mean

Answer: d

Explanation

The standard error of the mean (SEM) is a statistic that may be applied to data where multiple samples have been collected from a given population. Consider a hypothetical population of 100 000 subjects. A sample of 100 is analysed. From this data, a mean and a standard deviation may be calculated. If the task is repeated with another sample of 100 subjects, a second (and hopefully similar) mean and standard deviation will be generated. If multiple samples (of 100 subjects in our case) are taken then it will be observed that the means of these multiple samples form a distribution of their own. This distribution needs descriptive terms of its own and the SEM is the term applied to its spread about the mean-of-means. The more samples that are taken, the more we can be confident that the mean of them approximates to the true population mean and the SEM becomes narrower (because it is the product of the standard deviation and the reciprocal of the square root of the sample size). The SEM may *not* be applied to actual sample data (for example, in order to give the appearance of narrower spread of data) – the standard deviation must be used for this. 95% confidence intervals should be calculated via $x \pm 1.96$ SEM (where x is the sample mean) although this is all too often misquoted.

Question 283: Risk of recurrent myocardial ischaemia

Two patients have been admitted with acute coronary syndrome and require escalation of therapy. However, there is currently only one critical care bed available. In assigning priority for admission, which of the following, considered in isolation of other factors, is LEAST likely to contribute to the patient being at high risk of a further cardiac ischaemic event?

a) That the patient had taken regular aspirin in the seven days leading up to hospital admission
b) That the patient had a serum creatinine of 220 micromol/L on admission to hospital
c) That the patient had a sinus tachycardia of 120 bpm on admission to hospital
d) That the patient is a hypertensive smoker
e) That the patient is 70 years old

Answer: d

Explanation

A cardiac ischaemic event includes one or more of death, myocardial infarction or recurrent myocardial ischaemia. It is clearly important to be able to risk stratify patients admitted with myocardial ischaemia into low and high risk groups in order to optimise their in-patient management. There are two major risk-assessment algorithms that have been developed to do this, the Thrombolysis in Myocardial Infarction (TIMI) risk score and the Global Registry of Acute Coronary Events (GRACE) risk model. In the TIMI risk score patients with three or more of seven variables fall into a high-risk group. The seven variables are: age of more than 65, three or more risk factors for atherosclerosis (including diabetes mellitus, active smoker, family history, hypertension, hypercholesterolemia), known coronary artery disease, two or more episodes of angina chest pain in the 24 hours prior to admission, the use of aspirin in the seven days prior to admission, elevated cardiac troponin or CK- MB and ST-segment elevation of 0.05 mV or more. The GRACE risk model uses eight variables: age, Kilip class (a measure of severity of heart failure with myocardial infarction), systolic arterial pressure, ST-segment deviation, serum creatinine, elevated cardiac troponin or CK-MB, heart rate and whether or not the patient had a cardiac arrest during presentation. The categories are added together to give a total score and then applied to a reference nomogram to give the patient's risk (see reference below). There is no evidence that one algorithm is better than the other at identifying high-risk patients. Both low- and high-risk patients being treated for an acute coronary syndrome should receive, in the absence of contraindications, aspirin, anti-anginal medication (beta blocker, nitroglycerin or calcium channel antagonist), an anticoagulant, clopidogrel and a statin. In the high-risk patient, consideration should be given to early coronary angiography with or without revascularisation, if appropriate.

Reference

Hillis LD, Lange RA. Optimal management of acute coronary syndromes. *N Engl J Med* 2009; **360**(21): 2237–40. Online at www.outcomes-umassmed.org/grace (Accessed 1 December 2009)

Question 284: P-POSSUM scoring

In the calculation of a P-POSSUM score, which of the following physiological parameters is NOT used?

a) Systolic BP
b) White cell count
c) Serum creatinine
d) Serum sodium
e) Glasgow Coma Score

Answer: c

Explanation

POSSUM stands for Physiological and Operative Severity Score for the enUmeration of Mortality and Morbidity. First developed in the early nineties, its use is increasing in popularity as medical culture moves further towards accurate assessment of outcome measures and informed patient choice. The original POSSUM score was made up of twelve physiological and six operative parameters. These parameters were then assigned a weighted value and entered into an equation to give a morbidity and mortality expressed as a percentage. The original POSSUM was felt to overestimate mortality in low-risk groups and at the extremes of age. P-POSSUM uses the same parameters as used in the original POSSUM entered into a slightly different equation. There have been a number of other modifications to the original POSSUM allowing more accurate risk prediction for certain types of surgery, e.g. colorectal (CR-POSSUM), vascular (vascular-POSSUM) and oesophageal (O-POSSUM).

P-POSSUM physiological parameters are as follows: age, evidence of cardiac failure, evidence of dyspnoea, ECG abnormalities, systolic BP, pulse rate, haemoglobin, white cell count, urea, sodium, potassium and Glasgow Coma Score.

P-POSSUM operative parameters are as follows: operation type, number of procedures, operative blood loss, peritoneal contamination, malignancy status, CEPOD class.

Reference

Risk Prediction in Surgery website. Online at www.riskprediction.org.uk (Accessed 1 December 2009)

Question 285: Cognitive dysfunction in the older patient

Which one of the following statements is NOT a criterion of the abbreviated mental test?

a) Name of hospital
b) Recognition of two people (e.g. a doctor and a nurse)
c) Name a pencil and a watch
d) Recall an address
e) Name of monarch

Answer: c

Explanation

Postoperative cognitive deficit (POCD) is a frequently overlooked sequela of anaesthesia for the older patient. It may have multifactorial predispositions in a patient, will be precipitated by surgery and perpetuated by the unfamiliar ward environment and lack of detection. It is as likely with regional as general anaesthesia. The Association of Anaesthetists of Great Britain and Ireland recommends that all anaesthetists should be familiar with, and be able to perform, simple tests of cognitive function. The abbreviated mental test is one such tool, which tests basic orientation and cognition and scores a patient out of ten. It does not involve language tasks such as identifying objects, which are included in the Folstein Mini-Mental State Examination (maximum score 30).

References

AAGBI Working Party. Anaesthesia and peri-operative care of the elderly 2001. Online at www.aagbi.org/publications/guidelines/docs/careelderly01.pdf (Accessed 1 December 2009)
Dodds C, Allison J. Postoperative cognitive deficit in the elderly surgical patient. *Brit J Anaesth* 1998; **81**(3): 449–62.

Question 286: Practicalities of one-lung ventilation

Regarding the practicalities of one-lung ventilation, which one of the following statements is TRUE?

a) During one-lung ventilation the clamp must be placed on the patient side of the universal connector of the unventilated lung and the catheter mount to that side must be open to air
b) A left-facing double lumen tube does not allow one-lung ventilation of the right lung
c) Size of double lumen endotracheal tubes can be estimated by considering patient weight
d) The depth of insertion of a double lumen endotracheal tube in an adult male is commonly 29 cm
e) At least 2 mL of air should be put in the bronchial cuff to prevent pendelluft ventilation

Answer: d

Explanation

During one-lung ventilation the clamp must be placed on the catheter mount to the unventilated lung and the catheter mount to that lung disconnected. The arrangement described in Option (a) would result in a large leak from the breathing system and significant hypoventilation of the ventilated lung, if not complete absence of ventilation. A left- or right-facing double lumen tube may ventilate either the right or left lung. A left-facing double lumen tube is preferred to avoid the challenge of aligning the right upper lobe bronchus with the side hole of the right-facing tube. In fact there are very few absolute indications for using a right-facing tube. The size and depth of double lumen tubes is best judged from the patient's height, not weight. For an adult male of 170 cm height a 39 French tube at 29 cm would be a sensible starting point. For every 10 cm (of patient height) below this, a sequentially smaller sized tube should be selected and depth reduced by 1 cm. For a patient of 180 cm height, a 41 French tube might be inserted to 30 cm. Alternative tube sizes must be available and the depth fine tuned for optimal positioning. The bronchial cuff should be inflated with the minimal volume of air that will prevent the ventilation of one lung interfering with that of the other. This may be as little as 1 mL. Pendelluft describes the situation where lung units have different compliance or resistance (and hence time constants), such that emptying of one region of lung may result in the distension of another region rather than egress of gas through the trachea. Thus gas passes 'to and fro' rather than 'in and out'.

Question 287: Collapsing pulse

A 73-year-old patient requires emergency laparotomy. During their preoperative assessment they are noticed to have a collapsing pulse. Which of the following conditions is LEAST likely to be the cause of this finding?

a) An undiagnosed patent ductus arteriosus
b) Hyperthyroidism
c) Mixed aortic valve disease
d) Haemoglobin 8.2 g/dL
e) Temperature 38.5 °C

Answer: c

Explanation
A collapsing or 'water hammer' pulse is classically seen in patients with aortic regurgitation (AR) although it is sometimes seen in patients with a hyperdynamic circulation (e.g. thyrotoxicosis, Paget's disease, anaemia or pyrexia). Mixed aortic valve disease will not give a collapsing pulse because the stenotic valve prevents the rapid retrograde flow that would otherwise be responsible for the nature of the pulse. A patent ductus arteriosus may be entirely asymptomatic or may present with shortness of breath, tachyarrhythmias, cardiomegaly and a continuous machine-like murmur as well as a collapsing pulse. The most common cause of AR in developing countries is rheumatic heart disease with clinical presentation in the second or third decade. In the developed world, severe AR is most frequently due to diseases that are either congenital (e.g. bicuspid aortic valve) or degenerative (e.g. anuloaortic ectasia) and presentation is usually between the fourth and sixth decades. Severe AR is clinically more often observed in men than in women. In addition to the collapsing pulse, the regurgitant diastolic flow combined with an increase in systolic stroke volume causes a widened pulse pressure. Aortic regurgitation is unique among valvular heart disease as it causes both left ventricular volume overload and pressure overload. Due to a late increase in left atrial pressure symptoms, features such as dyspnoea and angina usually develop slowly. General aims in the anaesthetic management of a patient with AR should include prevention of bradycardia, adequate volume loading, low systemic vascular resistance and maintenance of myocardial contractility.

Reference
Enriquez-Sarano M, Tajik AJ. Clinical practice. Aortic regurgitation. *New Engl J Med* 2004; **351**(15): 1539–46.

Question 288: Intratracheal drugs

An intravenous drug abuser has been brought into the emergency department (ED) in cardiac arrest secondary to ventricular fibrillation resistant to DC cardioversion. Assistance from the intensive care team is sought. The patient has had his trachea intubated, without drugs, by the paramedics; however, they and the ED physicians have been unable to secure intravenous access. The following drugs may be given via the intratracheal route EXCEPT which one?

a) Adrenaline
b) Lidocaine
c) Amiodarone
d) Naloxone
e) Atropine

Answer: c

Explanation

Intratracheal drug administration is suboptimal by virtue of its unpredictability. Theoretically absorption is intra-alveolar so the drug must be diluted up to around 10 mL with 0.9% saline and vigorously injected into the endotracheal tube. Alternatively, an infusion line may be introduced into the endotracheal tube as far as the carina and the preparation injected through this. Hyperventilation should follow to encourage intra-alveolar dispersion. There is no consensus on necessary dose due to the variable absorption, but encountered dose ranges are: adrenaline 1 to 5 mg, lidocaine 50 to 100 mg, naloxone 0.4 to 5.0 mg, atropine 1 to 3 mg. Although amiodarone might be useful here, in a case of persistent ventricular fibrillation resistant to DC cardioversion, intrapulmonary amiodarone (in rats) causes rapid inflammation and prompt fibrosis so cannot be administered via the intratracheal route.

Reference

Maddocks J, Yurdakök M, Erdem G. Intratracheal drugs. *Lancet* 1988; **331**: 1276–7.

Question 289: Harmful drugs in the intensive care unit

A sick septic patient is admitted to the intensive care unit (ICU) and at day two, the following drugs can be found on his drug chart. Which of them is statistically MOST LIKELY to cause him harm during his stay on the ICU?

a) Noradrenaline
b) Morphine
c) Gentamicin
d) Propofol
e) Insulin

Answer: a

Explanation

In 2008, a review of 12 084 incidents reported to the National Patient Safety Agency in a previous six-month period were reviewed. Drug-related incidents producing harm were identified. In this study, the drug most commonly reported in a critical care environment was morphine. However, relatively fewer of these reports were thought to have actually caused patient harm. There were 55 incidents of harm with noradrenaline followed by 48 with insulin.

Reference

Thomas A, Panchagnula U. Medication-related patient safety incidents in critical care: a review of reports to the UK National Patient Safety Agency. *Anaesthesia* 2008; **63**(7): 726–33.

Question 290: Carotid endarterectomy

Regarding awake carotid endarterectomy, which one of the following statements is TRUE?

a) Superficial and deep cervical plexus blocks are necessary for regional anaesthesia in the awake patient undergoing carotid endarterectomy
b) It is common to use an intermittent bolus sedation technique during clamping of the carotid
c) One advantage of the awake technique is that it obviates the need for a shunt
d) Agitation is common and should prompt reassurance of the patient
e) Chronic obstructive pulmonary disease may be a relative contraindication to the awake technique

Answer: e

Explanation

Of paramount importance during carotid endarterectomy is maintaining cerebral perfusion pressure and adequate oxygen delivery to all regions of the cerebrum throughout the procedure. Despite various technologies that allow us to infer this in the anaesthetised patient it is arguable that there is not one as reliable as being able to monitor the awake patient's cerebration during the operation. The advantages and disadvantages of awake carotid endarterectomy makes a good short answer question. Many vascular anaesthetists use just a superficial cervical plexus block along with surgeon infiltration of local anaesthetic intra-operatively. An intermittent bolus technique is ill advised, especially while the carotid is clamped, because a reduction of conscious level might be falsely attributed to this where cerebral hypoperfusion is the culprit (or vice versa). The awake technique alerts us to the need for a shunt but does not obviate it. Agitation is a common manifestation of cerebral hypoperfusion and should prompt further assessment. Management of agitation including reassurance should occur only once ischemia has been eliminated. The anaesthetist would usually consider regional anaesthesia in a patient with COPD in whom a general anaesthetic might pose a higher risk. The converse is sometimes true with carotid endarterectomy. The patient must be able to lie still and fairly flat without moving or coughing unpredictably. Many patients with COPD may not satisfy this requirement. A continuous infusion technique for sedation may lead to carbon dioxide retention with a sudden large gasp disrupting surgery. Also the phrenic nerve block associated with cervical plexus block may cause an unacceptable degree of respiratory embarrassment.

Question 291: Autonomic dysreflexia

Eight months following a road traffic accident in which a 30-year-old man sustained a spinal cord injury, the same patient presents for surgery to treat a urethral stricture. Regarding potential autonomic dysreflexia (AD), the following statements are true EXCEPT which one?

a) A blood pressure of 120/80 mmHg would be inconsistent with a diagnosis of AD
b) Injuries below the sixth thoracic vertebra (T6) and incomplete spinal cord lesions are less likely to lead to AD than lesions above T6 and complete spinal cord lesions

c) Signs include flushed, sweaty skin above the level of the lesion and cool, pale skin below this level

d) Both tachycardia and bradycardia are commonly seen during an episode of AD

e) The most common triggers for episodes of AD are stimulation of the lower urinary tract or bowel distension secondary to faecal impaction

Answer: a

Explanation

Autonomic dysreflexia usually occurs following complete or incomplete spinal cord injury above the level of T6. It may also occur following lower spinal cord lesions but symptoms are much milder. Presenting symptoms include headache, sweating above the level of the injury, nasal congestion, malaise, nausea and blurred vision. Signs include flushed, sweaty skin above the level of the lesion and cool, pale skin below this level. Blood pressure is elevated but it is important to note that resting blood pressure is usually lower following spinal cord injury, hence a blood pressure of 120/80 mmHg would still be consistent with a diagnosis of AD. During episodes of AD systolic blood pressures and diastolic blood pressures as high as 300 and 220 mmHg respectively have been reported. Reflex bradycardia secondary to vagal stimulation is often seen but tachycardia is also common. Autonomic dysreflexia is caused by spinal reflex mechanisms that remain intact despite the patient's injury, and is precipitated by a noxious stimulus that produces an afferent impulse generating a generalised sympathetic response. Stimulation of the lower urinary tract and bowel distension secondary to faecal impaction account for the majority of precipitants. With lesions at or above the T6 level, the splanchnic vascular bed becomes involved, which provides the critical mass of blood vessels required to cause the elevation in blood pressure. In a person without spinal cord injury, descending inhibitory pathways would respond to the rise in blood pressure and modulate the sympathetic response. However, the injury to the spinal cord prevents such signals from descending to the sympathetic chain. The end result of this unopposed sympathetic activity is peripheral and splanchnic vasoconstriction. During labour and delivery, the risk of autonomic dysreflexia in patients with lesions at or above T6 may be up to 90%. The early use of neuraxial blocking techniques reduces this risk considerably.

Reference

Blackmer J. Rehabilitation medicine: 1. Autonomic dysreflexia. *Can Med Assoc J* 2003; **169**(9): 931–5.

Question 292: Neonatal neurological physiology

Regarding neonatal physiology, which one of the following statements is TRUE?

a) A neonate has low levels of endorphins compared to adults

b) A neonate has mature neuromuscular junctions by two weeks of age

c) A neonate has reversed direction of flow of CSF compared to adults

d) A neonate has blunted parasympathetic reflexes

e) A neonate has poor sympathetic response to bleeding

Answer: e

Explanation

The physiology of groups such as the elderly, the pregnant or neonates is a rich source of questions for the examiner. There is therefore no getting away from learning all the important differences of the major body systems. Neonates have high levels of endorphins and encephalins. They have immature neuromuscular junctions, poor sympathetic response to bleeding and brisk vagal reflexes.

Question 293: Osmolality

Regarding osmolality, the following statements are true EXCEPT which one?

a) Raoult's law applies to one of the colligative properties of solutions
b) Plasma osmotic pressure is approximately 7 atmospheres
c) One mole of a substance dissolved in one kilogram of solvent will produce a freezing point depression of 1.86°C
d) Plasma osmolality may be estimated from a patient's urea and electrolytes, and their blood glucose
e) An osmolality gap may be observed following transurethral resection of the prostate

Answer: c

Explanation

When a solute is added to a solvent, it predictably alters the solvent's physical characteristics. It will cause a depression of vapour pressure and freezing point and an elevation of its boiling point and osmotic pressure. These are called the colligative properties of solutions. Raoult's law simply states that the depression in solvent vapour pressure is proportional to the molar concentration of added solute. An osmole refers to the number of osmotically active particles liberated in solution *not* the molar concentration of the solute. For example the molar concentration of a bag of 0.9% saline is 154 mmol/L, but as the ionic compound NaCl dissociates into two moieties (Na^+ and Cl^-), the osmolality of the solution is 308 mOsm/kg. Note that osmolality is per kilogram of solvent. Osmolarity (osmoles per litre of solution) is less useful clinically given the huge range of molecular sizes in plasma. Osmolality may be estimated ($2 \times [Na^-] + [Urea] + [Glucose]$) or measured using any of the colligative properties of solutions, although most practically it is done via measurement of depression of the freezing point. One osmole of a substance dissolved in one kilogram of water will produce a freezing point depression of 1.86 °C, a boiling point elevation of 0.52 °C, a vapour pressure decrease of 0.04 kPa and an osmotic pressure of 2300 kPa (or 23 atmospheres!). It can be seen now that plasma osmolality of around 300 mOsm/kg is indeed around 7 atmospheres ($0.3 \times 2300 = 690$ kPa). Avoid confusion with plasma oncotic pressure which is about 3.3 kPa (25 mmHg) and used with Starling forces calculations. Absorbed glycine during transurethral resection of the prostate causes an osmolality gap.

Question 294: Acid–base management during cardiopulmonary bypass

Regarding acid–base management during cardiopulmonary bypass, which one of the following statements is TRUE?

a) The solubility of carbon dioxide decreases as the temperature decreases
b) The 'alpha' of alpha-stat pH management refers to the alpha-globin subunit of haemoglobin
c) On cardiopulmonary bypass without correction, as the temperature falls, the pH of the blood falls
d) In alpha-stat management, carbon dioxide must be added to the bypass circuit
e) In pH-stat management, the arterial blood gas values are corrected for the temperature the patient was when they were taken

Answer: e

Explanation

During cardiopulmonary bypass (CPB) a degree of therapeutic hypothermia is employed. Henry's law states that at a given temperature the quantity of gas dissolved in a liquid is directly proportional to the partial pressure of the gas in equilibrium with that liquid solvent. As temperature falls the solubility of a gas in a liquid increases. If the solvent is in contact with the gas to be dissolved then as the temperature drops a greater quantity of gas dissolves – the content increases and the partial pressure remains the same. If the solvent is in a closed container without contact with the gas in question, then as the temperature falls the content remains the same. However, a proportion of the gas previously exerting a gas tension now dissolves and its partial pressure falls. This is the case in vivo, which can be considered akin to this closed container as basal metabolic rate contributes an unchanging and finite quantity of carbon dioxide to the blood.

Recalling the determinants of blood pH it follows that as temperature falls and $PaCO_2$ falls, pH rises.

$PaCO_2$ is an important determinant of cerebral blood flow, while pH is important for satisfactory enzymatic function. In essence, which of these we prioritise determines our choice of alpha-stat or pH-stat management during the hypothermia of CPB. The gas electrodes in the arterial blood gas analyser are held at 37 °C. In pH-stat measurement a correction factor is used to compensate for the temperature of the patient (and therefore sample), then carbon dioxide is added to the CPB blood to render the pH 7.4 at that body temperature – total body carbon dioxide increases. Cerebral autoregulation is lost and cerebral blood flow becomes directly proportional to the cerebral perfusion pressure. Cerebral blood flow is greater than with alpha-stat and micro-emboli risk is higher. In alpha-stat management there is no correction for patient temperature. It is assumed that if the $pH:PaCO_2$ ratio is acceptable at 37 °C then that ratio is acceptable at whatever the temperature it was taken. This retained ratio means enzyme activity is maintained. Cerebral autoregulation is preserved (although the graph is down- and left-shifted).

In most cases, alpha-stat management is used. Alpha refers to the alpha imidazole group on the intracellular protein histidine. Its degree of ionisation remains constant despite a change of temperature.

Question 295: Poisoning

A 35-year-old woman is admitted confused and vomiting to the emergency department following ingestion of a quantity of unknown tablets. The critical care team is called because of the following blood gas result:

pH 7.55; pO_2 19.02 kPa; pCO_2 2.53 kPa; HCO_3^- 18 mmol/L.
Of the following drugs, which has MOST LIKELY been ingested?

a) Paracetamol
b) Dothiepin
c) Aspirin
d) 3,4-methylenedioxymethamphetamine (MDMA)
e) Cocaine

Answer: c

Explanation

The blood gas shows a mixed picture of a respiratory alkalosis and a metabolic acidosis. This is classically seen in salicylate overdose. The metabolic acidosis is due to a number of mechanisms including ketoacidosis via the stimulation of lipolysis, the uncoupling of oxidative phosphorylation and hence increased hydrolysis of ATP producing more H^+ and interference with the tri-carboxylic acid cycle. The respiratory alkalosis is due to the direct stimulation of the respiratory centre. The clinical features of salicylate poisoning depend on the dose ingested. Severe overdose may lead to respiratory depression and even apnoea when the blood gas result will obviously be different. Neurological features include agitation, confusion, tinnitus, lethargy and coma. Pulmonary oedema may occur, which is non-cardiogenic in origin. Cardiovascular instability may be due to dysrhythmias especially those related to hypokalaemia. Nausea, vomiting and abdominal pain are common. Salicylate levels may be misleading as absorption of aspirin can be slow, so plasma salicylate concentration may continue to rise for several hours. Also, plasma salicylate level tends not to correlate well with clinical severity, particularly at extremes of age. Despite this, the clinical severity of poisoning is low below a plasma salicylate level of 500 mg/L (3.6 mmol/L). Activated charcoal can be given within one hour of ingesting more than 125 mg/kg of aspirin. Treatment with intravenous sodium bicarbonate may be given to enhance urinary salicylate excretion (forced alkaline diuresis). Haemodiafiltration may be useful in severe salicylate poisoning, for example in the presence of a severe metabolic acidosis.

Question 296: Prophylaxis following splenectomy

A 50-year-old lady has undergone emergency splenectomy following a road traffic accident. Regarding her follow-up care the following statements are correct EXCEPT which one?

a) She should receive pneumococcal vaccination against *Streptococcus pneumoniae* approximately two weeks after her splenectomy
b) If not previously immunised she should be vaccinated against *Haemophilus influenzae* type B
c) Influenza vaccination is recommended for her on a yearly basis
d) She should be immunised against *Neisseria meningitidis*
e) She should receive ongoing prophylactic antibiotics to reduce the chance of serious infection with *Staphylococcus*

Answer: e

Explanation
Reduced post-splenectomy levels of opsonins, splenic tuftsin and immunoglobulin (IgM) (which promote phagocytosis of particulate matter and bacteria), as well as the loss of the spleen's ability to mechanically filter blood, hamper the body's ability to clear some infecting organisms. Post-splenectomy patients are at particularly increased susceptibility to infection from encapsulated organisms, some Gram-negative rods, protozoa and possibly some yeasts. The predominant infecting organisms are pneumococcus (50 to 90% of all infections), *Neisseria meningitidis* and *Haemophilus influenzae* hence vaccination against all three of these is recommended. The risk of infection is highest in young children, particularly in those with sickle cell disease. In addition to vaccinations, antibiotic prophylaxis against *Streptococcus* (group B streptococcus is another example of an encapsulated organism) is currently recommended for life. Immunisation should ideally take place two weeks before planned splenectomy but in the emergency setting should happen approximately two weeks after. Timing of vaccine administration following splenectomy is, however, open to debate. Of concern is the patient's immunogenicity in the peri-operative period and their impaired immune function while critically ill. The patient's present state of health should be considered prior to the administration of post-splenectomy vaccines. In patients with moderate to severe acute illness, vaccination should be delayed until the illness has resolved. This minimises adverse effects of the vaccine, which could be more severe in the presence of illness or could confuse the patient's clinical picture (such as a post-vaccine fever).

Reference
Davies J, Barnes R, Milligan D. Update of guidelines for the prevention and treatment of infection in patients with an absent or dysfunctional spleen. *J Royal Coll Phys Lon* 2002; **2**(5): 440–3.

Question 297: Pulmonary aspiration

A patient aspirates their stomach contents on emergence from anaesthesia while lying supine. They receive mechanical ventilation on ICU and are successfully weaned and extubated but still need supplementary oxygen. At day 12, they develop raised inflammatory markers, a temperature of 39.5°C and evidence of pulmonary abscesses on their plain chest radiograph. Which one of the following is the MOST LIKELY site of their abscess?

a) Superior segment of the right lower lobe
b) Superior segment of the lingular
c) Superior segment of the left lower lobe
d) Posterior basal segment of the right lower lobe
e) Lateral segment of the right middle lobe

Answer: a

Explanation
This question tests knowledge of the anatomy and orientation of the tracheobronchial tree. Aspirate tends to pool in the dependent segment therefore the likely site of abscess depends on the patient's position at time of aspiration and consideration of into which of the segmental bronchi gravity might direct the aspirate. This is only a probability of course, but the question asks for the *most likely* site. In the supine position aspiration tends to favour the superior segment of the right lower lobe. If in the right decubitus position, aspiration will most likely affect the posterior segment of the right upper lobe (or sometimes quoted as the lateral segment of the right middle lobe). In the left decubitus position the lingular is the most likely destination and if the patient is erect, one would expect pooling in the posterior basal segment of the right lower lobe.

Question 298: Postoperative urinary retention

The following features would place a patient at risk of postoperative urinary retention EXCEPT which one?

a) Male gender
b) 500 mL intravenous infusion of Hartmann's solution during knee arthroscopy
c) Previous history of severe bradycardia under anaesthesia
d) Open reduction and mesh repair of inguinal hernia
e) Intravenous midazolam sedation in recovery

Answer: b

Explanation
Postoperative urinary retention (POUR) is the inability to void in the presence of a full bladder. The incidence has been reported as anything from 5 to 70%. As fewer patients are now catheterised in the peri-operative period it has become increasingly important to be able to recognise and treat POUR. It is therefore useful to understand who might be at higher risk of POUR. Patients over 50 years old have a 2.4 times greater risk of POUR than under 50s, and males have a 1.6 times greater risk than females. Patients having hernia repair or anorectal surgery or who have previously had pelvic surgery

are at risk. Pre-existing obstructive urinary symptoms or the presence of neurological diseases such as alcoholic neuropathy, a cerebral or spinal lesion or diabetes also put the patient at risk, as does preoperative treatment with α- or β-blockers. Intraoperative risk factors include intravenous anticholinergic agents, intravenous infusion of more than 750 mL of fluid to patients having high-risk operations, long duration of surgery and spinal or epidural blockade. Features of a spinal making it particularly high risk include using high-dose, long-acting local anaesthetic or using opioids that are hydrophilic (such as morphine), have high mu-receptor selectivity or are at a high dose. Features of an epidural that make it high risk for POUR include site of insertion (lumbar higher risk than thoracic), using long-acting local anaesthetic, hydrophilic or mu-receptor selective opioids, or using epidural adrenaline. Post-operatively, risk of POUR is increased by having a bladder volume of >270 mL on arrival in the recovery room, receiving sedative medication (e.g. midazolam) or receiving analgesia via continuous epidural infusion or a patient-controlled epidural device. The previous history of bradycardia would increase the patient's likelihood of POUR by increasing the likelihood of administration of prophylactic or therapeutic anti-muscarinic drugs.

Reference
Baldini G, Bagry H, Aprikian A, Carli F. Postoperative urinary retention: anesthetic and perioperative considerations. *Anesthesiology* 2009; **110**(5): 1139–57.

Question 299: Non-heart beating organ donation

A patient has been accepted for non-heart beating organ donation (NHBD). Which of the following organs cannot be successfully transplanted if the patient dies 90 minutes after withdrawal of active treatment?

a) Heart valves
b) Corneas
c) Liver
d) Skin
e) Kidneys

Answer: c

Explanation
Non-heart beating organ donation (NHBD) is not new, as the first cadaveric organs to be transplanted were retrieved as NHBDs. Initially considered as marginal donors, improved techniques of organ preservation and assessment of function before transplantation have resulted in outcomes (certainly in the case of kidney transplants) to rival those achieved after transplantation of organs from heart beating donors. Recently the number of organs that can be used following NHBD increased with reports of successful liver, pancreas and lung transplantations. Currently, for liver transplantation to occur, the donor must die within an hour of withdrawal of treatment (two hours for renal transplantation). The decision to abandon organ donation is determined by the need to limit the warm ischaemic time and by the availability of an operating theatre and retrieval team. Tissues that can be donated include corneas and sclera, heart valves, bone, tendons, menisci and skin. Tissue can be retrieved up to 24 hours after circulatory arrest except for heart valves, which can be retrieved up to 48 hours after circulatory arrest.

Reference
Intensive Care Society. Guidelines for adult organ and tissue donation. Online at www.ics.ac.uk/icmprof/downloads/Organ%20&%20Tissue%20Donation.pdf (Accessed 1 December 2009)

Question 300: Urea: creatinine ratio

A 67-year-old, 75 kg woman requires anaesthesia for a total knee replacement. Her admission blood results are reviewed. Some of them are as follows: urea 15.1 mmol/L; creatinine 77 micromol/L; haemoglobin 8 g/dL.

Which of the following represents the LEAST likely cause?

a) Regular non-steroidal use over the past six months
b) Chronic renal failure secondary to hypertension and non-insulin dependent diabetes mellitus
c) That she is on medication for treatment of cardiac failure
d) That she has been taking prednisolone, 20 mg daily, for the last six months
e) A history of alcohol excess, known hepatic cirrhosis and oesophageal varices on endoscopy

Answer: b

Explanation

A number of clinical situations may cause an elevated urea:creatinine ratio (UCR). These include dehydration, cardiac failure, diuretic therapy (hence Option (c) is true), gastrointestinal haemorrhage and high protein intake. Steroid therapy and other causes of increased protein catabolism (e.g. SIRS and sepsis) may also increase the UCR. Conversely a low UCR is caused by a low protein diet, pregnancy, liver failure or overzealous hydration. In chronic renal impairment and established acute renal failure the urea and creatinine should rise in parallel. The other part to this question is the low haemoglobin (Hb). Insidious gastrointestinal bleeding can elevate the UCR and direct questioning should elicit evidence of change in stool colour. A history of alcohol excess, known hepatic cirrhosis and oesophageal varices could result in either a high or a low UCR depending on the cause of the low Hb as it could be nutritionally related or due to gastrointestinal haemorrhage.

Index